Advances in Computer Vision and Pattern Recognition

For further volumes:
http://www.springer.com/series/4205

Marek R. Ogiela · Tomasz Hachaj

Natural User Interfaces
in Medical Image Analysis

Cognitive Analysis of Brain and Carotid
Artery Images

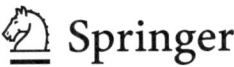 Springer

Marek R. Ogiela
AGH University of Science
  and Technology
Kraków
Poland

Tomasz Hachaj
Pedagogical University of Kraków
Kraków
Poland

Series editors
Sameer Singh
Rail Vision Europe Ltd.
Castle Donington
Leicestershire
UK

Sing Bing Kang
Interactive Visual Media Group
Microsoft Research
Redmond, WA
USA

ISSN 2191-6586
ISBN 978-3-319-37700-1
DOI 10.1007/978-3-319-07800-7
Springer Cham Heidelberg New York Dordrecht London

ISSN 2191-6594   (electronic)
ISBN 978-3-319-07800-7   (eBook)

Printed on acid-free paper

Springer is part of Springer Science+Business Media (www.springer.com)

Preface

Contemporary methods classified as image recognition techniques and computer vision systems have been developing very rapidly in many domains. They are used in advanced hardware technologies as well as in a series of methodologically complex algorithmic solutions allowing diverse images recorded by computer systems to be visualized, classified, and analyzed. Such techniques are also increasingly applied in practice, not just to help solve complicated scientific problems of interpreting complex images: they have been implemented and are accessible to a broad group of users. Among the many usage areas of methods related to computer image recognition techniques, which attract a lot of interest due to the possibility of their broad use in practical applications, we can also list such subjects as the analysis of complex images and scenes aimed at of their semantic interpretation, techniques for reconstructing 3-D images and visualizing them in augmented reality environments, as well as advanced methods of recognising images used in man–machine interfaces.

The most recent discoveries and state-of-the-art technical solutions from the above fields are of great importance for the further development of advanced computer vision and image recognition systems. Their invention required solving many major, very difficult problems of image algebra, cognitive image interpretation, and creating a technology for 3-D rendering, and thus creating 3-D images and virtual objects with which the user can interact in an augmented reality environment. The development of image recognition methods in the above areas went so far that we now have innumerable practical applications of such techniques and methods, available in almost every facet of life (sports, science, leisure, work, etc.), scientific disciplines (IT, medicine, geology, chemistry, natural science, automation and robotics, etc.), or areas of human activity (e.g., space research, oceanography, weapon design, defence, and security of both the state and individuals).

The available image recognition technologies and algorithms can also be analyzed from the scientific, theoretical perspective. This perspective should also lead us to appreciate the solutions available in this area: in recent years, the capabilities of such systems have come close to the perceptual analysis of images which is achieved only by the vision systems of primates (including mainly humans). This requires not only with the ability to record stereo-vision and 3-D images but also to perceptually analyze them or understand the meaning of a given image or scene.

Although the capabilities of computer image analysis that have appeared recently do not work as well as the processing of visual information in the human visual system yet, it seems that soon we might see technical solutions with abilities close to the most advanced biological vision systems. This research area is still open and related to research on neuro-biological and psychological cognitive processes, as well as technological attempts to construct an artificial brain that could be used to build cognitive humanoid robots [1].

The topics of this monograph will contribute to similar, interesting schools of research on modern systems of image recognition and their practical applications. This book will present selected topics, both theoretical and practical, from this broad area of contemporary IT.

Within the scope of practical applications of advanced Image Analysis methods, we will try to show some important, practical uses of such techniques to analyze selected medical images, and in particular of the brain and carotid arteries. In this area, we will discuss the complete methodology of processing, analyzing and interpreting diagnostic results of example computed tomography images. With regards to practical applications, we will also discuss an innovative method of recognizing gestures and motions which can obviously be used widely in areas associated with analyzing medical images, but can also find its application in similar fields, e.g., as a fully functional man–machine interface.

In this monograph, we will also try to get the reader interested in selected topics of theoretical and methodological nature. For this purpose, we will not only discuss selected methods and techniques of image analysis and recognition, but also present significant problems related to new approaches and computational paradigms in the field of computer-based image understanding and semantic image analysis. Such capabilities have appeared after the development of techniques for cognitively analysing of image patterns, which the authors spend many years on [2, 3]. The presentation of such topics will constitute an interesting supplement to the practical applications discussed in this book.

However, it is worth noting that both the presented theoretical subjects and practical solutions are open in nature and can be improved by researchers wishing to make their own contribution to the development of these methods, or to improve the operation of the algorithms presented in the following chapters. This is why the described solutions will be accompanied by example source codes of the implemented algorithms, and also broad literature allowing the reader to extend their knowledge of the area of interest to them.

As this book is interdisciplinary in nature, on the one hand presenting advanced algorithms for image recognition and on the other their use to analyze the images of the brain and carotid arteries, but also because it describes not just practical methods but also advanced theoretical formalisms, we can briefly state that it will touch upon the following subjects:

1. Discussing and defining methods of perceptual image analysis based on the existing processing and the recognition algorithms [2, 4].
2. Indicating the possibility of using cognitive image analysis for the semantic interpretation of medical images [1].
3. Developing a methodology for computer-based semantic analysis of brain and carotid artery perfusion images [5, 6].
4. Developing effective algorithmic and implementation solutions for visualising selected 3-D structures [7].
5. Developing the GDL (Gesture Description Language) technology as an innovative solution for Natural User Interfaces [8].

These subjects will be discussed in six subsequent chapters of this monograph, including five main chapters and the summary.

The Preface talks about the entire topical scope of this book and the directions of contemporary scientific research on image recognition and cognitive vision systems. We will also present the areas of scientific research conducted by the authors, dealing with techniques of advanced analysis and recognition of images.

The lengthy first chapter reviews selected methods of initial image analysis, major classification techniques including a list of holistic and syntactic methods, and introduces to techniques of semantic image analysis. This chapter also contains source codes of example implementations of selected image processing methods.

Chapter 2 presents the idea behind the semantic analysis of images, based on the resonance processes. It defines the cognitive resonance model and the methods of its implementation using image languages. The possibilities of conducting a semantic analysis are illustrated with medical samples of diagnostic images showing brain perfusion maps and computer 3-D reconstructions of carotid vessels.

Chapter 3 presents the authors' original approach to the semantic analysis of two types of medical images. The first of them is the analysis and detection of lesions in the blood perfusion of brain tissue, portrayed in CT (computed tomography) images. For these images, the complete examination methodology is presented, which allows lesions be detected and their meaning interpreted. The second example is the ability to make 3-D reconstructions of carotid arteries aimed at diagnosing morphological changes of these structures and detecting brain ischemia conditions. For both cases of images analyzed, example results produced by the developed algorithms are presented, and the codes of example procedures making it possible to conduct such analyses are given.

Chapter 4 deals with techniques for creating 3-D visualizations and 3-D rendering. It presents a series of notions from image algebra and techniques for 3-D transformations of images. It also gives examples of hardware implementations of such methods, as well as the source codes of the proposed data visualisation methods.

Chapter 5 discusses the currently available interfaces for image communication between humans and computers with their use in practical applications and mobile devices, but it also presents an innovative GDL technology. The authors of this monograph have proposed the GDL technology which allows users not only to communicate with computers, but also supports sophisticated analyses of human motions and gestures, e.g., during navigation, behavioral analyses, the psychological interpretation of gestures, and also in physical (exercise) therapy.

The last chapter of this monograph contains a summary of the authors' significant research achievements in the field of advanced image recognition techniques and their practical applications. The summary will also chart the possible further research directions in which this discipline can be developed.

References

1. Ogiela L, Ogiela MR (2012) Advances in cognitive information systems. Cognitive systems monographs, vol 17. Springer, Berlin Heidelberg
2. Ogiela L, Ogiela MR (2009) Cognitive techniques in visual data interpretation. Studies in computational intelligence, vol 228. Springer, Berlin Heidelberg
3. Hachaj T, Ogiela MR (2011) A system for detecting and describing pathological changes using dynamic perfusion computer tomography brain maps. Comput Biol Med 41(6):402–410. doi: 10.1016/j.compbiomed.2011.04.002
4. Duda RO, Hart PE, Stork DG (2001) Pattern classifications. Willey, New York
5. Hachaj T, Ogiela MR (2012) Framework for cognitive analysis of dynamic perfusion computed tomography with visualization of large volumetric data. J Electron Imaging 21(4), Article Number: 043017, doi: 10.1117/1.JEI.21.4.043017
6. Ogiela MR, Hachaj T (2013) Automatic segmentation of the carotid artery bifurcation region with a region-growing approach. J Electron Imaging 22(3), Article Number: 033029, doi: 10.1117/1.JEI.22.3.033029
7. Hachaj T, Ogiela MR (2012) Visualization of perfusion abnormalities with GPU-based volume rendering. Comput Graph-UK 36(3):163–169. doi: 10.1016/j.cag.2012.01.002
8. Hachaj T, Ogiela MR (2014) Rule-based approach to recognizing human body poses and gestures in real time. Multimedia Syst 20:81–99. doi 10.1007/s00530-013-0332-2

Contents

Chapter 1
Image Processing, Pattern Recognition, and Semantic Understanding Techniques

The development of image processing and analysis technology as well as the constant efforts of scientists trying to find more ways of extracting important information from analyzed images have produced scores of various algorithms for processing, analyzing, recognizing, and even understanding the meaning of image patterns available to us today. Nowadays, image analysis techniques and systems are applied very broadly. These applications include areas such as analyzing satellite photographs of the Earth's surface or astronomical images of outer space, microscopic images of material samples, geological structures, or even living organism tissues. We can now see the use of such techniques for personally identifying people, detecting their emotions, analyzing their behaviour, and recognizing their gestures and motions [1–5]. Many applications can also be found in defence, the analysis of metabolic processes of plant and animal cells, and even in such fields as antique book analysis. One can thus see that IT techniques constituting the area of computer vision allow us not only to acquire the images to be analyzed from various recording equipment, but also to improve, assess, and classify them, and even interpret their meaning.

It is these subjects that will form the topic of this chapter, whose subsequent paragraphs will discuss in order the three most important groups of methods and algorithms used by modern image analysis systems in more detail. These groups of methods are as follows:

- Image processing—groups techniques of image preprocessing, which usually allow the quality of the analyzed images to be improved or certain significant objects of interest for further analysis to be extracted from the entire complex image (e.g., during its classification) [6–10].
- Pattern classification—a group of methods which allow certain significant features of the entire image or its selected elements to be identified and used for classification, by indexing them as objects which are members of certain previously defined classes [11–14].
- Image understanding—analysis methods aimed at determining the meaning of a given image by analyzing its semantics. Such techniques are very advanced and can be used only for images which contain meaning, e.g., various medical images [15–22].

M. R. Ogiela and T. Hachaj, *Natural User Interfaces in Medical Image Analysis*,
Advances in Computer Vision and Pattern Recognition,
DOI: 10.1007/978-3-319-07800-7_1,
© Springer International Publishing Switzerland 2015

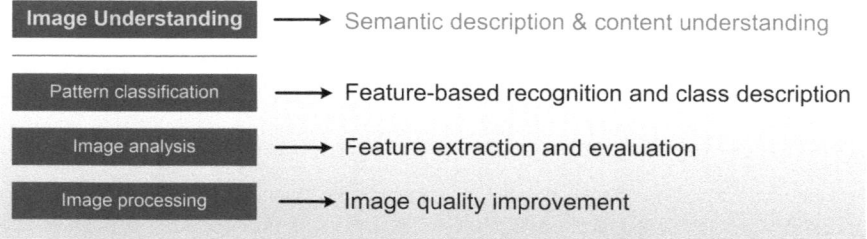

Fig. 1.1 Dependencies of various stages of the image analysis and interpretation process

The links and interdependencies between various stages and techniques of image analysis are shown in Fig. 1.1.

The recognition methods listed above will be presented in greater detail in subsequent subsections of this book. It is only worth noting that all of the three aforementioned stages of computer image processing are being applied more and more often, which makes them significant for the entire field of computer vision. However, these techniques were invented at various stages in the development of computer-based image recognition methods and are characterized by various complexity and sophistication. In general, image preprocessing methods were the first techniques to be developed and used in computer image analysis. Today, they are still very frequently used to analyze simple images (whose preprocessing may already mean recognizing a certain object), but they are also utilized in analyzing more complex ones, where they allow the image quality to be improved or individual elements to be identified, and these elements are then holistically analyzed. As image processing techniques improved, methods of recognizing and classifying these images also appeared. We now have many types of such methods which will be discussed in the subsections below. The most recent of the listed types of methods are those for computer image understanding. They have been developed relatively recently and are used to analyze images—i.e., semantics. Obviously not all kinds of images can contain layers of semantics, and for those that do not, their analysis ends when they are classified to one of the known classes of objects. Computer image understanding methods, on the other hand, can be used to analyze complex patterns, scenes, video recordings, or to analyze behaviors. They are also frequently used to analyze various medical images [11, 16, 18], and lower down in this book they will be discussed in the context of supporting the diagnostics of, and analyzing brain and carotid artery images [23–28]. These techniques have now become very useful tools to support and streamline the work of physicians of various specializations, because after the images have been processed and their semantics analyzed, the diagnostician can have a much better view of the details of interest in the examined organ and processes taking place in it, and as a result can take a better and more reliable diagnostic decision, supported by a computer executing advanced analysis of the meaning of the given image.

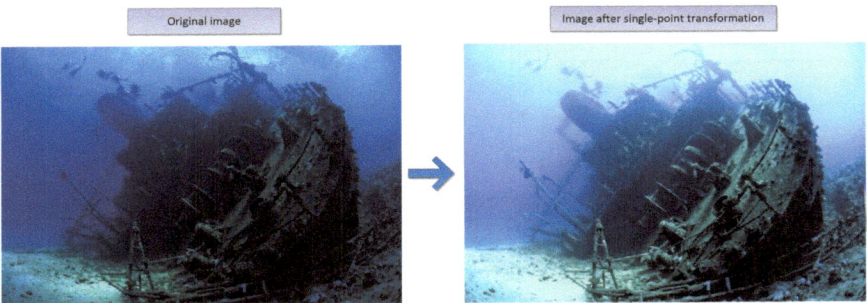

Fig. 1.2 An example of using single point operations to improve the legibility of an image of an underwater wreck

1.1 Image Enhancement and Basic Processing Methods

This subsection briefly presents the most popular techniques of image preprocessing. Of the many different techniques and methods of image processing, this subsection presents only those that are used the most frequently and that have been confirmed as very useful in this regard in many practical cases. Obviously, when considering various methods of processing an image, it is more convenient to refer to its raster interpretation as a two-dimensional function of gray levels or the color palette of the selected color space model.

1.1.1 Single Point Processing

The simplest class of computer techniques for image processing includes methods which execute single point operations, i.e., methods for processing an image following the rule of modifying a single pixel of the image taken from the original image. It is easy to see that this simple operating principle practically rules out obtaining additional information from the context (neighborhood) of the analyzed pixel. Single point operations are often useful, particularly in situations in which we want to improve the quality of images with poor contrast by the appropriate selection of colors or gray levels. An example of improving the legibility of an image is shown in Fig. 1.2.

During image analysis, single point operations can be combined with other contextual operations (e.g., segmentation techniques), allowing only those fragments of an image which contain the information needed for the classification to be selected for their further analysis. The remaining details will then be deleted from the image. If automatic techniques of image recognition or understanding are used, the above approach can be successfully utilized to simplify the entire analysis process.

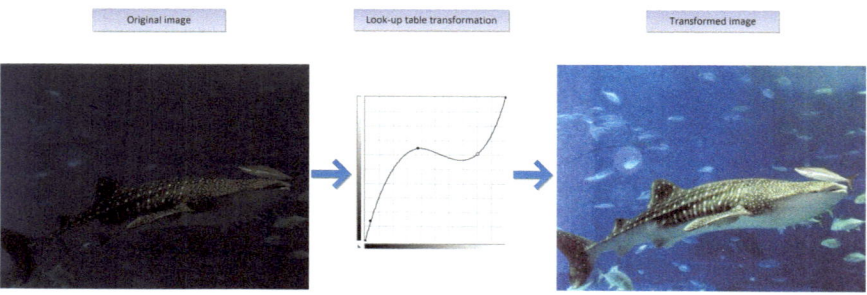

Fig. 1.3 Executing a transformation given by any function

It is worth noting that the main advantage of single point transformations is the speed of their execution. Even if the point operation that is executed is very complex, its values have to be calculated only as many times as there are pixels in the image. Consequently, even for images containing millions of pixels this will take only fractions of a second. In this regard, the execution of context transformations described in the following subsection is worse.

The range of single point transformations described in the literature is very broad, and in addition it is possible to use transformations in which the function modifying the values of individual pixels is freely set by the user (Fig. 1.3). Such freely defined transformations are usually executed using a technique called *the look up table*.

In practice, it is not always easy to determine which transformation will extract the desirable features from a specific image or will allow the objects looked for to be isolated, so it is sometimes worth using certain standard solutions for this purpose or predefined functions which can very precisely reveal material elements of the image.

One of such effective techniques is the histogram equalization method. This method first produces a histogram of the original image, i.e., a graph showing the result of counting how many times pixels of specific gray levels or colors appear in the image (Fig. 1.4).

Because a histogram allows us to obtain a lot of valuable information about the distribution of colors in the image, it often also allows us to determine what transformation the examined image should be subjected to, so that what is poorly visible in it is exposed better and more clearly. For this purpose, the histogram must be equalized, which practically means that the higher the value in the histogram the more distant it should be from other values shown on the histogram. The use of similar operations for all extreme values of the histogram allows the colors from the entire color palette to be evenly distributed. In the output image, this also produces a better contrast of the image and a better exposition of those fragments of it which were not clearly visible originally.

Figure 1.5 shows examples of applying the histogram equalization operation to selected images.

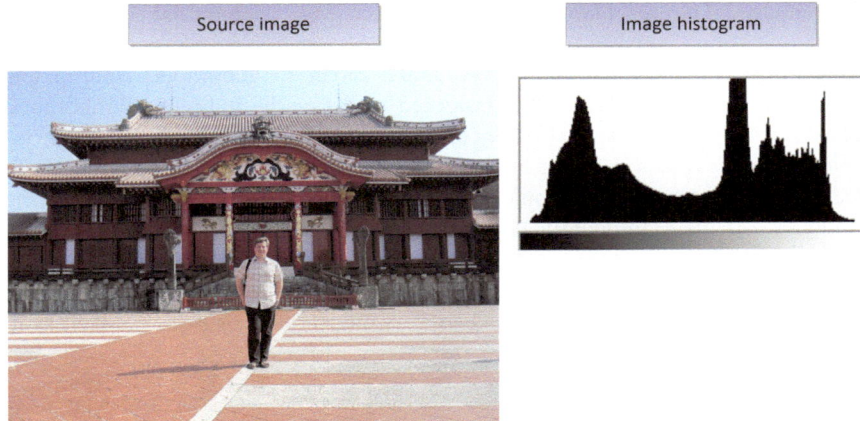

Fig. 1.4 An example image and its histogram

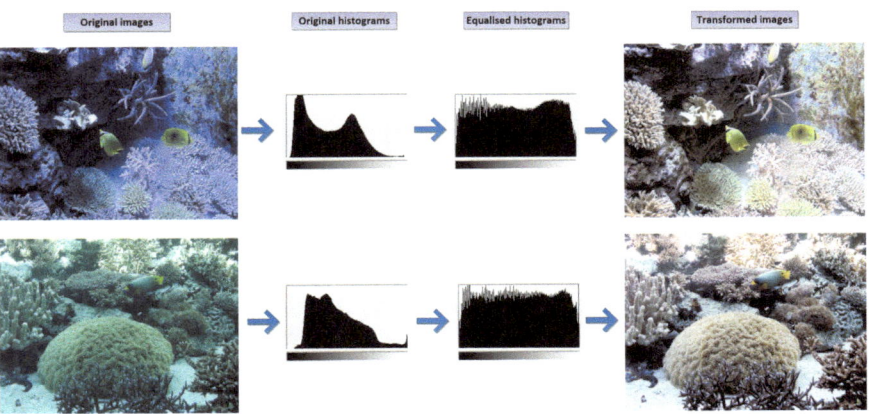

Fig. 1.5 Histogram equalization operation

1.1.2 Context Image Processing Methods

Quite a few operations currently performed on images are characterized by the fact that in order to determine the value of one point of the output image, one has to make calculations based on many points of the source image. A context operation related to a certain pixel of the output image thus consists in determining the value of a function whose arguments consist in the values of pixels with the same location in the source image as the pixel for which the calculations are executed, and the values of points surrounding it. The value calculated using the appropriately defined function can be taken as the new value of the considered pixel in the output image. The neighborhood usually taken into account when executing context operations consists of points surrounding the point undergoing the processing. Such points determine the so-called direct neighborhood (four pixels whose edges adjoin the currently considered pixel) or the indirect neighborhood (points touching it with their edges or corners). Computer analysis may use various neighborhood schemes defining only direct neighbors, or masks containing both direct and indirect neighbors. Context operations, and particularly various filtering techniques, are very frequently used in image processing and analysis. Unlike single point operations, they significantly change the contents of the image, including the geometry of objects visible in it. They can be used to effectively eliminate certain undesirable elements such as interference or noise, as well as to expose certain information within the image (e.g., edges).

1.1.2.1 Linear Filtering

Image filters are the most frequent context operations. Filters are divided into linear and nonlinear. A filter is classified as linear if the function φ which it executes meets two linearity conditions:
it is additive

$$\varphi(f + g) = \varphi(f) + \varphi(g) \tag{1.1}$$

and uniform

$$\varphi(\lambda f) = \lambda \varphi(f), \lambda \in \Re \tag{1.2}$$

where: φ—the function executed by the filter, f, g—images filtered.
    The linear filters most frequently used in practice are those which also meet the condition of invariability relative to a shift. If this condition is fulfilled, every point of the image which is subjected to the operation of this filter will be transformed in the same way.
    The operation of filters used for the linear filtering of images is most frequently based on the convolution operation. It consists in executing the following operation for every point of the image identified by the coordinates x and y:

$$f'(x,y) = \sum_{(i,j) \in M} f(x+i, y+j) \cdot W_{i,j}, \tag{1.3}$$

where:
    $f(x, y)$—represents the value of the pixel of the source image with the coordinates x and y;
    $f'(x, y)$—represents the new value of the output image pixel;
    i, j—indexing variables defining the interior of the window or the convolution mask W, which at the same time constitutes the neighbourhood M of the point (x, y).

It is worth noting that values of image pixels that have specific interpretations as gray levels or color values of specific points of the image most often have the form of positive integers from a strictly defined interval of values (e.g. [0, 255] for gray-scale images or 2^{24} for color ones). However, the results of calculations described by the above formula defining the values of convolution $f'(x, y)$ do not always have to meet these conditions. For example, if we use low-pass filtering, all coefficients $W_{i,j}$ are positive integers of different values, and then the maximum value that the convolution function $f'(x, y)$ can take may significantly exceed the boundary value for a single pixel. The situation is similar for high-pass filtering, where the convolution window coefficients $W_{i,j}$ are integers, both positive and negative, which in practice means that the output value $f'(x, y)$ can be either positive or negative.

Hence we can see that when executing filtering (both low-pass and high-pass), it is necessary to adjust the calculated value $f'(x, y)$ and bring it down to the permissible interval before it is accepted as the new value of the pixel of the output image. The correction formula may be defined in various ways, but it is most often executed as simple scaling.

The type of transformation that is executed on an image as a result of the operation of the above convolution operator depends on the value of coefficients $W_{i,j}$ defined by the adopted convolution mask. Having defined the values of coefficients $W_{i,j}$, we obtain a tool which can be considered, in particular, to represent a linear filter acting on the entire processed image.

Linear filters are divided into low-pass and high-pass. Low-pass filtering means that signal components of low frequencies are allowed to pass through the filter, while high-frequency components (usually noise) are stopped by the filter. High-pass filtering means that high-frequency components are selectively let through the filter (i.e., the elements in which the signal changes quickly and suddenly are amplified).

In two-dimensional images, convolution filters can act symmetrically or can be directional. In the case of low-pass filters, their directional operation is usually offset as a result of adopting sets of coefficients $W_{i,j}$ with central symmetry, whereas for high-pass filters, the directional operation of the filter is sometimes intentionally used to obtain certain special effects in the processed image, e.g., to detect the edges of objects in a specific location.

Low-pass Filters

If the convolution mask of linear filters is filled out with only positive values of coefficients, we obtain a class of low-pass filters. The more important applications of low-pass filters include de-noising an image, making it fuzzy or smoothing it. In this case, simple averaging filters are usually used, which can have masks presented in Fig. 1.6.

As a result of applying such filters to an image, one can indeed eliminate or significantly reduce minor noise present in that image, and smooth certain edges. Minor brightness changes in a given area will also be eliminated. Unfortunately, this filter also causes undesirable effects, such as the fuzzy contours of objects visible in the image and a poorer recognition of their shapes.

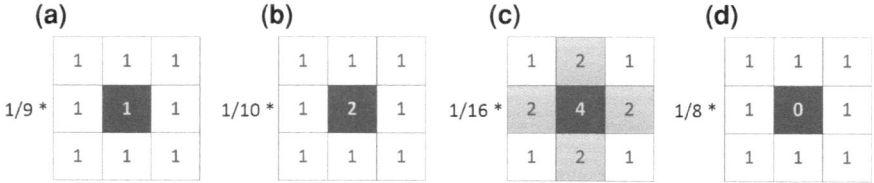

Fig. 1.6 Example masks of low-pass filters. **a** a simple averaging filter, **b** an averaging filter with a more strongly amplified central point, **c** an averaging filter with an even more strongly amplified central point and its direct neighbourhood, **d** an averaging filter with a weakened central point of the filter mask

Fig. 1.7 Roberts directional gradient masks

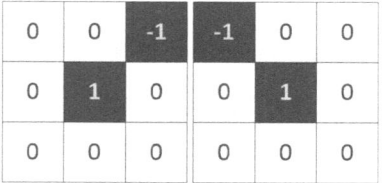

In order to reduce the negative effects of averaging filtering, filters with an amplified central point of the mask or also its direct neighborhood can be used (Fig. 1.6b, c). Such values mean that the original value of the pixel has a greater influence on its filtered value in the output image. Sometimes filters are also used whose mask is not amplified in the central point, but, on the contrary, it weakens the influence of this point on the final result of the filtering. An example of such a mask can be seen in image Fig. 1.6d.

As the presented examples show, low-pass filters can have variously defined functions for modifying the value of individual image pixels during the transformation from the source image to the output image. However, they also have one common feature: while removing noise from the image, they simultaneously reduce its contrast and can thus eliminate some of the significant information about the edges or the texture of selected areas or objects in the image. Consequently, such filters are used in the way defined for the specific analysis of various types of images and their effects are usually combined with procedures that compensate for making the image fuzzy.

High-pass Filters

The second important class of filters are high-pass filters used for segmenting elements responsible for quick changes of brightness in the image, for example, contours and edges. In general, such operations are referred to as amplifying object edges in the image. One can say that high-pass filters work by differentiating the signal. The simplest example of such a filter is the so-called Roberts gradient, whose filter masks are shown in Fig. 1.7.

This filter emphasizes the distinguished directions of edges, but because it includes positive and negative coefficients in its mask, the output image may contain

Fig. 1.8 A set of level 5
Robinson masks generating
image gradients of various
directions

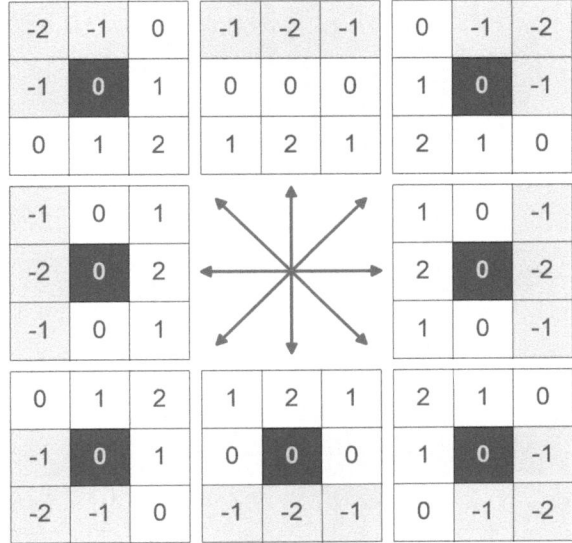

pixels with positive or negative values exceeding the set values resulting from the adopted representation of the color palette used. Consequently, to obtain the correct image, one has to take into account the absolute values of pixels, or scale the image. The Roberts gradient is directional in nature, which causes lines of certain orientation to be amplified, the orientation depending on the mask applied.

Similar directional gradients or corner detection gradients [9] are used to analyze various images in order to detect and describe the edges of the analyzed structures or objects. Figure 1.8 shows an example set of masks for Robinson filters which detect edges running in specific directions (the place where a specific mask is located on the diagram shows which directional structures are detected by this mask).

The effect of the operation of Robinson masks shown in Fig. 1.8 is shown in Fig. 1.9. These examples are demonstrated on an example image in which it is easy to see the effects of the operation of individual directional gradients.

The aforementioned high-pass filters use the convolution operation to determine the first derivatives of the image signal, which allows the contours of objects visible in the image to be identified along a certain, defined direction. However, it is frequently necessary to detect all contours and edges in the image, regardless of the direction in which they run. In order to detect all edges, it is thus convenient to use an operator which determines the value of the second derivative of the image. Examples of convolution masks allowing all edges to be detected are shown in Fig. 1.10.

In summary, it can be said that depending on the type of filtering used, the same image can look very different: this supports various directions of its analysis and

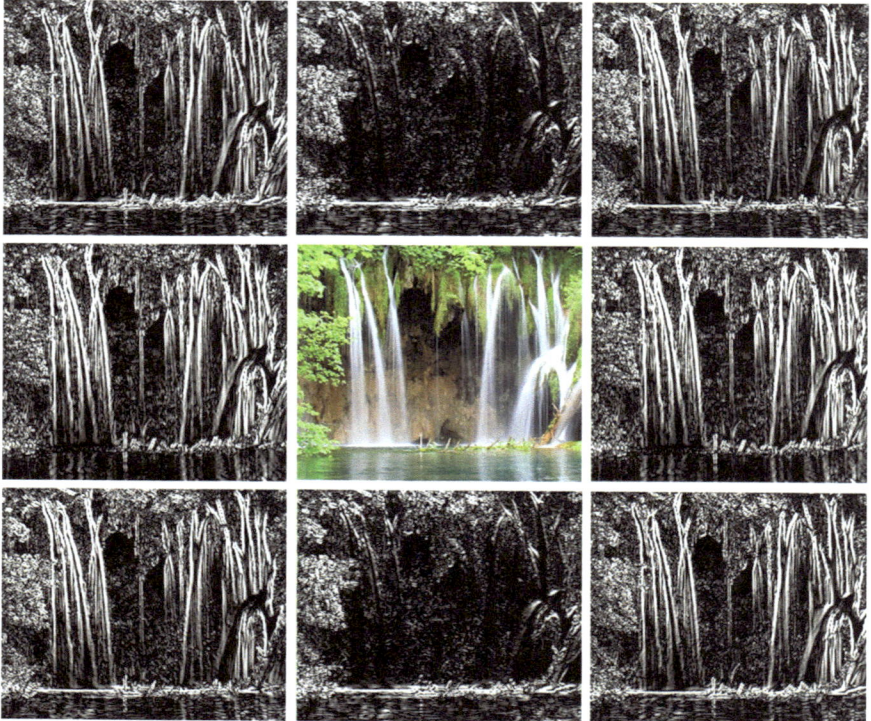

Fig. 1.9 The effect of the operation of Robinson directional gradients whose masks are shown in Fig. 1.8. The original image being processed is in the *center*

0	-1	0
-1	4	-1
0	-1	0

-1	-1	-1
-1	8	-1
-1	-1	-1

-2	1	-2
1	4	1
-2	1	-2

Fig. 1.10 Example masks of filters detecting edges—Laplacians

makes it possible to amplify or, on the contrary, suppress certain of its specific features. More examples of image analysis with the use of such filters and effects of their operation are available in [20].

Fig. 1.11 Effects of noise removal using median filtering. An example noisy image on the *left*. An image after median filtering with the use of a 3 × 3 mask on the *right*

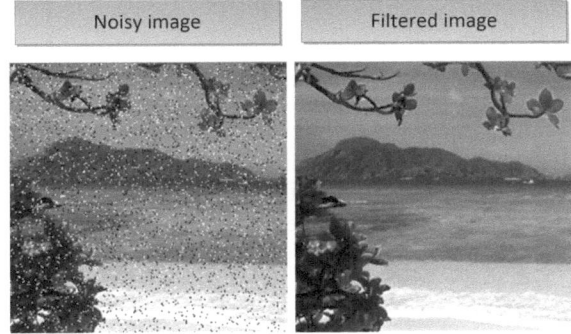

Noisy image   Filtered image

1.1.2.2 Nonlinear Transformation

Another important class of filters are nonlinear filters which make use of various nonlinear transformations of signals, and which can be used to perform filtering of the image more complex than that done with linear filters. One of the simpler ways of nonlinear image transformation is to use the so-called combined filters. Their operation consists in using two gradients in perpendicular directions, and then performing a nonlinear combination of the results produced by applying these gradients. The operation of this filter yields results better than linear filtering does, and in the case of amplifying contours in the image, for instance, produces a very clear image with amplified contours regardless of the direction of those contours.

Nonlinear filters are used in image analysis to produce the following effects:

- Damping noise and other distortions found in the image. In this case, the filter usually operates based on the median of the brightness of points surrounding the processed pixel.
- Amplifying certain elements of the image which are consistent with the pattern given by the specified structural element or neighborhood. A specific point is amplified or de-amplified depending on whether its neighbourhood meets certain conditions, e.g. logical ones.

Median Filtering

One example of a nonlinear filter is the widely used median filter, which makes it possible to very radically remove minor noise observed in the image [5, 7, 9]. The median filter is classified to filters of very severe operation, because even extreme values of distorted pixels, which significantly deviate from the average for a given region of the image, have no influence on the value obtained on the output of the filter. An example of the operation of the median filter is shown in Fig. 1.11.

In practice, a median filter leaves no trace of the removed salt and pepper noise, whether eliminating dark noise visible on a bright background or the opposite. The main advantage of median filtering is that it does not degrade the sharpness of object edges found in the filtered image. It is also worth noting that this filtering does not introduce new values into the image, so there is no need to additionally scale signal amplitudes assigned to individual pixels after it has been completed.

The disadvantages of median filtering can include a slight erosion of small objects or fragments of the image. This type of erosion is very desirable for all small details of the image, particularly those found on the edges of objects, which can be treated as noise by the median filter. Another disadvantage of the median technique is that the filtering is very time-consuming due to the necessary repeated execution of color value sorting operations for points found in the filter window. Median filtering is most frequently used to eliminate noise from the image. Figure 1.11 shows an example use of a median filter to eliminate noise from an image.

Fast Implementation of Median Filtering

If a median filter is to be used to filter the signal represented by an integer matrix, its fast implementation can be used. In the fast implementation of the median filter, value sorting in the filter window is replaced by finding a median in the table of the window pixel histogram. Finding a median in a sorted table is linearly complex. When calculating the value of the histogram for the subsequent window position, the previously found histogram can be used. We take the old histogram and delete values found in the column or the row, which is no longer covered by the window of the new histogram, and we add the values from the new column or row. The filter windows starts from the top left corner of the image, moves to the right and then, after reaching the maximum right position, moves one row down. Then the filtering proceeds to the left until it reaches the maximum left-hand side position. The window is shifted right and left along lower and lower rows until the entire image has been filtered. Figure 1.12 shows the first few steps of the fast median filtration algorithm.

Morphological Operators

A special class of nonlinear image transformations which help obtain images with features better suited for their interpretation comprises morphological transformations. The fundamental concept in morphological transformations is the so-called structural element of the image. This is usually a certain section of the image (a mask) with one central point distinguished. The most frequently used structural element is a circle with the radius of one unit, where, due to the discrete nature of the raster making up the image in the computer, the notion of the circle can be modified as appropriate to the form of a square or hexagonal mesh [8, 9].

The general operating algorithm of a morphological transformation is as follows:

- The structural element is shifted all over the image and for each point of the image, the points of the image are compared to the selected structural element
- In every point of the image, a check is made whether the real configuration of image pixels in the neighborhood of this point is consistent with the model structural element
- If the pattern of image pixels is found to comply with the template of the structural element, the defined operation is executed on the examined point.

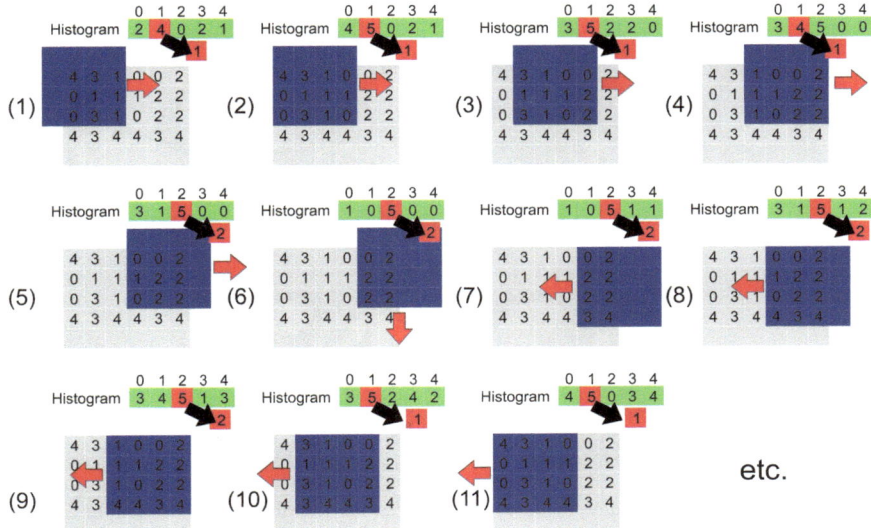

Fig. 1.12 The first 11 steps in a fast median filtration of an example six-pixel-wide matrix with a 4 × 4 pixel filter. The filtered matrix is *gray*, the filter window *blue*, and the histogram *green*. The median is marked in *red* on the histogram. *Red arrows* show the direction of subsequent filter window shifts

Morphological transformations are very popular in applications for processing and the simple analysis of technical, geological, and medical images, because these transformations can be used to execute very subtle actions on the analyzed images, which is sometimes very important for obtaining the final result [6–9].

Selected morphological operations will be briefly discussed below. The first one is erosion.

To define the erosion operation, it is assumed that there exists an irregular area A and a circle C with the radius R, which will constitute the structural element. The center of the circle C is adopted as the center point of the structural element. Then the erosion of figure A by the element C can be defined as follows:

> The eroded figure is the set of all centers of circles with the radius R which are completely contained inside the area A [8, 9].

The erosion thus defined can also be treated as the so-called minimal filter, i.e., a filter which assigns the lowest of the values of the neighbors of each point to this point [9]. Erosion is a very effective method for removing minor noise, which sometimes appears as artifacts on the edges of objects. Unfortunately, one of the features of erosion is the irrevocable removal from the image of certain small objects which could be significant and contain information important from the

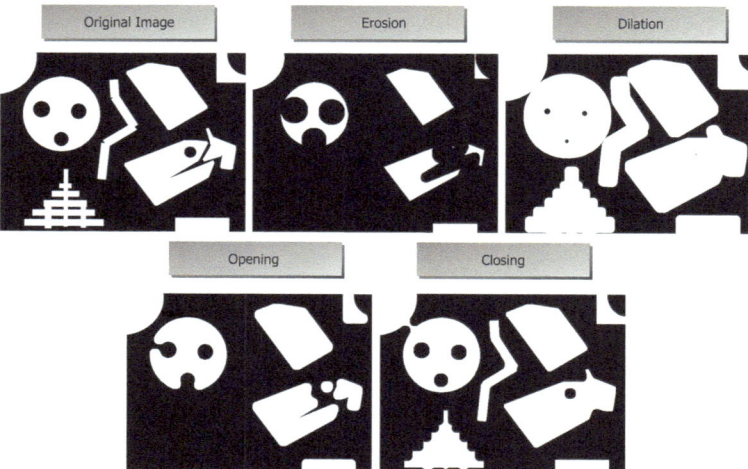

Fig. 1.13 The results of the morphological transformations described in this section for a binary input image

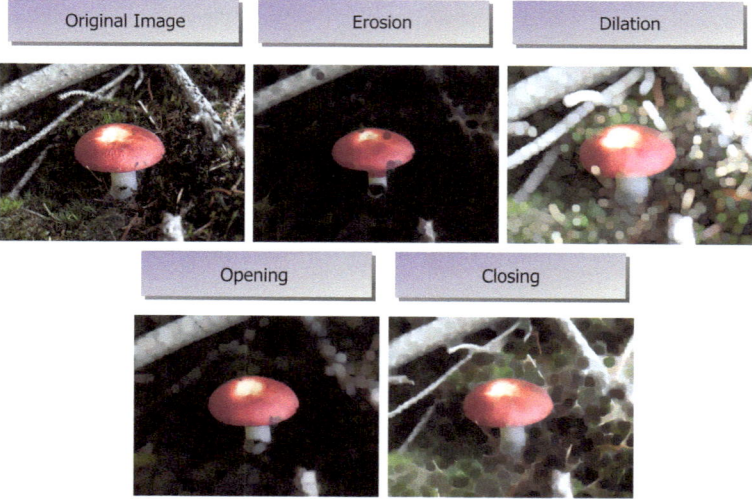

Fig. 1.14 The results of the morphological transformations described in this section for a color input image

point of view of the identification and the further analysis of the image. Examples of erosion effects are shown in Figs. 1.13 and 1.14.

The second basic morphological operation for image analysis is dilation. Unlike erosion, dilation does not reduce the area of the analyzed object but may increase it. To define the dilation operation, it is assumed that there exists an irregular area

A and a circle *C* with the radius *r*, which will form the structural element. Then, the dilation of figure *A* by element *C* may be defined as follows:

> The dilated figure is a set of the centers of all circles C for which at least one of their points overlaps any point of the original figure.

In practice, the dilation operation acts as maximal filter, i.e., a filter which assigns the highest of the values of the neighbors of each point of the considered neighborhood to this point [9]. Examples of the effects of dilation are shown in Figs. 1.13 and 1.14.

The above two basic morphological operations, i.e., erosion and dilation, have a significant drawback when used alone. They significantly change the surface area of the transformed images. Erosion reduces it and dilation increases it. To eliminate this drawback, two other transformations have been introduced, which are the combination of erosion and dilation. These are the image opening and closing operations which can be defined as follows:

$$\text{opening} = \text{erosion} + \text{dilation}$$

$$\text{closing} = \text{dilation} + \text{erosion}$$

Figures 1.13 and 1.14 show the results of applying the above morphological operations to, respectively, a binary and a color image.

Thinning and Skeletonization Techniques

Another very important morphological transformation is the thinning or skeletonization operation [8, 20]. Skeletonization is an operation which allows axial points of figures to be distinguished in the analyzed image. A more formal definition says that the skeleton of a figure is a set of all points which are equidistant from at least two points belonging to the edge of the figure.

In the computer analysis of structures which are characterized by complex shapes or major morphological changes, it may be beneficial to skeletonize the examined structures in order to identify shape changes useful for further analyses [8, 20]. Thinning with the use of a structural element consists in applying this element to each point of the image in such a way that the central point overlaps the analyzed point, and then executing one of two possible operations:

- Either leave the examined point unchanged; or if the structural element does not overlap with its neighborhood
- Change the value of the point to the value of the background if the structural element fully fits the neighborhood of the analyzed point.

The thinning processes can be executed iteratively until the stage at which subsequent steps do not produce significant changes in the image.

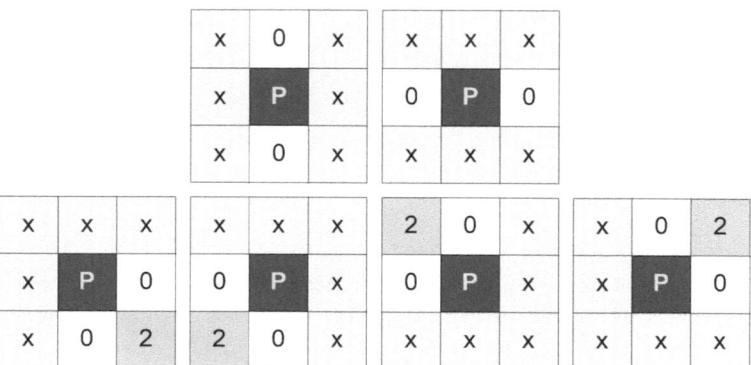

Fig. 1.15 Neighbourhood patterns for skeletal points of an image in the Pavlidis method

Skeletonization represents a special case of the thinning process. Skeletonization should produce a centerline (a skeleton line) of the thinned object, which is equidistant from the external edges and one unit thick.

The skeletonization algorithm should meet the following conditions:

- The skeleton should retain the continuity and reflect the shape of the original object
- The skeleton should be centrally located and equidistant from external object edges
- The algorithm should not cause excessive object erosion so that end points of the skeleton are detected as quickly as possible, and thus the line characterizing the object is not excessively shortened relative to the actual length of the structure which is to be represented by this skeleton;
- The skeleton should be independent of small perturbations of the processed object's external edge, while noise and other external objects should have no impact on the skeleton shape.

Structures portrayed in images can be skeletonized using, for example, the Pavlidis skeletonization algorithm, because a lot of studies of actual images have shown it to be one of the best among the many known thinning algorithms in terms of the properties and the quality of the skeleton it produces [8].

The way it works is that it removes any point P belonging to the thinned object from the image if the following criteria are met:

- P is an edge point (which means that at least one of its direct neighbors is a background point);
- P is not an end point;
- The neighborhood of the point P does not correspond to any neighborhood pattern defining skeleton points of the object, which are shown in Fig. 1.15.

In Fig. 1.15 P represents the point currently considered, and the value 0 represents points of the image background, while 2 represents skeleton points. Point P is a skeleton point if at least one of each group of points X is different from the background, i.e., it belongs to the object or is already a skeleton point represented by 2.

The main advantage of this algorithm is that it generates continuous, very regular and small skeletons which are one unit wide and centrally located. In addition, the generated lines are only slightly shortened at the ends of the analyzed structure, unlike in many other frequently used algorithms. From the perspective of the effectiveness of further analysis, another very important advantage is that the Pavlidis algorithm leaves the fewest artifacts in the form of apparent side branches of the skeleton, which are produced during the skeletonization of small irregularities of the original structure's contours.

The skeleton of a figure obtained through the thinning operation is much smaller than the figure itself, but fully reflects its basic topological properties. The analysis of skeletons of figures later makes it possible to execute the following image analyses:

- Object classification based on their shapes;
- Identifying the orientation of elongated objects;
- Separating objects that have stuck together;
- Drawing the centerline of elongated objects or tubular structures.

Many interesting examples of the use of skeletonization methods and thinning algorithms for objects can be found in [19, 20].

Filling Holes and Labeling

In some cases, the desirable end effect of image transformation is to generate a binary mask which can be used to determine areas which one would like to detect in the analyzed image. The mask is sometimes nonuniform and inside the area delineated by its nonzero edges it contains background pixels with zero values which can be called "holes." If these holes are undesirable (for example they are the effects of input image noise), the simplest way of removing them is to use a transformation called hole filling. As a result of it, all background pixels which are surrounded by the edges of objects are replaced with objects pixels, thus increasing the size of the mask.

The second useful transformation executed on binary images is called labeling. As a result of labeling, every pixel of the image is given a label defining the object found in the image to which this pixel belongs. Objects are defined as disjointed groups of pixels which are not background. If the pixel does not belong to any object (is a background pixel), it will not be labeled. The disjointedness of objects is most often examined using the direct neighborhood or the indirect neighborhood as defined in Sect. 1.1.2. Figure 1.16 shows the effects of employing both aforementioned transformations.

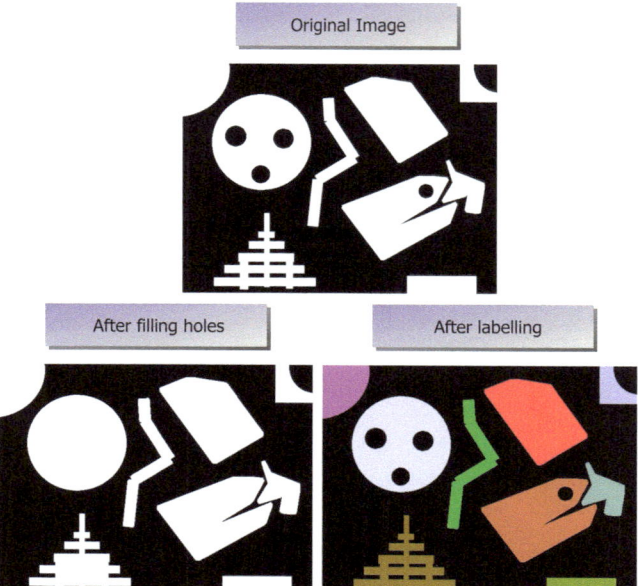

Fig. 1.16 Example results of the hole filling and labeling algorithms. The binary input image is at the *top*, *white* pixels make up objects, *black* pixels are the background. *Bottom left* the input image with filled holes. On the *right*: the input image after the labeling operation. Pixels corresponding to individual labels have been colored with randomly generated colors using a look up table

1.1.3 Other Nonlinear Transformations

Nonlinear image transformations can also be executed without regard to the neighborhood of a given point, and then they are not context operations. There are very many important image processing procedures, which make use of complex pixel transformation functions without taking into account the neighborhood of the examined point of the image. Such methods also include various techniques of image segmentation or image transformation into other coordinate systems.

Image Segmentation Techniques

A class of nonlinear methods that is very important from the perspective of image processing comprises image segmentation or binarization algorithms. Segmentation usually represents the first step at the stage of the preliminary analysis of images, which allows significant elements of the image to be extracted, while at the same time suppressing the unnecessary background elements. Its purpose is to significantly reduce the amount of information contained in the image and to remove components which are immaterial from the point of view of the semantic analysis. The segmentation process consists in converting the entire scope of the color palettes or the grayscale of a given image into an image that is composed of only two colors, represented in a binary form. Most frequently, it is possible to use several binarization methods including the simplest methods of standards thresholding as well as advanced techniques aimed at segmenting complex visualizations. Among the simplest binarization methods, it is worth noting the so-called binarization with lower or upper threshold. They are defined as follows:

- Lower threshold binarization:

$$I' = \begin{cases} 0; I(m,n) \leq a \\ 1; I(m,n) > a \end{cases} \tag{1.4}$$

- Upper threshold binarization:

$$I' = \begin{cases} 0; I(m,n) \geq a \\ 1; I(m,n) < a \end{cases} \tag{1.5}$$

where:

$I(m, n)$—point brightness in the source image;

$I'(m, n)$—the value of the appropriate point of the output image, coming from a two element set (depending on the convention this may be $\{0, 1\}$ or e.g. $\{0, 2^{24}\}$, where 24 is the number of image bits);

a—the preset binarization threshold.

When this method is used, it is necessary to select the binarization threshold. One of the easiest techniques for selecting such as threshold consists in the previously mentioned histogram analysis techniques [6, 7, 9], as the histogram shows the distribution of the number of image points having a specific value of colors or graylevels. In this approach the value of the binarization threshold is frequently set based on the local minima of the histogram function.

Figure 1.17 shows an example image and its histogram, as well as the result of executing a simple threshold for the color level determined on the histogram.

In the case of images in which the objects have brightness levels significantly different from the elements of the image background, methods as simple as single threshold binarization may produce satisfactory results. Unfortunately, in the majority of cases they leave too many immaterial elements, which is frequently the reason to look for other, more advanced and oriented methods. These slightly more advanced binarization methods make it possible to segment images of a more complex structure.

Generally, the appropriate segmentation method should be selected depending on the type of image processed as well as the expected results and its subsequent analysis. For a given type of image, not every segmentation method may turn out

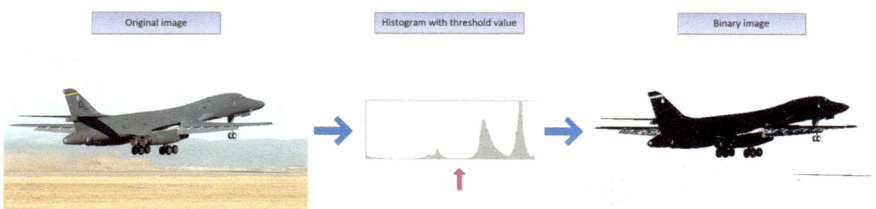

Fig. 1.17 An example color image together with the histogram on which the binarization threshold has been marked

right, whereas the results of various segmentation algorithms can frequently be combined, using masking and logical operations on binary images. Such combinations frequently produce satisfactory results [6, 9].

However, because segmentation is frequently strongly connected to binarization, it is worth remembering that the following binarization techniques can be distinguished:

Segmentation by Thresholding
Segmentation by thresholding consists in defining a threshold value, that is a certain graylevel or color, which marks the border between the image background and objects. As a result of this process all image points whose brightness is below the threshold value get, for example, the value of zero, while points with a brightness equal to the threshold value greater get the maximum value. This type of binarization can be executed with two or more threshold values. If there are two threshold values, the points whose brightness is between the threshold values get the logical value of one and are classified as the object, while the remaining points receive the logical value of zero and are considered the background. The threshold values can be selected experimentally, for example on the basis of an analysis of the input histogram, or automatically, by a computer program, based on certain heuristics. The segmentation of color images by the creation of chromatic masks constitutes a special type of thresholding segmentation, where three monochromatic images corresponding to primary colors are extracted from a color image, and then the threshold values are determined for each channel separately. The points whose brightness in each channel falls between the threshold values are given the logical value of 1, whereas the remaining points—zero.

Segmentation by Edge Detection
Segmentation executed by detecting edges is a method which consists in setting the values of image edge gradients, which can be done, among others, using top pass filters whose operation results in amplifying all edges of objects or only directional edges. An image obtained this way is not a pure binary image, but the edges have a certain color or gray-level distribution. To unambiguously identify the edges of objects, it is necessary to define the criteria according to which points of the image belong to the edges of the object. Such criteria include an analysis of

the brightness gradient value differences in a specific neighborhood of every point. If this difference is greater than a certain threshold value, the point is considered to belong to the object border. For these methods, such parameters as the size of the area of the neighborhood considered and the threshold value of gradients which will be used to locally describe image contrasts can be defined. Every area whose contrast is greater than the threshold value is treated as an object and is given the logical value of one. Such activities aimed at detecting edges are frequently called the dynamic segmentation or adaptive segmentation. It should be noted that following such as segmentation process, only the borders of structures will have been identified, without keeping their interiors [9].

Binarization by Area Growing
Segmentation by area growing consists in connecting points or fragments of an image into larger areas. The operation of this method consists in finding pixels around the selected starting pixels, which former pixels meet a specific similarity condition. This condition may relate to the brightness, color, texture, etc. When a given point meets the defined condition, it is attached to the area and the points neighboring it are checked against the similarity criteria, and if they meet it, they are added to the selected area. If none of the neighboring points of the area meets the condition, the area growth stop stops. The appropriate number of starting points is selected depending on the number of areas into which the image is to be divided [9].

Segmentation Using Neural Networks
Images can also be segmented using a properly trained neural network, which can accept, as input data, a fragment of the image and a set of features determined for the fragment. On the output, this network generates the number of the class to which a given fragment or point of the image has been assigned (background or object). Feedforward MLP networks, unsupervised learning Kohonen networks and Hopfield recurrent networks are those most frequently used [9, 20].

Hough Transform in Image Processing
In an analysis of image processing techniques, it is also worth mentioning the Hugh transform [9]. This transform was proposed in 1962 by Paul Hugh and allows selected image features to be extracted [9]. It represents a special case of the Radon transform, known since 1917 and equivalent to the Hough transform as far as binary images are concerned. The main task of this transform is to extract regular sets of points forming lines, circles, curves, etc., from an image. When analyzing the idea behind the Hough method for the simplest example of detecting a straight line in an image, a set of co-linear points should be identified in the image using the following formula:

$$\lambda_0 = \{(x, y) \in R^2 : y - ax - b = 0\} \qquad (1.6)$$

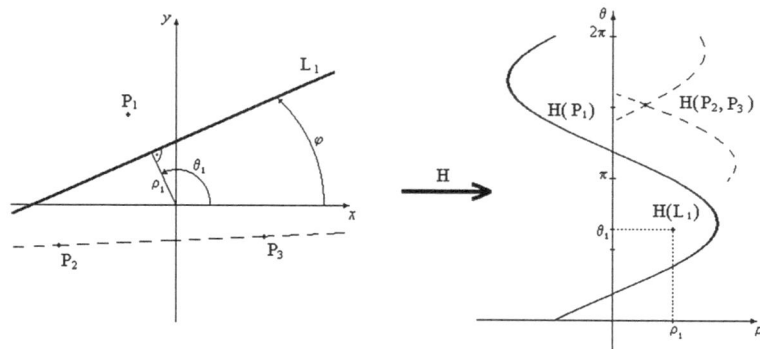

Fig. 1.18 A graphic notation of the Hough transform. An example mapping the straight line *L1* and the points *P1*, *P2* i *P3* from the Cartesian plane to the Hough plane. **a** Cartesian space, **b** Hough transform space [20]

where *a* and *b* are parameters characterizing the straight line. The solution of this equation is a set of points on a plane, and this set's characteristic feature is that for one point we can obtain a set of co-linear points in the parameter space. As a result, it is possible to identify all straight lines running through a given point, and then to select those lines which could cause the pixel looked for to be activated. The identification of the appropriate straight lines is strictly connected with the notion of the reverse projection which consists in analyzing every active pixel of the image in order to identify these straight lines.

Figure 1.18 shows the graphic notation of the Hough linear transform. This transform maps a Cartesian plane to a two-dimensional plane of parameters (ρ, Θ) describing straight lines (the Hough plane). The straight line from the Cartesian plane is mapped to a single point on the Hough plane, with the coordinates of this point unambiguously identifying this straight line. On the Hough plane, the point from the Cartesian plane becomes a sinusoid curve determining a pencil of lines running through this point. This is described by the following formulas:

$$x \cdot \cos \theta_0 + y \cdot \sin \theta_0 = \rho_0 \;\longrightarrow\; (\rho_0, \theta_0)$$
$$(x_0, y_0) \;\longrightarrow\; x_0 \cdot \cos \theta + y_0 \cdot \sin \theta = \rho, \; 0 \leq \theta < 2\pi \qquad (1.7)$$
$$\text{for } 0 \leq \theta \leq 2\pi, \; \rho \geq 0$$

These relationships produce the following characteristic: the intersection point in the Hough space of two curves constituting the transforms of two different points of the Cartesian space describes the straight line running through these two points in the Cartesian space.

Using this transform to process digital images consists in finding a point in the transformed image in which a large number of curves representing points of the Cartesian space intersect. This point may mean that the original image contains a straight section belonging to a straight line mapped to a point of the Hough space. This point is the point of intersection of sine waves in the transformed image— Fig. 1.18.

Several types of Hough transforms are distinguished, the main ones being as follows:

1. fast Hough transform;
2. probabilistic Hough transform;
3. randomized Hough transform;
4. hierarchical Hough transform;
5. fuzzy Hough transform; and
6. variable resolution transform.

Practical problems most frequently solved using the Hough method can include not only identifying straight lines, but also curves, arcs, polygons, circles, or ellipses, and in addition the use of this method for 3D images is considered.

The Hough transform has many advantages. Since every point of the image is treated independently, the transform can be executed using parallel calculations and multiprocessor systems. This method is relatively resistant to image noise (because it quantizes the values of angles and distances between straight lines), and therefore can identify even partly deformed objects. Even if only between 10 and 20 % of pixels from an image are given, the transform is often still able to detect an object as well as circles, spheres, and ellipses in the image.

1.2   Image Classification and Recognition Techniques

The second very important group of image analysis techniques comprises identification and classification algorithms. These methods enable the computer recognition of analyzed objects and their categorization to the appropriately defined classes of patterns. In very general terms, image recognition consists in determining whether various types of patterns or objects belong to certain previously, a priori defined classes. Recognition can be performed based on principles and rules determined by the type of objects being recognized and dependent on specific characteristics of the image. Rule-based recognition can be used for only relatively simple problems. In the case of many other tasks where there is no a priori information about the rules according to which these or those objects (and their images) belong to specific pattern classes, the only information that can be used by the classifying algorithm is contained in the so-called training sequence, i.e., a sequence of patterns comprising objects whose correct classification was known before [12, 20, 21]. The need to refer to a training set means that the task of image recognition becomes extremely interesting as an example of a problem requiring induction reasoning to be carried out by the computer. In practice this means that the computer recognizing images must, to some extent, learn to recognize new images based on examples presented to it previously.

The key to training image recognition algorithms is generalization, which means that such an algorithm is able not only to collect knowledge based on the patterns provided to it, but additionally, after completing the training, can recognize completely new images which had not been included in the training sequence: as a result of this, it can be used in practice to recognize completely new patterns.

During the recognition of relatively simple images containing repeatable objects which are not significantly different one from another (for example, when recognizing printed characters), recognition is possible with the use of a simple analysis of the image as such: e.g., by way of comparing it to a stored pattern. This method is called template matching. In the case of many classes of complex images, the varied nature of objects which can be subject to recognizing requires a recognition process whose preliminary stage is to detect significant features characteristic for the given images. After that stage, this recognition process consists in analyzing the detected features and ends in an attempt to take a decision, i.e., to classify the image to one of the previously defined object classes [12, 20].

The development of image recognition methods started in the early period of artificial intelligence method build-out in the 1950s. The first practical implementations of image recognition techniques were based on neural network systems created by Rosenblatt in 1968. These systems were based on a structure of several levels of artificial electronic neurons containing computational data, premises collected during the learning process and supporting the recognition, as well as output systems which took final decisions.

By today, many image recognition methods have been developed and tested. The first to appear were the so-called classical image recognition methods based on metrics in the feature space, also called the minimum-distance methods. Their forerunner was the Nearest Neighbor (NN) method [12, 14, 20, 21], which will be presented lower down in this chapter. This method was simple, but often prone to failure, so various modifications of it were developed, namely algorithms insensitive to errors in the training sequence, such as the k-NN method or the j_N-NN method. These methods are still frequently used today, because they offer highly accurate object recognition, though at the cost of large requirements for storage that is taken up or the time taken by the computations.

Other types of classical image recognition methods which appeared in addition to minimum-distance techniques were the approximation and probabilistic methods. All together, they form the so-called holistic image recognition methods. They are characterized in greater detail lower down in this chapter. They represent a completely different approach to building an object classification algorithm, yet one which in many cases produces similar results and a similar recognition effectiveness as minimum-distance methods, albeit with a much smaller load on the recognition system, both in terms of the memory used and the computing time.

In the case of complex images, the effectiveness of classical recognition methods is poor, particularly when they are recognizing patterns composed of many objects. This problem was solved by the appearance of the second important

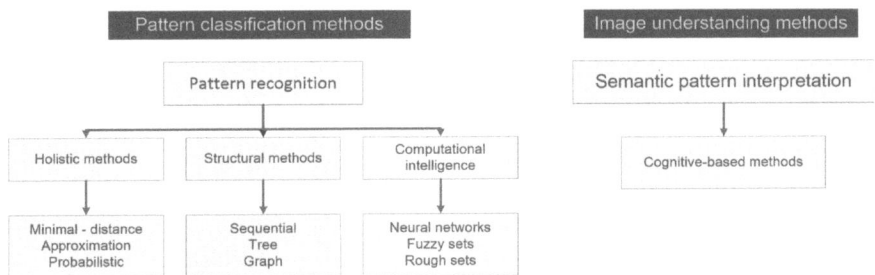

Fig. 1.19 The general classification of image recognition and understanding methods

class of methods, i.e., syntactic and structural methods, which make use of mathematical linguistic formalisms [17, 21, 22, 29].

The development of image recognition techniques was also connected with the increased intensity of research on neural networks and the ability to use them to classify patterns, which occurred in 1980.

At that time, several very effective, formal and heuristic methods of training multilayer neural networks were proposed, which allowed patterns to be recognized by way of imitating examples from the so-called training set, subsequently generalized to patterns which had not been presented during the training, but which were to some extent similar to the training ones. However, the applicability of neural networks to analyzing and classifying complex images is limited because the image itself (particularly a high resolution one) cannot be fed as a whole to the input of a neural network, while attempts to train networks to recognize images using image features (extracted during preprocessing) have not demonstrated any significant advantage of this technique over techniques based on the previously mentioned holistic methods.

As a result of the introduction of the above methods, there are now many different ways of identifying various types of patterns and of automatically classifying images. Figure 1.19 shows a general classification of methods for recognizing images and new techniques of computer image understanding [21, 22].

Further subsections characterize selected techniques for recognizing and semantically analyzing images. Methods using neural networks, decision-making methods and syntactic methods based on the use of formal languages will be discussed in particular detail.

1.2.1 Holistic Methods of Pattern Recognition

This presentation of various techniques for recognizing images will start with a discussion of holistic methods. In these methods, images are recognized by executing an algorithm allowing the analyzed patterns to be classified based on certain distinguished features of the image [12, 21]. This algorithm can be written in the form of a general mapping:

$$\mathbf{R} : \mathbf{I} \rightarrow \mathbf{r} \cup \{r_0\}, \tag{1.8}$$

where:

I—the set of images being recognized

r—defines the set of classes of recognized objects

r_0—represents a neutral recognition, i.e., the lack of a decision.

In particular, the mapping R can be executed as the composition of three independent recognition stages given by the following, subsequent mappings:

$$R = D \bullet C \bullet B, \tag{1.9}$$

where:

B—is the pattern reception function (of an analysis-oriented at identifying features);

C—is a function describing the membership of vectors of features describing patterns in individual classes;

D—is the decision-making (classification) function which supports the unambiguous assignment to a recognized class or generates a message that this classification cannot be completed.

The first stage in recognizing any object is to measure significant features of the objects being recognized. This measurement defines the perception function given in the following form:

$$B : I \rightarrow X, \tag{1.10}$$

where X—represents the feature space.

The ability to identify significant features makes it possible to transform the recognized objects $d \in I$ to n-dimensional points of the X feature space. The elements of this space are n-element vectors $\underline{x} = (x_1, x_2, \ldots, x_n) \in X$ describing the most important parameters of the recognized objects.

The feature vector having been defined, the next stage in the recognition process is to determine whether the unknown object $d \in I$ belongs to particular classes. This process consists in calculating the values of the so-called functions of membership of all the considered classes. This stage of the recognition process is defined by the following mapping:

$$\mathbf{C} : \mathbf{X} \rightarrow \Re^{\mathbf{N}}, \tag{1.11}$$

where $\Re$—a set of real numbers and N—the number of recognized classes

In order to execute this mapping, the defined feature vector $\underline{x}$ (determined by the perception function) should be used to calculate the values of the membership function one after another for every recognized pattern. The values of these functions define the measure of the membership of an unknown object d in individual classes, so they are real numbers. As the quantity of these numbers that have to be identified is equal to the quantity of the considered classes, the result of mapping C is a set N of such numbers, and this is formally recorded as an element of an N-dimensional space of real numbers $\Re^N$.

The ultimate stage in image recognition is to take the final decision on the correct recognition (or the inability to recognize), using the mapping:

$$\mathbf{D} : \Re^N \rightarrow \mathbf{r} \cup \{r_0\} \tag{1.12}$$

The classification function D is used to take the decision that a given object $d \in I$ (described at this stage by the feature vector $\underline{x}$) is a member of the class

$i \in r$ for which the value of the appropriate membership function is the greatest. All these stages are detailed in the book [21].

1.2.1.1 Metrics-Based Methods of Pattern Recognition

The discussion of examples of image recognition methods will start with minimum-distance methods in which the membership functions are related to the notion of the distance in the image feature space. Consequently, this space must be equipped with the appropriate metric so that such distances can actually be determined. As there are many relationships which fulfill the axioms of metrics, the author of the recognition method is completely free in choosing and using the appropriate metric. It should be noted, however, that in practical uses of minimum-distance methods the effectiveness of the method often strongly depends on the selected metric, which has a huge impact on the results obtained [12, 14, 21].

In minimum-distance methods, the concept of recognizing and classifying unrecognized patterns consists in selecting the number of the class to which the pattern closest (according to the adopted metric) to the object currently being recognized belongs as the correct recognition. Minimum-distance methods are based on assumptions related to the geometry of the feature space. Hence, if points corresponding to objects of various classes aggregate together into clear concentrations or clusters, it makes sense to use the values of the distance when taking the decision to classify a new pattern.

The Nearest Neighbor (NN) Method
The simplest of the minimum-distance methods is the NN method. The decision-making rule of the NN algorithm assumes that a new object will be put in the class to which the object of the training sequence located closest to it in the feature space belongs (Fig. 1.20).

The advantage of this method is its simplicity, but its significant drawback is its computational complexity which reaches high values if the training sequence consists of a large number of elements.

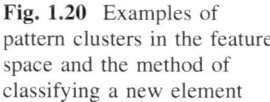

Fig. 1.20 Examples of
pattern clusters in the feature
space and the method of
classifying a new element

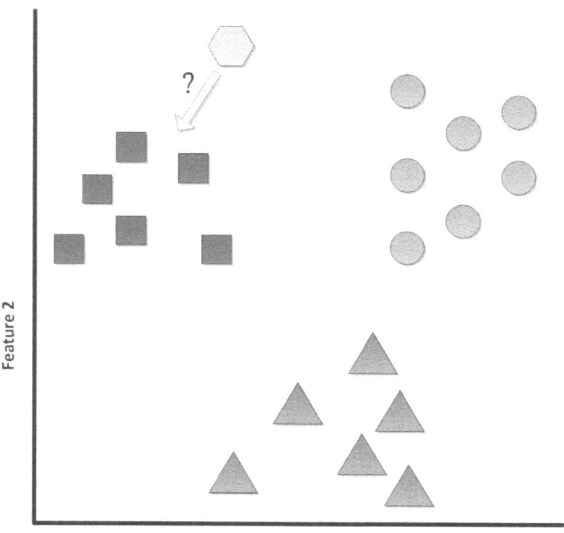

The k-Nearest Neighbors (k-NN) Method

Because the classical NN method is very sensitive to errors in the training sequence, if the membership of even one element from the training sequence is determined incorrectly, its entire neighborhood will be incorrectly classified and assigned to the same group as the previously incorrectly classified element of the training sequence.

In order to minimize the number of wrong classifications, methods are introduced in which the decision is taken based on a greater number of objects from the training sequence, located the closest to the object of unknown membership. Assuming that there are k of those objects, this method is called k-NN. In this method, the value k is used as the parameter whose choice determines the characteristics of the method. This parameter is chosen arbitrarily, as a certain small natural number.

In this method, the classification process is executed in such a way that after determining the value k for pattern being recognized, the values of the distance from all elements of the training sequence are calculated. Then, the training sequence is arranged in the order of the increasing distance from the newly recognized pattern, and subsequently k initial objects of this sorted training sequence are selected. At the end, the new pattern is classified to the class which is most numerously represented among the considered k elements closest to it in the entire training sequence.

The characteristics of the j_N-NN algorithm are similar to the k-NN method. The former algorithm, in essence, is about determining that an unknown object is a member of the class to which the j_Nth subsequent element of the U training sequence belongs according to the rules described for the k-NN.

When characterizing minimum-distance algorithms we can state that they are frequently used in practice because of their simplicity and intuitiveness as well as their high effectiveness. However, they have some drawbacks, namely their high computational complexities and storage requirements. These methods require storing the entire training sequence and require calculating the distance between the object being recognized and all elements of the training sequence in order to select the object's k nearest neighbors.

1.2.1.2 Approximation-Based Methods

The second broad class of holistic methods are the approximation ones. In these methods, the functions of pattern membership of particular classes are expansions into series against a defined family of base functions which form an ordered family [12, 14]. The coefficients of this expansion are treated as weights which allow a specific membership function to be determined for each of the classes considered. These coefficients are important in that, for the preset family of base functions, the job of defining the decision-making rules for particular classes is replaced with the job of determining the values of weighs of a finite expansion of the membership function into a series of base functions.

Because the expansions of membership functions are finite, it is obvious that to identify all membership functions, it suffices to identify only $N*m$ values of coefficients (N is the number of classes whereas m is the number of base coefficients) which are the only information that has to be stored during the subsequent recognition. When contrasted with the necessity of storing the entire training sequence in the minimum-distance methods, this is a major simplification.

Linear Approximation Techniques
Once we have defined the base family of functions, the training sequence can be used to determine the values of weighing coefficients of the expansion of membership functions. Under special assumptions, these functions allow the membership function to be expanded into a linear function.

Once we have such a function, we can easily derive the rules of identifying the weighing coefficients, because they can be determined based on an optimization aimed at minimizing the error made by the classifier when separating individual classes. In this recognition case, the optimal membership function is defined for classes which are to be separated linearly in the feature space.

In practice, we are never certain whether the considered classes are linearly separable, so it makes sense to try to use this method as the first in a sequence, but one has to be ready for the necessary, precise verification of the result and replacing the membership function with nonlinear functions if the classifier generates too many errors.

The benefits of using linear membership functions are as follows:

- The recognition algorithm is simple, while the membership function itself is easy to compute.
- The number of elements which must be stored is the lowest possible and it is sufficient to store $N*(m + 1)$ weighing coefficients of the expansion of membership functions.
- The training algorithm is simple to execute and boils down to just determining the values of expansion coefficients based on the training sequence.

What is interesting is that the formula defining the membership functions can also be interpreted as the simplest description of a neuron's operation. Here, the human ability to recognize objects serves as a kind of pattern for the recognition tasks considered in practice. This subject is more broadly elaborated on in the chapters below which deal with neural networks.

Nonlinear Transformations in Region Separation

The linear function method described above was based on using a linear approximation of the expansion of the membership function into a finite sequence of base functions. However, such an expansion of the membership function may sometimes not enable obtaining satisfactory recognition results due to the shapes of clusters of objects in the feature space. Yet, it turns out that the linear expansion formula makes it possible to generate separating planes of any shape, and not only shaped as hyperplanes like in the case of linear approximations. For example, the use of second degree polynomials as base functions makes it possible to obtain ellipsoids, paraboloids, hyperboloids and any combinations thereof as the separating structures. It also turns out that the number m of the coefficients present in the expansion of the membership function also influences the recognition effectiveness (the correct separation of classes in the feature space). There is a theorem about the link between the number of weights determined and the probability of a correct recognition [10, 12]. This theorem says that if there are problems with recognition and the m is increased, this will contribute to getting better results. It therefore makes sense to adopt a recognition method based on a membership function of the following general form:

$$C^i(\underline{x}) = \sum_{v=0}^{m} V_v^i \varphi_v(\underline{x}) \tag{1.13}$$

where

C^i—is the function of membership of the ith class

V_v^i—are expansion coefficients of the membership function calculated for the ith class

$\varphi_v(\underline{x})$—are base functions

For this function, the training process (namely finding the weights V_v^i) is conducted similarly to that for linear functions, but with the difference that one specifies the transformation of the n-dimensional feature space into a straightening m-dimensional space in which the areas belonging to various classes, which are not linearly separable in the feature space, can be separated with hyperplanes. The details of this operation can be found in [10, 21].

This clearly shows that as the dimension m of the space increases, so does the probability of a correct recognition. However, it should be borne in mind that the m should be increased in such a way as to introduce components which significantly add new information. These can be additional features of images, but they can also be new transformations executed on the feature space.

Support Vector Machines
Methods consisting in separating regions or clusters of objects using linear or nonlinear classifiers mainly follow the principle that vectors of features describing new objects being classified should be of the smallest possible dimension. The job of recognizing patterns using a feature vector is in this case executed for the smallest possible number of features characterizing the researched image. A slightly different approach can be seen in Support Vector Machines (SVM) methods. The SVM technique consists in preprocessing data in such a way that patterns can be presented using feature vectors of a high dimension, usually much higher than the originally considered feature space. If the right non-linear mapping, which will allow a sufficiently high dimension to be achieved, is used, all data (e.g., from two categories, but not linearly separable in the original feature space) can always be separated by the appropriate hyperplane in a space of a suitably greater dimensionality, in which it will be possible to separate them linearly, but using a hyperplane of the appropriately higher dimension. To do this, however, it becomes necessary to train the SVM so that it would find a plane separating the classes that has the greatest margins (i.e., distances between the hyperplane and the instances of two classes located closest to one another) but still allows the analyzed patterns to be correctly classified [10, 12]. It is assumed that the greater the margin, the better the generalization of the classifier. The distance between any hyperplane and the transformed pattern is given with a certain, permissible margin. The purpose of this approach is to find the weight vector which maximizes the value of the margin b. As the target vector can be changed arbitrarily and still indicate the correct hyperplane, the restriction $b||a|| = 1$ is imposed. The solution considered to be correct should also minimize the value $||a||^2$. Support vectors are the transformed patterns for which the above relationship is true. The patterns are then equidistant from the produced hyperplane and are treated as training samples, which identify the optimum separation of the hyperplane dividing individual classes. Such patterns are the most useful and provide the most information in the classification process [10].

The first step in training an SVM is to select nonlinear functions which will transform the input patterns into a space of a new (higher) dimension. This is frequently imposed top-down, but if this information is missing, one can use a Gaussian function, for instance, or another family of well-parametrized functions. The dimensionality of the space being transformed can be as high as desired, but is usually restricted by the computing capacity. More information about SVMs is available in [10, 12].

1.2.1.3 Probabilistic Methods of Pattern Recognition

Probabilistic methods can also be included in the classical (holistic) image recognition methods. Such recognition algorithms can be divided into supervised and unsupervised methods. Recognition is supervised when it refers to patterns preset previously (the training sequence). This type of recognition can, in turn, be subdivided into smaller groups of methods such as:

- Maximum probability method;
- Bayesian method;
- Minimum-distance classifier (previously described);
- Entropy criterion.

Unsupervised recognition takes place without reference to known patterns, which are not available in this case. This group of methods can be split into subgroups, including;

- K-means grouping;
- Vector quantization;
- Hierarchical clustering.

Statistical image recognition methods assign patterns to the most probable classes. The decision-making rules (classification functions) can be created in many ways here. What is usually taken into account are the values of the classification error as well as the transformation known from the assumptions and associated with the given probability class $P(c_i)$ for the conditional probability $P(c_i|x)$, where x is an n-dimensional feature vector.

In image recognition by statistical methods it is assumed that the probabilities $P(x|c_i)$ and $P(c_i)$ are known for every class. The set of training samples is frequently also given. They represent the type, the features and the basic classes. For the classifier to be able to recognize new objects, only the problem of training it arises. If the probability density function is unknown, we encounter a problem with determining its parameters. The Bayesian method is one of the ways of determining this probability density function (PDF) based on available experimental data described by the feature vector and corresponding to training sample patterns. Every PDF density function can be characterized by the appropriate set of parameters.

The one most frequently used is the Gaussian function characterized by average values and a covariance matrix defined for each class c_i included in the training dataset. This technique is called the parametric estimation. Two methods exemplify parametric estimations, namely the maximum probability method and the Bayesian method [10, 12–14].

The maximum probability method assumes that the parameters searched for are constants, but unknown. It finds the best parameters which raise the probability of obtaining the given learning set. The Bayesian method, on the other hand, uses the training set to update the learning set conditional on the density function of

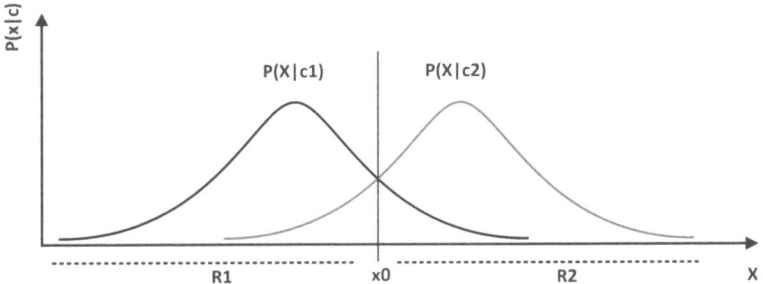

Fig. 1.21 A diagram of a Bayesian rule classification

unknown parameters. The training set allows a priori information to be replaced with experimentally determined density functions.

Bayesian Method

The Bayesian decision-making theory is the fundamental statistical method used to classify images. This technique is based on the assumption that the problem of taking a decision is formulated in a probabilistic way and significant parameters of statistical distributions are given. The best method of illustrating this topic will be to present it using the example of two separable classes c_1 c_2. The a priori probabilities that these classes will occur are defined as $P(c_1)$ and $P(c_2)$ and are known from the assumptions from the moment they can be distinguished from the available training set. We also know the probability density distribution functions $P(x_i|c_i), i = 1, 2$.

$P(x_i|c_i)$ can be called the conditional probability function c_i referring to the feature vector x_i.

By referring to the Bayesian rule, we obtain the relationship for the *posteriori* probability

$$P(c_i|x) = \frac{P(x|c_i)P(c_i)}{P(x)} \tag{1.14}$$

where $p(x)$ is the probability density x, to which the following formula applies:

$$P(x) = \sum_{i=1}^{2} P(x|c_i)P(c_i) \tag{1.15}$$

For each vector x, the total *posteriori* probability is equal to 1.

The Bayesian classification is easiest discussed for two classes c_1 c_2. The following rules then apply:

If $P(c_1|x) > P(c_2|x)$, then x is determined for c_1

If $P(c_1|x) < P(c_2|x)$, then x is determined for c_2

Figure 1.21 shows two equally probable classes and their probability density functions $P(x|c_i)$. The vertical line marks the threshold dividing the one-dimensional feature space into two regions R1 and R2. Based on the Bayesian rule, all values x belonging to R1 are determined for the class c_1, and the values x belonging to R2 are determined for the class c_2.

The probability of making a decision error can be calculated using the formula below.

$$P(\text{error}) = \int_{-\infty}^{x_0} P(x|c_2)P(c_2)\mathrm{d}x + \int_{x_0}^{+\infty} P(x|c_1)P(c_1)\mathrm{d}x \qquad (1.16)$$

The classification error is the lowest when features are divided into two regions R1 and R2 as follows:

$$\text{R1}: \; \mathrm{P}(c_1|\mathrm{x}) > \mathrm{P}(c_2|\mathrm{x}) \qquad (1.17)$$

$$\text{R2}: \; \mathrm{P}(c_2|\mathrm{x}) > \mathrm{P}(c_1|\mathrm{x}) \qquad (1.18)$$

Obviously, the presented line of reasoning for two classes can be generalized for any M number of classes $c_1, c_2,..., c_m$. Then, the feature vector x is assigned to class c_i if the following is true:

$$P(c_i|x) > P(c_j|x) \, \forall j \neq i \qquad (1.19)$$

Every time an object is assigned to some class, there is a risk of a wrong recognition being made. The method of identifying wrong recognitions is given by the (alleged) loss function. Let $L(i, j)$ be the loss (cost) resulting from the wrong classification of an object to class i, if it really is a member of class j. Under these assumptions, the ability to assess a wrong classification is achieved by defining the alleged loss function $L(i, j)$ where $i, j = 1, 2,..., M$. This function $L(i, j)$ is equal to zero if the feature vector x is assigned to the right class and is greater than zero in the opposite case, i.e. $L(i, j) > 0$, if x is classified to class c_j and not to its right class c_i. If wrong classifications are considered in terms of the losses incurred, the conditional loss parameter $R_i(x)$ of the classification of x to the ith class can be defined as:

$$R_i(x) = \sum_{j=1}^{M} L(i,j)P(c_j|x) \qquad (1.20)$$

or in other terms

$$R_i(x) = \sum_{j=1}^{M} L(i,j) \frac{P(x|c_j)P(c_j)}{P(x)} \tag{1.21}$$

For practical applications, the following are assumed: $L(i, j) = 0$ for $i = j$ and $L(i, j) = 1$ for $i \neq j$.

The above conclusions and definitions yield a slightly modified Bayesian classification according to which the feature vector x is assigned to the class c_i for which $R_i(x)$ is the minimum.

Maximum Entropy Criterion
If the probability density functions are unknown, we can estimate them using parameters such as the entropy, by aiming to maximize it. The definition of entropy comes from Shannon's information theory [30] and for image recognition applications it determines the randomness measurement of feature vectors. The entropy H for the probability density function $p(x)$ is given by the following formula:

$$H = - \int_X p(x) \ln p(x) dx \tag{1.22}$$

It should also be assumed that $p(x)$ is unknown, but certain boundary data (average values, variances) is known.

To understand this better, it is worth illustrating it with an example.

Let us assume that the random variable x is different from zero for $a \leq x \leq b$ and is equal to zero outside this interval. We wish to determine the maximum entropy of its probability density function. In this sense, we need to determine the maximum of the above formula for entropy assuming that:

$$\int_a^b p(x) dx = 1 \tag{1.23}$$

Using Lagrange multipliers, we obtain the equivalent form [10, 12]

$$H_L = - \int_a^b p(x)(\ln p(x) - \lambda) dx \tag{1.24}$$

The derivative H_L for $p(x)$ is given by the formula

$$\frac{\partial H_L}{\partial p(x)} = - \int_a^b \{(\ln p(x) - \lambda) + 1\} dx \tag{1.25}$$

By equating the above equation to zero we get

$$\hat{p}(x) = \exp(\lambda - 1) \tag{1.26}$$

The assumptions indicate that $\exp(\lambda - 1) = \frac{1}{b-a}$. Consequently, we will get the value of the looked for probability $p(x)$ for which entropy reaches its maximum from the formula

$$p(x) = \begin{cases} \frac{1}{b-a} & a \leq x \leq b \\ 0 & \text{else} \end{cases} \tag{1.27}$$

It is then easy to notice that the requirement to obtain the maximum entropy of an unknown probability distribution $p(x)$ is met when $p(x)$ is a uniform distribution over a certain interval.

Nonparametric Estimation Methods

Unlike in parametric methods of estimating the function of probability density distributions, in the nonparametric estimation we have little data we can use directly. In the majority of image recognition jobs, we have no information about the probability density functions associated with classes, so they have to be estimated directly based on the data. There are many methods based on the nonparametric estimation. Some consist in estimating the density function $p(x|c_i)$ based on trial patterns. If results obtained in this manner turn out to be good, they can be added to the optimum classifier. Another way is to estimate directly from the a posteriori probabilities $P(c_i|x)$. This is a method better connected to nonparametric decision-making procedures, which omit probability estimation and execute decision-making functions straight away.

The most useful and popular nonparametric estimation methods are as follows [12, 14]:

- Histogram method
- Parzen windows
- k-Nearest Neighbor
- Potential function method.

The Histogram Method

The histogram method can be cited as an example of nonparametric estimation. It is the best and the most popular method of estimating probability density functions. Almost no theoretical premises are needed to use it, but to get reliable results, we do need a relatively large sample with a set of data allowing the required statistics to be built. For a simple one-dimensional example, the x axis is split into h-long intervals, and then the probability of sample x contained in each interval is approximated for this interval.

Fig. 1.22 The histogram
method

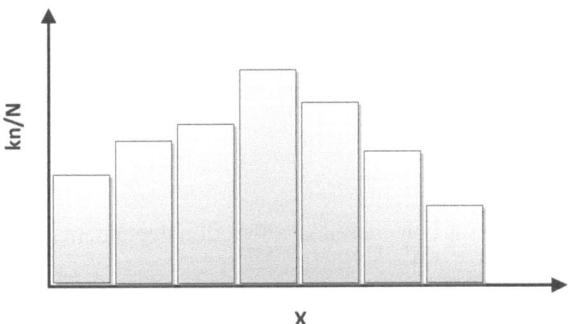

Let N be the total number of samples and k_N be the number of samples
belonging to a certain interval. The probability of respective classes is then given
by the formula $P \approx k_N/N$.

This method of proceeding is shown in Fig. 1.22.

It is conceptually simple to generalize this method of proceeding to a multidimensional case, but because the number of intervals for which the values of k_N
should be determined grows quickly in multidimensional spaces, this method is of
rather marginal practical utility.

Parzen Windows

A more useful nonparametric estimation technique is the Parzen windows method
[10, 12]. It is the most significant of nonparametric methods. To understand it
better, let us consider a simple, one-dimensional case in which the purpose is to
estimate the value of the density function $p(x)$ at point x. To do this, we have to
determine the number of samples N_h which are found within a certain interval
around point x, i.e., within the interval $[x - h, x + h]$. These values must be
determined for each point x and then divided by the total number of feature vectors
M and the length of the interval, i.e., by the value of $2h$. This procedure gives us an
estimated value of the density function looked for at point x.

$$p(x) = \frac{N_h(x)}{2hM} \tag{1.28}$$

We select the following as the supporting function K:

$$K = \begin{cases} 0.5 & |m| \leq 1 \\ 0 & |m| > 1 \end{cases} \tag{1.29}$$

Having made the substitutions, we obtain:

$$p(x) = \frac{1}{hM} \sum_{i=1}^{M} K\left(\frac{x - m_i}{h}\right) \tag{1.30}$$

with the *i*th component of the sum equal to zero if the value of m_i exceeds the interval $[x - h, x + h]$, and this leads to the following form of the relationship:

$$\gamma(x, m) = \frac{1}{h} K\left(\frac{x - m}{h}\right) \tag{1.31}$$

If $p(x)$ is considered as a function dependent on the number of samples, we get: $p(x) = p(x, M)$

Parzen proved that estimating the value of p for $M \to \infty$ is free of variances if $h = h(M)$ and $\lim_{M \to \infty} h(M) = 0$.

In practice, if we only have a finite number of samples, the appropriate values M and h have to be chosen. It is good to start by initially estimating the value of h, and then to try changing to minimize the possibility of an error of classification occurring. In theory, a high M is needed to obtain better recognition effectiveness, but in practice a large number of points needlessly increase the computational complexity of the entire classifier.

1.2.2 Structural Methods of Pattern Classification

Regardless of their complexity and sophistication, the holistic methods discussed in previous subsections of this book are not very effective in some cases. This is particularly noticeable during analyses of very complex images for which the number of classes is large, resulting in a significant increase of the dimension of the feature space necessary for describing the patterns. However, such limitations do not apply to syntactic methods of image recognition which use formalisms of mathematical linguistics [17, 21, 22].

In the syntactic approach, the image is divided into smaller subimages, which can be recognized using holistic methods when treated as independent units, or which can be further divided until certain elementary image units, defined a priori in these methods, are obtained. If these smaller subimages are still highly complex, this division operation is continued until it produces picture primitives. These picture primitives are indivisible elements of the image which we assume to exist and to be definable for a given class of images.

Hence, in syntactic methods, before we start the recognition proper, we have to distinguish picture primitives which we will use to describe more complex patterns, and we should also define the relations between these primitives. The most frequent way of distinguishing picture primitives is to segment the image using methods such as: edge detection with gradient operators or operators of template matching described in the subsections above. Identifying patterns is an extremely important stage because, when recognizing images, we treat the former as independent subimages. Consequently, composing the entire image from sub-images is a condition of its correct recognition.

Apart from defining picture primitives, another important element in the syntactic approach to recognizing a given image is to identify the relations between such picture primitives. This is because relations determine the correct composition of the image, and thus its right recognition. The character of relations also constitutes a very important criterion for the basic classification of syntactic image recognition methods.

Syntactic image recognition methods are classified into three main formal methods. The first group, developed the earliest, comprises *sequential methods* [21, 22, 29]. More complex ones described below are called *tree methods* and *graph methods* [21, 22].

The earliest group of methods to be developed was the sequential methods in which the image is described by a sequence of terminal elements, so in this case we distinguish only one type of relation that can exist between picture primitives. This relationship is sticking another element on, i.e., the so-called concatenation. Sequential languages are used to recognize and describe single (frequently very complex) objects in an image. Examples of such languages are: languages based on chain codes, image description languages, and shape feature description languages [21]. These languages are not capable of describing multiobject or multidimensional (e.g. 3D) images. This functionality is, however, offered by the more extensive tree or graph languages. Examples of interesting applications of sequential formalisms to analyze medical images are available in [16, 18, 19, 21].

More extensive linguistic formalisms with greater descriptive capacity are based on tree grammars. Tree methods are constructed based on tree languages and the two most frequently used types of their application are scene analysis and texture analysis. Scene analysis is a process for recognizing a 2D or 3D image in which objects that make it up have been distinguished and identified while relations between these objects have been described. Here, we distinguish two sets of picture primitives. The first is the description of objects making up the complex image, while the second is the description of relations between such objects [21].

The third class of grammars used in the syntactic recognition of images is graph grammars. Graph grammars are the descriptively strongest formalisms used to classify patterns. The use of graphs to describe 2D or 3D images is commonly found in literature [15]. Examples of the use of such methods can be found in [15, 21].

An interesting property of all methods of syntactic image analysis is that the classification of images with their use does not run just like in holistic methods, i.e., the recognition process is not divided into the stages of pattern reception, calculating the classification functions, and taking decisions. Here, the classifier is the appropriately constructed parser (syntax analyser) which enables determining whether the newly recognized object belongs to the language generated by the grammar defined for the considered object classes. In this case, training the classifier consists in correctly defining the rules of the formal grammar which should generally describe all possible cases of recognized patterns. Depending on the generating capacity of the grammars used, such methods can operate at various levels of detail, and by using additional functions or semantic procedures, they can also be used as techniques for the semantic analysis of image patterns. The subsections below present examples of such applications.

1.2.3 Neural Networks in Pattern Recognition

Neural networks also constitute an important class of image recognition and classification techniques. These methods are currently included among computational intelligence algorithms, so together with methods based on fuzzy sets and rough sets they form a separate class of image recognition algorithms [12, 14, 22]. The discussion of all such techniques exceeds the limits of this book, but this chapter will outline the most important types of neural networks which can be used for image recognition.

Neural networks are systems of many interconnected neurons processing information in parallel. To a limited extent, such neurons model the operation of real, biological neurons which make up the brain structures responsible, inter alia, for perception and consciousness, as well as for interpreting all other signals and stimuli coming from the outside world. Neurons are made up of the part with multiple inputs, i.e., the neural synapses, and the part constituting the single output, i.e., the axon.

The properties of individual neurons are determined by the weigh coefficients of synapses (called synaptic weights) which characterize every input of every numbered cell of the network, and an additional coefficient called the neuron threshold or bias.

The advantage of neural networks is their method of operation which is based on processing data in parallel and the ability to learn from the input data fed to the network. They can be used to execute certain tasks by appropriately controlling the connections between neurons and determining the synaptic weights. The process of weight determination consists in training the network and for every network type there is an algorithm allowing the network to be trained in a way that produces its desirable properties. Training algorithms can be divided into two types: These are supervised learning algorithms and unsupervised learning algorithms. In supervised learning, the input data and the correct results—the training samples—are fed to the network. This process is conducted by comparing the output data directly to the correct solutions previously fed into the network. Unsupervised learning occurs if the fed input data is free of patterns, or correct results serving to define the correct solution.

Regardless of the great variety of neural networks, all of them, in their basic structure, include the components below.

1. A finite number of neurons $x(1)$, $x(2)$,..., $x(n)$, every one of which has a specific method of action within the time interval t which is determined by its input signal $x_t(i)$, $i \in [1, n]$.

2. A finite number of connections between neurons $W = (w_{ij})$, where w_{ij} defines
    the weight of the connection between neuron $x(i)$ and neuron $x(j)$.
3. The function for aggregating the input signal of a neuron, of the following form:

$$\tau_t(i) = \sum_{j=1}^{n} x_t(j) w_{ij} \tag{1.32}$$

4. The activation function f for which τ is the input value yielding the next output
    signal (or another state) of the neuron

$$x_{t+1}(i) = f(\tau_t(i) - \theta) \tag{1.33}$$

where θ is the so-called threshold and f is a nonlinear function, e.g., of the sigmoid
type.

A neural network usually has a layered structure. The layers distinguished in it
are as follows: the input layer to which input signals are fed from the outside, and
the output layer whose signals may indicate the result value.

The network training process consists in presenting patterns from the training
sequence U to the network in K subsequent steps and in assessing the output
signals generated by the network against the pattern at which the network is to aim.

Synaptic coefficients change during the presentation of subsequent signals by
increment values which depend on the network training method [10, 12].

In order to identify the processes taking place in a single neuron during network
training, it is possible to define the value of the total neuron activation when the
kth element of the training sequence is presented:

$$\tilde{e}_{\lambda}^{k} = \sum_{v=1}^{n} V_v^{(\lambda)(k-1)} x_v^k + \theta \tag{1.34}$$

where

$V_v^{(\lambda)(k-1)}$ define the synaptic weights of individual neuron inputs λ;

x_v^k define the values of signals on individual inputs of the neuron λ;

θ is the bias for the neuron λ;

The obtained value of the total activation is linked to its input signal by the
selected nonlinear function [10, 12, 21].

Due to their characteristics, neural networks have found great use in solving
various problems associated with recognzsing and classifying images [10, 21, 31].

In the most general classification, three basic types of neural networks are
distinguished:

Recurrent Hopfield Networks

These are nonlinear networks with feedback, in which neurons work in such a way that the output of each one is fed (as feedback signal) to the inputs of all remaining neurons. These networks have various applications, but are most frequently used as forms of associative storage. Patterns of images stored in them correspond to stable states of nonlinear systems and to the local minima of functions representing network energy. The storage capacity, in other words the permissible number of image samples stored depends on the network size. The most popular recurrent networks are the Hopfield network and the Bidirectional Associative Memory (BAM) [12].

Multilayer Feedforward neural Networks

In these networks, information flows in one direction. These networks perform a nonlinear mapping of input and output signals (usually the signals have the form of multidimensional vectors both on the input and the output). The most popular feedforward networks area the MLP—MultiLayer Perceptron trained by methods with error back-propagation and the Radial Basis Functions (RBF) which uses the so-called radial neurons in its hidden layer.

Self-organizing Maps (SOM)

The operation of these maps is based on competitive learning. Output neurons compete with one another and the output signal is fed only to the winning neuron, though sometimes also to its closest neighborhood. These types of networks are exemplified by Kohonen maps and Adaptive Resonance Theory (ART) networks.

Networks most frequently used in the area of image recognition and classification are Kohonen maps, Hopfield networks and the multilayer perceptron, and these will be briefly described in the following subsections.

1.2.3.1 Kohonen Maps

The Kohonen map is also called the self-organizing feature map and is the most popular self-organizing map. The Kohonen map features the so-called competitive learning and the network itself is usually feedforward. Neurons are connected to all components of the N-dimensional input vector X. The weighs of neuron connections together create the vector $w_i = (w_{i1}, w_{i2}, \ldots, w_{in})$. Before learning occurs, the input signal vector X is normalized.

Once the map is activated by the vector X, a competition takes place and is won by the vector whose weights are the closest to the appropriate components of the activating vector. Thus, the winning vector w_w fulfills the relationship $d(X, w_w) = \min_{1 < i < n} d(X, w_i)$.

The distance between the vector X and the vector w is represented by $d(X, w)$. A topological neighborhood surrounding the winning vector $Sw(n)$ whose radius decreases in subsequent iterations is also assumed. Then, the process of adaptation occurs subsequently between the winning neuron and the neighboring ones whose weights are also modified in accordance with the Kohonen rule

$$w_i(n+1) = w_i(n) + \eta_i(n)[X - w_i(n)] \qquad (1.35)$$

$\eta_i(n)$ is the coefficient of the ith neuron from the neighborhood $Sw(n)$ and its value decreases along with the distance from the winning vector, while the values of neurons from outside its neighbourhood do not change.

The general form of the Kohonen map learning algorithm is as follows:

$$w_i(n+1) = w_i(n) + \eta G(i, X)[X - w_i(n)] \qquad (1.36)$$

The learning coefficient of each neuron i depends on its distance from vector X represented by the neighborhood functions $G(i, X)$. An example neighborhood function $G(i, X)$ can be defined as follows:

$$G(i,X)\begin{cases} 1 & \text{when } d(i, w) \leq \lambda \\ 0 & \text{else} \end{cases} \qquad (1.37)$$

$d(i, w)$ is the Euclidean distance between the winning neuron w and the ith neuron. The value λ defines the neighborhood radius which decreases over time. This neighborhood is called rectangular.

Another type of neighborhood found in Kohonen maps is the Gaussian neighborhood for which

$$G(i,X) = \exp\left(-\frac{d^2(i, w)}{2\lambda^2}\right) \qquad (1.38)$$

The Euclidean distance and the neighborhood radius determine the degree of adaptation of neurons from the neighborhood of the winning one. In practice, a Gaussian neighborhood turns out to be better, because it leads to better learning results and a better map organization [10, 12].

1.2.3.2 Hopfield Networks

Hopfield networks are recurrent networks forming associative storage (content-addressable memory). Such storage is usually presented as a system with feedback, which means that output signals of neurons are at the same time the input signals of the network as shown in Fig. 1.23. In the classical arrangement of a Hopfield network, the feedback of the neuron to its own output is ignored, as a result of which the weight matrix is symmetrical.

For a network to work as associative storage, it should be trained in a special way. For this purpose, the weights of individual neurons should be selected so that during the retrieval, the network is able to find the set of data closest to the testing vector. This process leads to the creation of an area of attraction of individual equilibrium points which correspond to the training data. In the case of a network with associative storage, there is a single vector or a set of vectors which establish

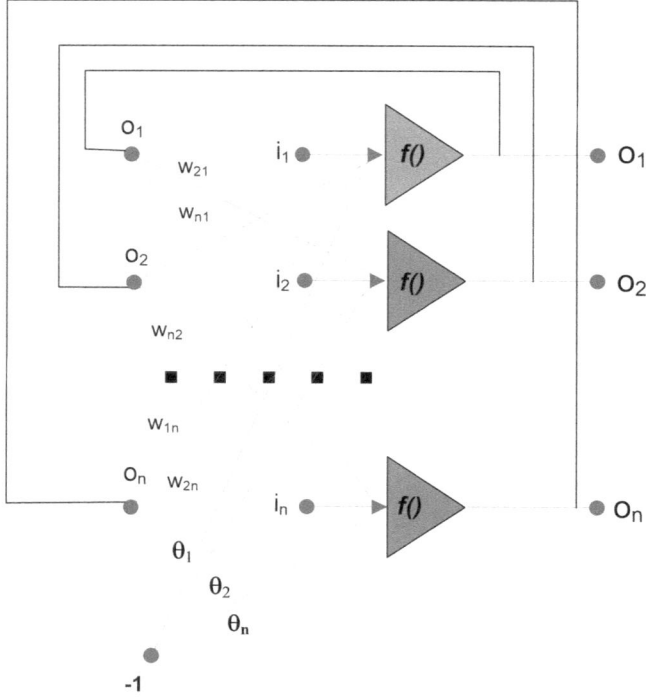

Fig. 1.23 A Hopfield network diagram

the location of individual attractors by learning. It is assumed that each neuron has
a signum-type activation function which takes the value of ± 1, as a result of which
the output signal of the ith neuron can be described by the following function:

$$O_i = \text{sgn}\left(\sum_{j=1}^{N} w_{ij}x_j + \theta_i\right) \tag{1.39}$$

It should also be assumed that the bias constant which defines the operation of
individual neurons is a component of the input vector X. If we ignore unit delays of
the network representing the synchronous mode of signal transmission, the relationships describing the network can be presented as follows (for the original
condition $O(0) = X$):

$$O_i(k) = \text{sgn}\left(\sum_{j=1,i\neq j}^{N} w_{ij}O_j(k - 1)\right) \tag{1.40}$$

We can distinguish two operating modes of a Hopfield network—the learning
mode and the retrieval mode. In the learning mode, the weights of connections are

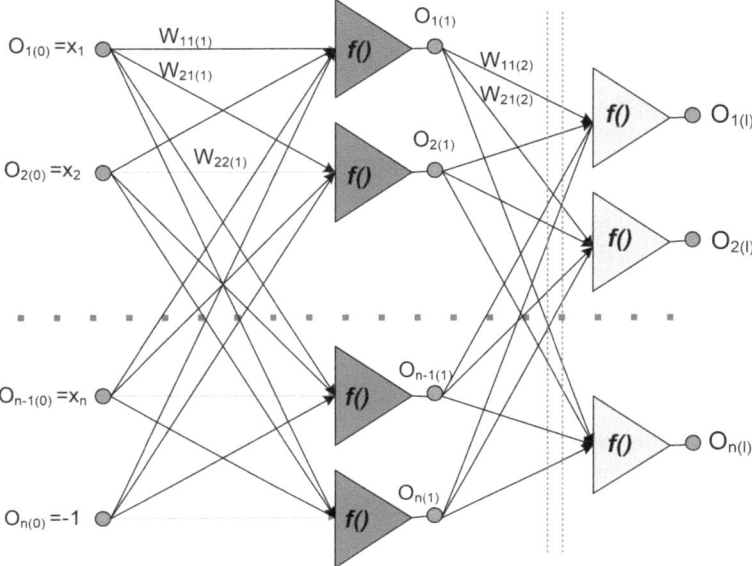

Fig. 1.24 A multilayer network diagram

picked based on pre-set training patterns. In the retrieval mode, assuming the initial condition of neuron $O(0) = X$ and with the set values of weights, an interim process occurs which ends at the defined local minimum where $O(n) = O(n-1)$. During the presentation of one training pattern X, changes will last until the above relationship is fulfilled for all neurons.

Associative storage implemented using a Hopfield network has correcting properties. If the presented test sample differs by a certain number of bits, the network can correct these differences and complete the classification process at the appropriate attractor. Associative storage has a certain capacity, understood as the maximum number of patterns stored and retrieved with a defined minimum error.

1.2.3.3 Multilayer Perceptron

Perceptrons are networks built of layers of regularly connected neurons. Every input of a neuron from a given layer is connected to the output of all neurons of the previous layer (Fig. 1.24).

There can be any number of neurons in each layer and any number of layers in the network. In a special case, a perceptron can be made up of a single layer and a single neuron, although in practical image classification jobs, multilayer perceptrons are used. Their first layer is called the input layer, the last one is the output layer, while the remaining ones are called hidden layers. There can be any number of hidden layers, but in practice no more than two are usually used because this cuts down the computation time.

A training method with error back-propagation is used to train networks featuring at least one hidden layer. This is one of the most popular methods of multilayer network training and has significantly broadened the range of applications of artificial neural networks. A model with error back-propagation is made up of at least three layers of neurons. The input and output layers contain the same number of neurons while the hidden layer is usually composed of a smaller number. The structure of this model does not include feedbacks. A network with any number of layers can be trained using the error back-propagation method, but at least two of these layers must have the initial weight values set. Weight values should be set in such a way that after the activation by a certain set of input vectors, the desired set of output vectors is obtained. This is done using training pairs, each of which contains an input vector and a corresponding output (or target) vector. The set of all pairs forms the training set. Before the training process can start, all weights must be initiated as small random numbers to avoid the possible saturation of neurons at a later stage. The training process itself consists in selecting a subsequent pair from the training set and feeding the activating vector to the network input. The state on the network output is then calculated and an error is determined between the value of the target vector and the value calculated on the input of the network. Subsequently, the values of network weights are set so as to minimize the error. This whole operation runs until the error for the entire set is small enough. The calculations are made layer by layer, starting with the output layer. After the recognition is completed, the final state representing the result is established on the output layer neurons.

1.3 Semantic Analysis and Content Understanding of Visual Patterns

The previous subsections discussed the algorithms that can be used to process, analyze and recognize images. This chapter, however, presents a new approach that the authors have been developing for several years, leading to understanding the meaning of the examined images, i.e., to determining their semantics.

Automatic image understanding is still a new research concept based on the use of advanced computational intelligence techniques and cognitive informatics [15, 21, 22, 32–34]. In this concept, we take advantage of cognitive reasoning mechanisms which are very different from all image recognition techniques described in previous subsections. These techniques represent a significant innovation compared to all known traditional image classification methods because they support automatic machine perception which reaches much deeper into the meaning of the information contained in the image than all the techniques proposed before. Typical recognition techniques are first used to arbitrarily collate a list of classes (categories) to which a considered object could belong, and then the entire image analysis is conducted so as to determine which class the considered object may be categorized to. In contrast to this very formal procedure, in the automatic under-standing of images we try to grasp the semantic significance of all details detected in the specific image as a result of analyzing it. In the case of medical images, this penetration of the substantive content of the image and the attempt to understand the nature of processes that have given the examined organ the appearance it has in the image (and not a different one) may lead, inter alia, to identifying the disease units to which the considered medical condition (the detected lesion) should be classified to. As a result, automatic understanding can be a very valuable tool in supporting diagnostic processes, described in the following chapters of this book.

The need for a new approach to the problem of understanding arose when IT tried to barge into this area. As we wanted to entrust more and more areas of our own information activities to computers, we have already repeatedly reached situations in which an apparently obvious and generally understood activity performed by men frequently and without paying much attention to its nature became really mysterious and difficult to define precisely when it had to be entrusted to machines. It is worth noting that typical IT activities, such as making calculations, processing text, col-lecting data, communicating, and sending information did not lead to such discus-sions and never gave rise to such problems. The current attempts to build an artificial brain, which would equip computers with the ability to intelligently execute difficult tasks usually requiring men to use their intellect, are leading to numerous scientific discussions and disputes [32, 33]. However, it seems that the very rapid development of computer technologies has brought us to the point at which we have to decide on such issues whose clarification will be of great value, both theoretical and practical. So is it possible to develop intelligent methods of computer understanding of images portraying complex situations or scenes from the surroundings?

It is quite obvious that such methods can yield measurable benefits. Typical computer applications available at present, even very sophisticated ones, are not even beginning to authentically understand the huge resources and streams of information recorded, stored, transmitted, and processed by computers.

This is why there is more and more talk of the need to develop—as a new field in computational intelligence—a technique for computer understanding of differ-ent information appearing in cyberspace. This need was first felt by specialists dealing with textual information analysis. The problem of semantic networks, of searching for information based on various ontologies, of the automatic translation of documents written in one language into other ones as well as of the automatic generation of summaries of long texts have unavoidably led to a need to reach deeper than just to the lexical layer of the texts considered. Having solved prob-lems of a syntactic nature resulting from the complex structure of natural language grammar, it became necessary to face the semantic aspect, the barrier between the sphere of meanings of specific information, which is so much richer and more difficult than the sphere of their signatures dealt with by semiotics.

Similarly, the authors of this work have introduced the concept of the automatic understanding of visual patterns, originally defined for medical images containing very rich layers of semantics into the world literature [21, 22]. This is important as visual patterns have not just a form, but also contents. The form may be modeled by computers using various digital image processing software. The form of an image can also be analyzed, with various parameters of objects visible in images being automatically determined, and also classified, for example, using the opportunities offered to everyone now by neural networks. On the contrary, we do not have similar software tools for determining the contents of an image.

Our vision system is extremely efficient in processing signals from our visual receptors because it very quickly generalizes image information to the form of a contextual conceptual map of the recognized objects and relationships between them. This form of scene description is called high level, in contrast to the low level representation formed by the set of impressions recorded by the eye's retina. The brain does not form subsequent versions of photographs of scenes from the world around us, but rather their models which define the meaning of the observed situation, and not its form. In computer systems we must also aim at extracting the substantive meaning of the acquired image, instead of using one algorithm after another to convert, with increasing sophistication, the sequence of values of subsequent pixels of the image which constitute the direct result of its acquisition.

The next part will discuss the fundamental notions associated with the automatic understanding of images, which will first be treated very generally, to structure and collate the appropriate notions, and then in greater detail.

It has already been mentioned that all techniques of the computer processing, analysis, and recognition of images do not exhaust the whole scope of tasks and problems which may appear in connection with using an image as a source of useful information. In this entire analysis process, the semantic interpretation of the data obtained is the most important, but also the hardest. At the present stage in the development of computer image analysis methods, it is only the knowledge collected in the recognizing system and the experience of the designers of such systems that are the key to the correct understanding, which is due to the fact that the examined image has this or that appearance.

Computer image processing can help describe significant features or shapes of the examined images, but it is difficult to answer the question of what follows from the fact that this or that is visible in the image.

Neither does the process of extracting and identifying the features of the image, which accompanies its automatic analysis and the attempts at its automatic classification, provide more than just some premises for the reasoning process which the system must conduct based on the collected knowledge. Without this content-related interpretation of analysis results and elements of the automatic classification, they are in fact all worthless, because the value of this or that image parameter or the class to which this or that object visible in the image can be classified is often immaterial. It is what follows from the fact that the object has been classified to a specific image class that is significant.

If you account for the possible interpretation problems caused by the constantly developing, but therefore also constantly changing, contemporary *image vision* technology, for the number of different objects and scenes inspected and for the many different ways these images can change, it is no surprise that computer vision needs urgent support from modern image understanding techniques.

Medical images have already been mentioned as an image type containing very large amounts of semantic information. The next part discusses *brain perfusion and carotid artery images.* Generally, however, one can note that as a result of the development of techniques and newer and newer forms of medical images, there is a growing demand for better and better computer aid techniques for the process of analyzing, interpreting, and recognizing all these new images. It is increasingly frequently expected that a modern medical system will not only acquire the image of the inside of a human body and present it as legibly as possible, but will also pre-analyze the image and draw the physician's attention to the elements which are most likely to carry diagnostically significant information. This means that the computer not only has to analyze the values of each of tens of millions of pixels in the image, but must also intelligently interpret them, suggesting what follows from them to the physician. This is, of course, a major challenge for IT specialists, who not only have to develop such new techniques of image analysis, but also to constantly upgrade them.

The ability to determine the semantics of images and penetrate deep into their substantive contents has come about due to two reasons.

The first is the ability to define a semantically oriented linguistic description of the contents of the analyzed image, i.e., a description based only on the properly conducted analysis of the graphic structures detected in the image and their interrelations. This analysis must be preceded by the correct image preprocessing, consisting in executing a sequence of the known filterings, segmentations, and transformations of the image, chosen so that they would extract components of the image material from the point of view of its interpretation, while limiting or completely eliminating technical noise and variability factors causing difficulties during this semantically oriented analysis.

The second is the ability to verify the semantically oriented description of the important contents of the image against the properly expressed semantic expectations and projections. Such semantic expectations are the result of a priori knowledge of the content or the meaning of the examined image. This means that the appropriate representation of knowledge, forming the key to the automatic understanding of images, is not universal and must be built separately for every class of images.

This is significant in that at the present stage of IT development, we can easily use computers to come to grips with the image form, but the contents of it still remain completely out of automation's reach. However, all processes of using vision information in practice and of searching for image information about a given subject in large databases of images confirm that in the case of an image, the form of information may in fact be only very loosely connected to its content. In particular, it often happens that images that are graphically completely different contain the same meaning. This is shown by Fig. 1.25 in which similar objects are portrayed by two images that are completely different in their form, but have very similar meanings.

However, if the form of an image is not identical to its contents, it is reasonable to develop new computational paradigms which could be used to understand images and which will be able to determine the semantic sense of an image tangled up in its complex form. It is precisely the techniques of automatic image understanding, described by the authors of this work also in other publications [21–25], that consist

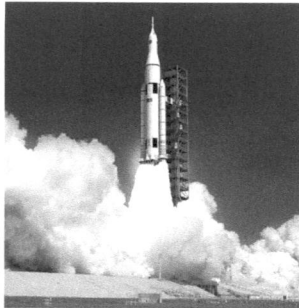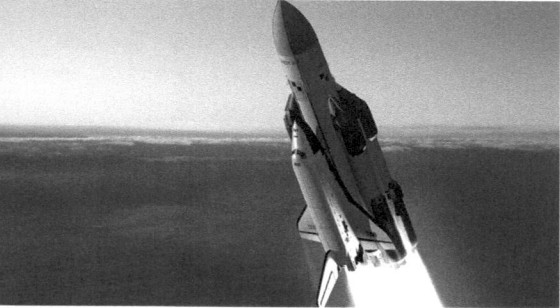

Fig. 1.25 Two images different in form, but with a similar semantic interpretation

of the computer extraction of a certain significant substantive meaning contained in the examined image, but in a tangled up form so it is not directly visible and obvious.

Thus the identification of the semantic meaning of images is possible thanks to advanced techniques of cognitive image analysis, which are presented in Sect. 2.5 and which constitute a significant enhancement of the existing methods of pattern processing and classification. Basic differences between image recognition methods and image understanding methods can be summarized as follows: in pattern recognition methods, we are usually dealing with a finite number of defined object classes to which a new element is categorized after its feature vector has been determined, and this is done using the appropriate classification function. In image understanding techniques, no finite number of recognized classes has to exist at all, while the correct determination of the semantic meaning of the image is independent of pattern classification criteria and can be done at various levels of detail [35–44].

1.4 Implementation of Selected Image Processing Methods

This section presents the implementation of selected image processing methods written in the C# language.

1.4.1 Approximation of a Two-Dimensional Gaussian Kernel Function

The two-dimensional Gaussian function is defined by the following formula:

$$g(x,y) = \frac{1}{\sigma^2\sqrt{2\pi}} \cdot e^{\frac{-1}{2}\cdot\left(\frac{x^2+y^2}{\sigma^2}\right)} \tag{1.41}$$

where σ (sigma) is the standard deviation.

The coefficients of a two-dimensional discrete Gaussian filter constitute an approximation of the above function.

```
/**
 * n - number of rows of kernel
 * m - number of columns of kernel
 * sigma - standard deviation
 * output - two-dimensional floating point approximation
 * of gaussian kernel
 * Example call:
 * double[][] kernel = CreateGaussianKernel(5, 5, 4);
 */
public static double[][] CreateGaussianKernel(int n, int m,
double sigma)
{
    double sigma2 = 2 * sigma * sigma;
    double denominator = 0;
    //Output kernel
    double[][] Kernel = new double[n][];
    for (int a = 0; a < n; a++)
            Kernel[a] = new double[m];

    double nHalf = (n - 1) / 2;
    double mHalf = (m - 1) / 2;
    double n1, n2, hg;

    int a1 = 0;
    int b1 = 0;
    //Main loop
    for (double a = -nHalf; a <= nHalf; a++)
    {
            n1 = a * a;
            b1 = 0;
            for (double b = -mHalf; b <= mHalf; b++)
            {
                    n2 = b * b;
                    hg = Math.Exp(-(n1 + n2) / sigma2);
                    Kernel[a1][b1] = hg;

                    denominator = denominator + hg;
                    b1 = b1 + 1;
            }
            a1 = a1 + 1;
        }

    for (int a = 0; a < n; a++)
            for (int b = 0; b < m; b++)
                    Kernel[a][b] = Kernel[a][b] / denominator;
    return Kernel;
}
```

1.4.2 *Two-Dimensional Discrete Convolution*

The program below implements formula (1.3).

```
/**
 *  Image - input grayscale image
 *  Kernel - kernel function with witch Image will be convolved
 *  output - result of two-dimensional discrete convolution
 *  Example call:
 *  //Image array is already initialized
 *  double[][] kernel =CreateGaussianKernel(5, 5, 4);
 *  double[][] output =ConvolutionFilter(Image, kernel);
 */
public static double[][] ConvolutionFilter(double[][] Image,
double[][] Kernel)
{
    int n = Image.Length;
    int m = Image[0].Length;
    //Output data
    double[][] ResultImage = new double[n][];
    for (int a = 0; a < n; a++)
            ResultImage[a] = new double[m];
    int nF = Kernel.Length;
    int mF = Kernel[0].Length;

    int nFHalf = nF / 2;
    int mFHalf = mF / 2;
    double result;
    int indexN, indexM;
    //Main loop
    for (int a = 0; a < n; a++)
            for (int b = 0; b < m; b++)
            {
                    result = 0;
                      for (int c = 0; c < nF; c++)
                          for (int d = 0; d < mF; d++)
                          {
                                  indexN = a - nFHalf + c;
                                  indexM = b - mFHalf + d;

                                  if (indexN < 0) indexN = 0;
                                  if (indexN >= n) indexN =
                                  n - 1;
                                  if (indexM < 0) indexM = 0;
                                  if (indexM >= m) indexM =
                                  m - 1;
                                  result += Kernel[c][d]
                                  * Image[indexN][indexM];
                          }
                    ResultImage[a][b] = (int)Math.Round(result);
            }

        return ResultImage;
}
```

1.4.3 Fast Implementation of a Median Filter

The operating principle of the program below is described in Sect. 1.1.2.2.

```
/**
 * Image - input grayscale image, data in table must
 * be non-negative integers
 * nW - number of rows of kernel
 * mW - number of columns of kernel
 * Output - Input image after median filtration
 * Example call:
 * //Image array is already initialized
 * double[][] Output = FastMedianFilter(Image, 5,5);
 */
public static double[][] FastMedianFilter(double[][] Image,
int nW, int mW)
    {
    //n,m - Image matrix dimension
    int n = Image.Length;
    int m = Image[0].Length;
    nW = nW - 1;
    mW = mW - 1;

    int leftnW = (int)Math.Floor((double)nW / 2);
    int rightnW = (int)Math.Floor((double)nW / 2) + (nW % 2);

    int leftmW = (int)Math.Floor((double)mW / 2);
    int rightmW = (int)Math.Floor((double)mW / 2) + (mW % 2);

    int a = 0;
    int b = 0;
    //Output data
    double[][] ResultImage = new double[n][];
    for (a = 0; a < ResultImage.Length; a++)
            ResultImage[a] = new double[m];
    //Determnie the size of histogram array
    int maxColorValue = 0;
       for (a = 0; a < n; a++)
            for (b = 0; b < m; b++)
                    if (Image[a][b] > maxColorValue)
                        maxColorValue = (int)Image[a][b];
    int[] Histogram = new int[maxColorValue + 1];
    //helper indices
    a = 0;
    b = 0;
```

```
int pstartN = a - leftnW;
int pstartM = b - leftmW;
int pstopN = a + rightnW;
int pstopM = b + rightmW;

int count = 0;

int startN = pstartN;
int startM = pstartM;
int stopN = pstopN;
int stopM = pstopM;

if (pstartN < 0)
{
        pstartN = 0;
        startN = 0;
}
if (pstartM < 0)
{
        pstartM = 0;
        startM = 0;
}
if (pstopN >= n)
{
        pstopN = n - 1;
        stopN = n - 1;
}
if (pstopM >= m)
{
        pstopM = m - 1;
        stopM = m - 1;
}

int pstartNreal = -1;
int pstopNreal = -1;
//Compute first histogram
for (a = 0; a <= pstopN; a++)
        for (b = 0; b <= pstopM; b++)
                Histogram[(int)Image[a][b]]
                = Histogram[(int)Image[a][b]] + 1;
//Compute size of the filter window
count = (pstartN - pstopN) * (pstartM - pstopM);

int deleteN;
int addN;
```

```
int startNreal;
int stopNreal;
int deleteM;
int addM;
//Loop through rows
for (a = 0; a < n; a++)
{
        startNreal = a - leftnW;
        stopNreal = a + rightnW;

        if (pstartNreal >= 0 && pstartNreal < n) deleteN
        = pstartNreal;
        else deleteN = -1;
        if (stopNreal >= 0 && stopNreal < n) addN = stopNreal;
        else addN = -1;

        startN = startNreal;
        stopN = stopNreal;
        if (startN < 0) startN = 0;
        if (startM < 0) startM = 0;
        if (stopN >= n)
                stopN = n - 1;
        if (stopM >= m)
                stopM = m - 1;
        //If it is not a first row, move filter window down
        if (a != 0)
                moveHistogramDown(Histogram, Image, startM,
                  stopM, deleteN, addN);
        pstartNreal = startNreal;
        pstopNreal = stopNreal;
        //Move window from left to right
        if (a % 2 == 0)
                //Loop through rows
                for (b = 0; b < m; b++)
                {

                startM = b - leftnW;
                stopM = b + rightnW;

                if (startM < 0) startM = 0;
                if (stopM >= m) stopM = m - 1;

                if (pstartM != startM && pstartM >= 0
                && pstartM < m)
                        deleteM = pstartM;
```

```
        else deleteM = -1;

        if (pstopM != stopM && stopM >= 0
        && stopM < m)
                addM = stopM;
        else addM = -1;

        //Compute histogramu
        count = (stopN - startN + 1)
        * (stopM - startM + 1);
        computeHistogram(Histogram, Image, startN,
        stopN, deleteM, addM);
        ResultImage[a][b] = computeMediana(Histogram,
         count);

        pstartM = startM;
        pstopM = stopM;
        }
//Move window from right to left
else
{
        //Loop through rows
        for (b = m - 1; b >= 0; b--)
        {

                startM = b - leftnW;
                stopM = b + rightnW;

                if (startM < 0) startM = 0;
                if (stopM >= m) stopM = m - 1;

                if (pstartM != startM && pstartM >= 0
                && pstartM < m)
                        addM = startM;
                else addM = -1;
                if (pstopM != stopM && pstopM >= 0
                && pstopM < m)
                        deleteM = pstopM;
                else deleteM = -1;

                //Compute histogramu
                count = (stopN - startN + 1)
                * (stopM - startM + 1);
            computeHistogram(Histogram, Image, startN,
            stopN, deleteM, addM);
```

```
                                 ResultImage[a][b]
                                 = computeMediana(Histogram, count);

                                 pstartM = startM;
                                 pstopM = stopM;
                          }
                }
        }
        return ResultImage;
}


/**
 * Helper function of FastMedianFilter
 */
private static void moveHistogramDown(int[] Histogram,
double[][] Image,
     int startM, int stopM, int deleteN, int addN)
{
     //Remove Image row values from Histogram
     if (deleteN >= 0)
             for (int a = startM; a <= stopM; a++)
                     Histogram[(int)Image[deleteN][a]] =
                             Histogram[(int)Image[deleteN][a]] - 1;
     //Add Image row values from Histogram
     if (addN >= 0)
             for (int a = startM; a <= stopM; a++)
                     Histogram[(int)Image[addN][a]] =
                             Histogram[(int)Image[addN][a]] + 1;
}


/**
 * Helper function of FastMedianFilter
 */
private static void computeHistogram(int[] Histogram,
double[][] Image,
     int startN, int stopN, int deleteM, int addM)
{
     //Remove Image column values from Histogram
     if (deleteM >= 0)
             for (int a = startN; a <= stopN; a++)
                     Histogram[(int)Image[a][deleteM]] =
                             Histogram[(int)Image[a][deleteM]] - 1;
     //Add Image column values from Histogram
     if (addM >= 0)
```

```
                for (int a = startN; a <= stopN; a++)
                    Histogram[(int)Image[a][addM]] =
                            Histogram[(int)Image[a][addM]] + 1;
}


/**
 * Helper function of FastMedianFilter
 */
private static int computeMediana(int[] Histogram, int count)
{
    double median = count / 2;
    for (int c = 0; c < Histogram.Length; c++)
    {
            //Count down number of histogram bars heights
            //until you reach the median
            count = count - Histogram[c];
            if (count <= median)
            {
                    return c;
            }
    }
    return 0;
}
```

1.4.4 Morphological Erosion

This program erodes a binary image. The operation of this algorithm is described in Sect. 1.1.2.2.

```
/**
 * Image - input "binary" image. Non positive value
 * is a backgroung.
 * Positve value is an object.
 * Element - array that represent the shape of structural element.
 * Output - two-dimensional binary image. Value zero
 * is a background.
 * Value 255 is an object.
 * Example call:
 * //Image array is already initialzied
 * //Array Element is already initialzied,
 * //for example it is 7x7 matrix
```

```
* //that have following values in rows:
* //[0,0,255,255,255,0,0]
* //[0,255,255,255,255,255,0]
* //[255,255,255,255,255,255,255]
* //[255,255,255,255,255,255,255]
* //[255,255,255,255,255,255,255]
* //[0,255,255,255,255,255,0]
* //[0,0,255,255,255,0,0]
* double[][] Output = Erosion(Image, Element);
*/
public static double[][] Erosion(double[][] Image,
double[][] Element)
{
    int n = Image.Length;
    int m = Image[0].Length;
    double[][] ReturnImage = new double[Image.Length][];
    //Output image
    for (int a = 0; a < Image.Length; a++)
    {
            ReturnImage[a] = new double[Image[0].Length];
            for (int b = 0; b < Image[0].Length; b++)
                    if (Image[a][b] > 0)
                            ReturnImage[a][b] = 255;
    }

    int nElement = Element.Length;
    int mElement = Element[0].Length;
    int centerNElement = (int)Math.Floor((double)nElement / 2)
    + 1;
    int centerMElement = (int)Math.Floor((double)mElement / 2)
    + 1;

    int rN = (int)Math.Floor((double)nElement / 2);
    int rM = (int)Math.Floor((double)mElement / 2);
    //Main loop
    for (int a = 0; a < n; a++)
            for (int b = 0; b < m; b++)
            {
                    //If this pixel belongs to border of an object
                      //but is not part of an object
                    if (ifErosionBorder(Image, a, b, n, m)
                    == true)
                            for (int c = -rN; c <= rN; c++)
                            if (a + c >= 0 && a + c < n)
                                    for (int d = -rM; d <= rM; d++)
```

```
                                    if (b + d >= 0 && b + d < m)
                                    if (Element[rN + c][rM + d]
                                    > 0)
                                    {
                                    ReturnImage[a + c][b + d] = 0;
                                    }
                        }
        return ReturnImage;
}


/**
 * Helper function of Erosion
 * Checks, if a pixel is a border of an object
 * but is not part of an object
 */
private static bool ifErosionBorder(double[][] Image, int a,
int b, int n, int m)
{
    if (Image[a][b] > 0) return false;
    if (a + 1 >= n || a - 1 < 0 || b + 1 >= m || b - 1 < 0)
            if (Image[a][b] == 0) return true;
                else return false;

    if (Image[a + 1][b] > 0 || Image[a - 1][b] > 0
    || Image[a][b + 1] > 0 || Image[a][b - 1] > 0)
            return true;
    if (Image[a + 1][b + 1] > 0 || Image[a + 1][b - 1] > 0
    || Image[a - 1][b + 1] > 0 || Image[a - 1][b - 1] > 0)
            return true;
    return false;
}
```

1.4.5 Morphological Dilation

This program dilates a binary image. The operation of this algorithm is described in Sect. 1.1.2.2.

```
/**
 * Image - input "binary" image. Non positive value
 * is a backgroung.
 * Positve value is an object.
 * Element - array that represent the shape of structural element.
 * Output - two-dimensional binary image. Value zero
 * is a background.
 * Value 255 is an object.
 * Example call:
 * //Image array is already initialzied
 * //Array Element is already initialzied, for example
 * //it is 7x7 matrix
 * //that have following values in rows:
 * //[0,0,255,255,255,0,0]
 * //[0,255,255,255,255,255,0]
 * //[255,255,255,255,255,255,255]
 * //[255,255,255,255,255,255,255]
 * //[255,255,255,255,255,255,255]
 * //[0,255,255,255,255,255,0]
 * //[0,0,255,255,255,0,0]
 * double[][] Output = Morphology.Dilation(Image, Element);
 */
public static double[][] Dilation(double[][] Image, double[][] El-
ement)
{
        int n = Image.Length;
        int m = Image[0].Length;
        double[][] ReturnImage = new double[Image.Length][];
        //Output image
        for (int a = 0; a < Image.Length; a++)
        {
                ReturnImage[a] = new double[Image[0].Length];
                for (int b = 0; b < Image[0].Length; b++)
                        if (Image[a][b] > 0)
                                ReturnImage[a][b] = 255;
        }

        int nElement = Element.Length;
        int mElement = Element[0].Length;
        int centerNElement = (int)Math.Floor((double)nElement / 2)
        + 1;
        int centerMElement = (int)Math.Floor((double)mElement / 2)
        + 1;

        int rN = (int)Math.Floor((double)nElement / 2);
        int rM = (int)Math.Floor((double)mElement / 2);

        //Main loop
        for (int a = 0; a < n; a++)
                for (int b = 0; b < m; b++)
                {
                //If this pixel belongs to border of an object
```

```
                        //and it is part of an object
                        if (ifDilationBorder(Image, a, b, n, m) == true)
                                for (int c = -rN; c <= rN; c++)
                                if (a + c >= 0 && a + c < n)
                                        for (int d = -rM; d <= rM; d++)
                                        if (b + d >= 0 && b + d < m)
                                                if (Element[rN + c][rM + d]
                                                > 0)
                                                ReturnImage[a + c][b + d] = 255;
                }
        return ReturnImage;
}


/**
 * Helper function of Dilation
 * Checks, if a pixel is a border of an object
 * and part of an object
 */
private static bool ifDilationBorder(double[][] Image, int a,
int b, int n, int m)
{
        if (Image[a][b] < 1) return false;
        if (a + 1 >= n || a - 1 < 0 || b + 1 >= m || b - 1 < 0)
        return true;
        if (Image[a + 1][b] <= 0 || Image[a - 1][b] <= 0
        || Image[a][b + 1] <= 0 || Image[a][b - 1] <= 0)
                return true;
        if (Image[a + 1][b + 1] <= 0 || Image[a + 1][b - 1] <= 0
        || Image[a - 1][b + 1] <= 0 || Image[a - 1][b - 1] <= 0)
                return true;
        return false;
}
```

1.4.6 Labeling

The operating principle of the program below is described in Sect. 1.1.2.2.

```
/**
 * Image - input "binary" image. Zero value is a background.
 * Nonzero value is an object.
 * connections - The variable n can have a value of either 4 or 8,
 * where 4 specifies 4-connected objects and 8 specifies
 * 8-connected objects.
 * numberOfLabels - returns number of labeled objects
 * detected by an algorithm.
 * Output - two-dimensional image, particular pixel
 * has either value zero
 * (when it is a background) or equals to number of object's
 * label.
 * Example call:
 * //Image array is already initialized
 * int numberOfLabels = 0;
 * double[][] Output = LabelImage(Image,8,out numberOfLabels);
 */
public static double[][] LabelImage(double[][] Image,
int connections, out int numberOfLabels)
{
    int n = Image.Length;
    int m = Image[0].Length;
    if (connections != 4 && connections != 8)
            connections = 8;
    //Output image
    double[][] LabelArray = new double[n][];
    for (int a = 0; a < Image.Length; a++)
            LabelArray[a] = new double[Image[0].Length];
    int labelIndex = 1;
    //Loop for each pixel
    for (int a = 0; a < n; a++)
            for (int b = 0; b < m; b++)
            //if pixel is not a bacground of Image
            //and was not yet labeled
            if (Image[a][b] != 0 && LabelArray[a][b] == 0)
            {
            //Begin labeling new object with label number
            //labelIndex
                    LabelImageArea(Image, a, b, n, m, LabelArray,
                     connections, labelIndex);
                    labelIndex++;
            }
    labelIndex--;
    numberOfLabels = labelIndex;
    return LabelArray;
}

/**
 * Helper function of LabelImageArea
 * Performs labeling of each pixel of an object.
 */
private static void LabelImageArea(double[][] Image, int a, int b,
```

```
    int n, int m, double[][] LabelArray, int connections,
int labelIndex)
    {
    //Stack with pixel indices for recursion
    int[][] RecursionArray = new int[n * m][];
    for (int c = 0; c < n * m; c++)
            RecursionArray[c] = new int[2];
    int recursionArrayIndex = 0;
    //Initialize stack with first pixel
    RecursionArray[recursionArrayIndex][0] = a;
    RecursionArray[recursionArrayIndex][1] = b;
    //While stack is not empty
    while (recursionArrayIndex >= 0)
    {
            a = RecursionArray[recursionArrayIndex][0];
            b = RecursionArray[recursionArrayIndex][1];
            recursionArrayIndex--;
            //If pixel was not yest labeled, label it
            if (LabelArray[a][b] == 0 || LabelArray[a][b] == -1)
                    LabelArray[a][b] = labelIndex;

            //Check 4-connected objects
            recursionArrayIndex =
            addRecursionLabelImageArea(Image, a + 1,
             b, n, m, LabelArray, RecursionArray,
            recursionArrayIndex);
            recursionArrayIndex =
            addRecursionLabelImageArea(Image, a,
             b + 1, n, m, LabelArray, RecursionArray,
            recursionArrayIndex);
            recursionArrayIndex =
            addRecursionLabelImageArea(Image, a - 1,
             b, n, m, LabelArray, RecursionArray,
            recursionArrayIndex);
            recursionArrayIndex =
            addRecursionLabelImageArea(Image, a,
             b - 1, n, m, LabelArray, RecursionArray,
            recursionArrayIndex);
            //Check 8-connected objects
            if (connections == 8)
            {
                    recursionArrayIndex =
                    addRecursionLabelImageArea(Image, a + 1,
                     b + 1, n, m, LabelArray, RecursionArray,
                    recursionArrayIndex);
```

```
                            recursionArrayIndex =
                            addRecursionLabelImageArea(Image, a + 1,
                             b - 1, n, m, LabelArray, RecursionArray,
                            recursionArrayIndex);
                            recursionArrayIndex =
                            addRecursionLabelImageArea(Image, a - 1,
                             b + 1, n, m, LabelArray, RecursionArray,
                            recursionArrayIndex);
                            recursionArrayIndex =
                            addRecursionLabelImageArea(Image, a - 1,
                             b - 1, n, m, LabelArray, RecursionArray,
                            recursionArrayIndex);
                }
        }
}


/**
 * Helper function of LabelImageArea
 * Checks if pixel was not yest labeled. If it was not,
 * adds it to stack.
 */
private unsafe static int addRecursionLabelImageArea(
double[][] Image, int a, int b, int n, int m,
double[][] LabelArray, int[][] RecursionArray,
int recursionArrayIndex)
{
        //If pixel is not inside Image borders
        if (a < 0 || b < 0 || a > n - 1 || b > m - 1)
                return recursionArrayIndex;
        //If pixel was not yet labeled
        if (Image[a][b] != 0 && LabelArray[a][b] == 0)
        {
                recursionArrayIndex++;
                RecursionArray[recursionArrayIndex][0] = a;
                RecursionArray[recursionArrayIndex][1] = b;
                LabelArray[a][b] = -1;
        }
        return recursionArrayIndex;
}
```

1.4.7 Filling Holes

The operating principle of the program below is described in Sect. 1.1.2.2.

```
/**
 * Image - input "binary" image. Pixel with values zero
 * is a background.
 * Positive value is an object.
 * Output - two-dimensional image. Value zero is a background.
 * Value 255 is an object.
 * Example call:
 * //Image array is already initialized
 * double[][] Output = FillHoles(Image);
 */
public static double[][] FillHoles(double[][] Image)
{
    int n = Image.Length;
    int m = Image[0].Length;
    int[][] FilledImage = new int[n][];
    int a, b;
    for (a = 0; a < FilledImage.Length; a++)
            FilledImage[a] = new int[m];
    //Stack with pixel indices for recursion
    int[][] RecursionArray = new int[n * m][];

    for (a = 0; a < n * m; a++)
    {
            RecursionArray[a] = new int[2];
    }
    int recursionArrayIndex = 0;
    //Inspect the first and last column
    for (a = 0; a < n; a++)
    {
            if (Image[a][0] == 0)
            {
                    FilledImage[a][0] = 2;
                    RecursionArray[recursionArrayIndex][0] = a;
                    RecursionArray[recursionArrayIndex][1] = 0;
                    recursionArrayIndex++;
            }
            if (Image[a][m - 1] == 0)
            {
                    FilledImage[a][m - 1] = 2;
                    RecursionArray[recursionArrayIndex][0] = a;
                    RecursionArray[recursionArrayIndex][1] =
                    m - 1;
                    recursionArrayIndex++;
            }
    }
```

```
//Inspect first and last row
for (a = 0; a < m; a++)
{
        if (Image[0][a] == 0)
        {
                FilledImage[0][a] = 2;
                RecursionArray[recursionArrayIndex][0] = 0;
                RecursionArray[recursionArrayIndex][1] = a;
                recursionArrayIndex++;
        }
        if (Image[n - 1][a] == 0)
        {
                FilledImage[n - 1][a] = 2;
                RecursionArray[recursionArrayIndex][0] =
                n - 1;
                RecursionArray[recursionArrayIndex][1] = a;
                recursionArrayIndex++;
        }
}
int iter = 0;
   recursionArrayIndex--;
   //While stack is not empty
//Find all pixels of background
//They have to be connected to initial points
//from RecursionArray
while (recursionArrayIndex >= 0)
{
        iter++;
        a = RecursionArray[recursionArrayIndex][0];
        b = RecursionArray[recursionArrayIndex][1];
        recursionArrayIndex--;
        //If not yet visited
        if (FilledImage[a][b] <= 0 || Image[a][b] == 0)
                FilledImage[a][b] = 2;
        //4-connected objects
        recursionArrayIndex = addRecursionFillHoles(Image,
        a + 1, b, n, m, FilledImage, RecursionArray,
        recursionArrayIndex);
        recursionArrayIndex = addRecursionFillHoles(Image, a,
         b + 1, n, m, FilledImage, RecursionArray,
        recursionArrayIndex);
        recursionArrayIndex = addRecursionFillHoles(Image,
        a - 1, b, n, m, FilledImage, RecursionArray,
        recursionArrayIndex);
        recursionArrayIndex = addRecursionFillHoles(Image, a,
```

```
            b - 1, n, m, FilledImage, RecursionArray,
        recursionArrayIndex);
}
//Output image
double[][] ReturnImage = new double[n][];
for (a = 0; a < n; a++)
        ReturnImage[a] = new double[m];
//If particular pixel is not a background pixel,
//it is an object interior so fill it
for (a = 0; a < n; a++)
        for (b = 0; b < m; b++)
                if (FilledImage[a][b] < 2)
                        ReturnImage[a][b] = 255;
    return ReturnImage;
}


/**
 * Helper function of FillHoles
 * Checks if pixel was not visited. If it was not,
 * adds it to stack.
 */
private static int addRecursionFillHoles(double[][] Image, int a,
int b, int n, int m, int[][] FilledImage, int[][] RecursionArray,
int recursionArrayIndex)
{
    //uses side effects and is not hermetic!!
    if (a < 0 || b < 0 || a > n - 1 || b > m - 1)
            return recursionArrayIndex;
    if (Image[a][b] == 0 && FilledImage[a][b] == 0)
    {
            recursionArrayIndex++;
            RecursionArray[recursionArrayIndex][0] = a;
            RecursionArray[recursionArrayIndex][1] = b;
            FilledImage[a][b] = -1;
    }
    return recursionArrayIndex;
}
```

References

1. Hachaj T, Ogiela MR (2012) Semantic description and recognition of human body poses and movement sequences with gesture description language. Commun Comput Inf Sci 353:1–8
2. Hachaj T, Ogiela MR (2013) Computer karate trainer in tasks of personal and homeland security defense. Lect Notes Comput Sci 8128:430–441
3. Hachaj T, Ogiela MR, Piekarczyk M (2013) Dependence of Kinect sensors number and position on gestures recognition with gesture description language semantic classifier. In: Ganzha M, Maciaszek L, Paprzycki M (eds) Proceedings of the 2013 federated conference on computer science and information systems (FedCSIS 2013), IEEE Catalog Number CFP1385 N-ART, IEEE Computer Society Press, Kraków, Poland, pp. 571–575. ISBN 978-1-4673-4471-5, 8–11 Sept 2013
4. Hachaj T, Ogiela MR, Piekarczyk M (2014) Real-time recognition of selected karate techniques using GDL approach. Adv Intell Syst Comput 233:99–106. doi:10.1007/978-3-319-01622-1_12
5. Hachaj T, Ogiela MR (2014) Rule-based approach to recognizing human body poses and gestures in real time. Multimedia Syst 20:81–99. doi:10.1007/s00530-013-0332-2
6. Bankman I (2009) Handbook of medical image processing and analysis. Elsevier, Burlington
7. Najarian K, Splinter R (2012) Biomedical signal and image processing. CRC Press, Boca Raton
8. Pavlidis T (2012) Algorithms for graphics and image processing. Springer, Berlin Heidelberg
9. Pratt WK (2014) Introduction to digital image processing. CRC Press, Boca Raton
10. Theis FJ, Meyer-Bäse A (2010) Biomedical signal analysis: contemporary methods and applications. The MIT Press, Cambridge
11. Bodzioch S, Ogiela MR (2009) New approach to gallbladder ultrasonic images analysis and lesions recognition. Comput Med Imaging Graph 33:154–170
12. Duda RO, Hart PE, Stork DG (2001) Pattern classifications. Wiley, New York
13. Suetens P (2009) Fundamentals of medical imaging. Cambridge University Press, New York
14. Theodoridis S, Koutroumbas K (2009) Pattern recognition. Academic Press, Burlington
15. Davis LS (2001) Foundations of image understanding. Springer, New York
16. Ogiela L (2008) Cognitive systems for medical pattern understanding and diagnosis. Lect Notes Artif Intell 5177:394–400
17. Ogiela L (2008) Syntactic approach to cognitive interpretation of medical patterns. Lect Notes Artif Intell 5314:456–462
18. Ogiela L (2009) UBIAS systems for the cognitive interpretation and analysis of medical images. Opto-Electron Rev 17(2):166–179
19. Ogiela L (2010) Cognitive informatics in automatic pattern understanding and cognitive information systems. Studies in computational intelligence, Vol 323. Springer, Berlin, pp 209–226
20. Ogiela MR, Bodzioch S (2011) Computer analysis of gallbladder ultrasonic images towards recognition of pathological lesions. Opto-Electron Rev 19(2):155–168
21. Ogiela L, Ogiela MR (2009) Cognitive techniques in visual data interpretation. Studies in computational intelligence 228, Springer, Berlin
22. Ogiela L, Ogiela MR (2012) Advances in cognitive information systems. Cognitive systems monographs 17. Springer, Berlin
23. Hachaj T (2012) Pattern classification methods for analysis and visualization of brain perfusion CT maps. Comput Intell Paradigms Adv Pattern Classif 386:145–170
24. Hachaj T, Ogiela MR (2010) Automatic detection and lesion description in cerebral blood flow and cerebral blood volume perfusion maps. J Signal Process Syst Signal Image Video Technol 61(3):317–328. doi:10.1007/s11265-010-0454-0
25. Hachaj T, Ogiela MR (2010) Augmented reality interface for visualization of volumetric medical data. Adv Intell Soft Comput 84:271–277 (Springer, Berlin Heidelberg)

26. Hachaj T, Ogiela MR (2011) Intelligent information system for interpretation of dynamic perfusion brain maps. Lect Notes Artif Intell 6591:406–415

27. Hachaj T, Ogiela MR (2011) CAD system for automatic analysis of CT perfusion maps. Opto-Electron Rev 19(1):95–103. doi:10.2478/s11772-010-0071-2

28. Hachaj T, Ogiela MR (2011) A system for detecting and describing pathological changes using dynamic perfusion computer tomography brain maps. Comput Biol Med 41(6):402–410. doi:10.1016/j.compbiomed.2011.04.002

29. Chomsky N (1988) Language and problems of knowledge, the Managua lectures. MIT Press, Cambridge

30. Shannon CE (1948) A mathematical theory of communication. Bell Syst Tech J 27:379–423, 623–656

31. Hachaj T, Ogiela MR (2013) Application of neural networks in detection of abnormal brain perfusion regions. Neurocomputing 122:33–42. doi:10.1016/j.neucom.2013.04.030

32. Albus JS, Meystel AM (2001) Engineering of mind: an introduction to the science of intelligent systems. Wiley, New York

33. Branquinho J (ed) (2001) The foundations of cognitive science. Clarendon, Oxford

34. Cohen H, Lefebvre C (eds) (2005) Handbook of categorization in cognitive science. Elsevier, The Netherlands

35. Ogiela MR, Ogiela U (2014) Secure information management using linguistic threshold approach. Advanced Information and Knowledge Processing. Springer, London

36. Hachaj T, Ogiela MR (2013) Real time area-based stereo matching algorithm for multimedia video devices. Opto-Electron Rev 21(4):367–375. doi:10.2478/s11772-013-0107-5

37. Hachaj T (2014) Real time exploration and management of large medical volumetric datasets on small mobile devices—evaluation of remote volume rendering approach. Int J Inf Manage 34:336–343. doi:10.1016/j.ijinfomgt.2013.11.005

38. Hachaj T, Ogiela MR (2011) Augmented reality approaches in intelligent health technologies and brain lesion detection. Lect Notes Comput Sci 6908:135–148

39. Hachaj T, Ogiela MR (2012) Visualization of perfusion abnormalities with GPU-based volume rendering. Comput Graph UK 36(3):163–169. doi:10.1016/j.cag.2012.01.002

40. Hachaj T, Ogiela MR (2012) Framework for cognitive analysis of dynamic perfusion computed tomography with visualization of large volumetric data. J Electron Imaging 21(4):Article Number 043017. doi: 10.1117/1.JEI.21.4.043017

41. Hachaj T, Ogiela MR (2012) Segmentation and visualization of tubular structures in computed tomography angiography. Lect Notes in Artif Intell 7198:495–503

42. Hachaj T, Ogiela MR (2012) Evaluation of carotid artery segmentation with centerline detection and active contours without edges algorithm. Lect Notes Comput Sci 7465:469–479

43. Ogiela MR, Hachaj T (2012) The automatic two-step vessel lumen segmentation algorithm for carotid bifurcation analysis during perfusion examination. In: Watada J, Watanabe T, PhillipsWren G (eds) Intelligent decision technologies (IDT'2012), vol 2, smart innovation systems and technologies, vol 16, pp 485–493

44. Ogiela MR, Hachaj T (2013) Automatic segmentation of the carotid artery bifurcation region with a region-growing approach. J Electron Imaging 22(3):Article Number 033029. doi: 10. 1117/1.JEI.22.3.033029

Chapter 2
Cognitive Methods for Semantic Image Analysis in Medical Imaging Applications

In the first part of this chapter, we will briefly discuss the foundations of selected imaging techniques making use of computed tomography (CT). We will focus on dynamic CT perfusion (CTP) and computed tomography angiography (CTA). Later, we will discuss some fundamentals of cognitive computer image analysis aimed at computer-aided diagnosis and semantic image description.

2.1 DICOM Standard

The Digital Imaging and Communications in Medicine Standard (DICOM) addresses multiple levels of the ISO OSI network model and provides support for the exchange of information on interchange media [1]. Its independence of the underlying network technology allows DICOM to be deployed in many functional areas of application, including but not limited to communication via Ethernet, virtual private networks, over dial-up, or other remote access connections. At the application layer, the services and information objects address five primary areas of functionality [1]:

- transmission and persistence of complete objects (such as images, waveforms, and documents);
- query and retrieval of such objects;
- performance of specific actions (such as printing images on film);
- workflow management (support of work lists and status information);
- quality and consistency of image appearance (both for display and print).

Commonly digitalized CT images constituting medical data are stored in DICOM Files [2]. A DICOM File is a file whose content is formatted according to the requirements of the DICOM Standard. In particular, such files contain File Meta Information and a properly formatted dataset. The dataset consists of data elements. Each data element is made up of the following fields:

M. R. Ogiela and T. Hachaj, *Natural User Interfaces in Medical Image Analysis*,
Advances in Computer Vision and Pattern Recognition,
DOI: 10.1007/978-3-319-07800-7_2,
© Springer International Publishing Switzerland 2015

Fig. 2.1 Schema of a DICOM data set structure consisting of multiple data element structures

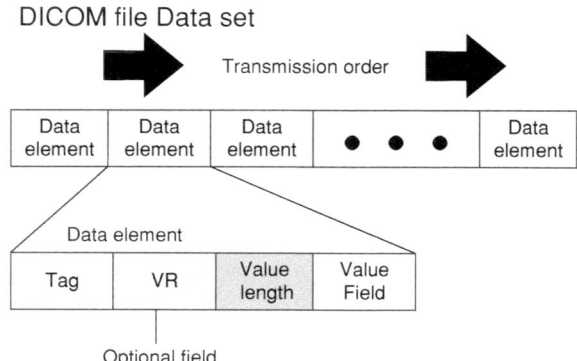

DICOM file Data set

- Data Element Tag representing the Group Number followed by the Element Number;
- Value Representation (VR)—only present in the two Explicit VR Data Element structures, it will not be discussed here;
- Value Length—containing the Explicit Length of the Value Field (or an Undefined Length in some special cases);
- Value Field—An even number of bytes containing the Value(s) of the Data Element.

Figure 2.1 presents a schema of the DICOM dataset structure that consists of multiple data element structures.

The information stored in the data element might, for example, comprise the date and time of data acquisition, the type of acquisition device, the imaging protocol, scaling parameters between digital image and real-world size, etc. Knowing the scaling parameters, we can measure the visualized structures for diagnostic purposes. Because of the DICOM file structure, dataset schema information about a particular patient will not be separated from his or her medical data.

2.2 Medical Practice in Computed Tomography Image Interpretation

Since its clinical introduction in 1991, volumetric CT scanning using spiral scanners has resulted in a revolution in diagnostic imaging [3]. In general terms, the capabilities of spiral CT can be expanded in various ways:

- to scan anatomical volumes with standard techniques at significantly reduced scan times,
- to scan larger volumes previously not accessible in scan times,
- to scan anatomical volumes with a high axial resolution (narrow collimation) to closely approach the isotropic voxel of high-quality datasets for excellent 3-dimensional post processing and diagnosis.

Computed tomography was the first diagnostic method that enabled the central nervous system (CNS) to be directly imaged. CT is often the first treatment of a patient with suspected CNS pathology, regardless of the fact that different tomography methods like Magnetic Resonance Imaging (MRI), Single-Photon Emission-Computed Tomography (SPECT), Positron Emission Tomography (PET) have already been introduced. The introduction of multidetector row-computed tomography (MDCT) has greatly improved the diagnostic capabilities of CT in neuroradiology. This applies mainly to examinations of the vascular structure, brain perfusion as well as the diagnosis of patients after trauma. Modern CT also 2D slices along any plane to be reconstructed at a resolution close to that of axial slices. It is also possible to create three-dimensional models of internal organs. If a radiocontrast agent is administered, it is possible to use CT to generate CTA images and computed tomography perfusion (CTP) maps.

The data generated by a contemporary CT scanner consists of a set of two-dimensional axial slices separated by some interslice distance. Each voxel in a slice represents a single Hounsfield unit value (normally 12-bit) of the tissue present inside a given volume. The Hounsfield unit (HU) scale is a linear transformation of the original linear attenuation coefficient measurement into one in which the radiodensity of distilled water at standard pressure and temperature (STP) is defined as zero, while the radiodensity of air at STP is defined as $-1,000$ HU [4]. Hounsfield units are used in medical imaging to describe the amount of X-ray attenuation of each voxel in the 3D image. In practice, these values are arranged on a scale from $-1,024$ to $+3,071$ HU, calibrated so that $-1,024$ HU is the attenuation produced by air and 0 HU is that produced by water, -120 by fat, $+40$ by muscle, and $+400$ or more by bone. The Hounsfield number of a tissue varies according to the density of the tissue; the higher the number, the denser the tissue. While describing CT images, a radiologist uses their knowledge of healthy human anatomy and known symptoms of various illnesses that they learned in their medical practice. Various applications provide them with two- and three-dimensional reconstructions of acquired data, volume measurements of tissues of interest, and HU values in a selected voxel or region. These descriptions, often accompanied by the results of other medical examinations, are used for the final diagnosis. Figure 2.2 presents several axial CT images (a fragment of a bigger volume) acquired for a single patient. Figure 2.3 shows a three-dimensional reconstruction with direct volume rendering of the same CT volume as in Fig. 2.2 [5–8]. We will discuss the direct volume reconstruction technique in Chap. 4 of this book.

2.3 Dynamic CT Perfusion Examination in Diagnostic Evaluation

Computed tomography perfusion (CTP) makes it possible to visualize structural, dynamic, and functional irregularities caused by ischemia, unlike CT which only shows static images of a patient's tissues. In neuroradiography, perfusion image

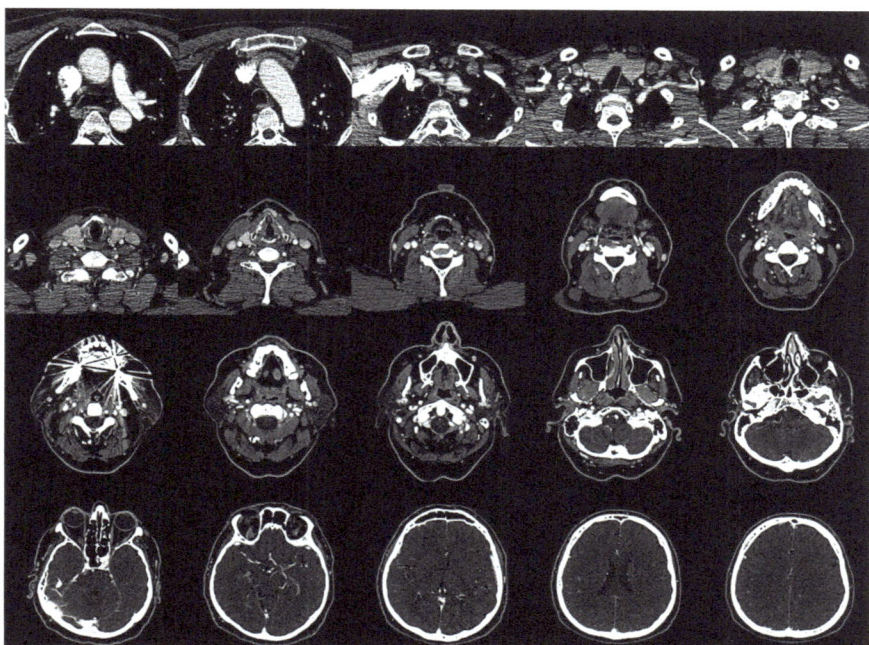

Fig. 2.2 Several CT images acquired for a single patient (the whole dataset includes 414 images). Pixels that represent voxel values are colored proportionally to HU (tissues with low HU values are *dark*, dense tissues are *white*)

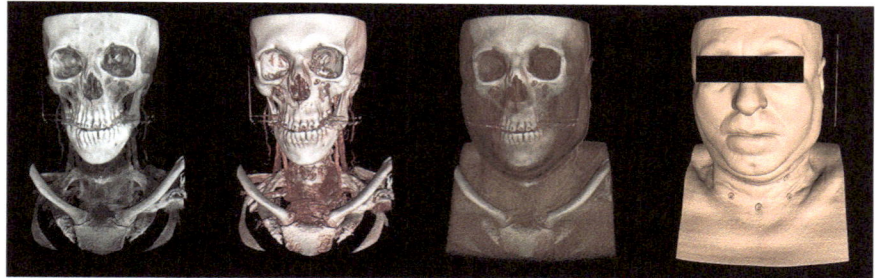

Fig. 2.3 A three-dimensional reconstruction made using the direct volume rendering technique of the same CT volume with a different range of densities enhanced by RGBA color values. From *left* pixels that represent voxel values colored proportionally to HU values (tissues with low HU values are *dark* and nearly transparent, dense tissues are *white* and opaque); bones and blood vessels are enhanced; opaque bones and semi-transparent skin and finally opaque skin (the identity of the person is hidden)

analysis (the terms "perfusion maps" and "perfusion images" are popularly used as equivalents) is currently used in cases of head injuries, epilepsy, vascular brain diseases, and especially to diagnose strokes [9] and brain tumors [10]. The basic principle of perfusion imaging is the repeated scanning of the same brain area while an intravenously injected bolus of a contrast agent passes through the patient's brain. The obtained scans must then be postprocessed to determine the set of quantity parameters, which are visualized in perfusion maps. The analysis of perfusion examination results (perfusion maps) is based on evaluating parameters important from a medical point of view. The most notable parameters are:

- CBF (cerebral blood flow)—the amount of blood (ml) that flows through 100 g of brain tissue in 1 min;
- CBV (cerebral blood volume)—the volume of blood (ml) that resides in cerebral capillaries and venules per 100 g of tissue;
- MTT (mean transit time)—the average time of contrasted blood flow through brain vascularity;
- TTP (time-to peak)—numbers proportional to the time until the bolus peak is reached, so higher numbers mean later bolus arrival.

2.3.1 Mathematical Model

A number of techniques have been developed during the past decades to evaluate cerebral perfusion [11]. The oldest used is Xe, a lipophilic radioactive tracer that easily diffuses through the blood–brain barrier. Stable xenon CT, however, requires excellent collaboration from the patient, as well as specialized and expensive equipment. It may occasionally be responsible for a decrease in the respiratory rate (yet without reported respiratory failure), headaches, nausea, vomiting, and convulsions [11].

The commonly used method for estimating brain perfusion parameters with CT is dynamic perfusion computed tomography. The theoretical basis of CT CBF measurement technique consists in the central volume principle, first discussed by Meier and Zierler [12], and later extended by Roberts and Larson [13]. Owing to the different possible path lengths that can be followed, blood elements flowing through the capillaries network of the brain will require different lengths of time (transit times) to travel from the arterial input to the venous outlet [14]. The average of all possible transit times through this capillary network is the MTT. The central volume principle relates CBF, CBV, and MTT in the following simple relationship:

$$\mathrm{CBF} = \frac{\mathrm{CBV}}{\mathrm{MTT}} \qquad (2.1)$$

In order to apply (2.1), we have to make the blood flow visible to a CT scanner. We can do this by injecting contrast material into the bloodstream. It is also

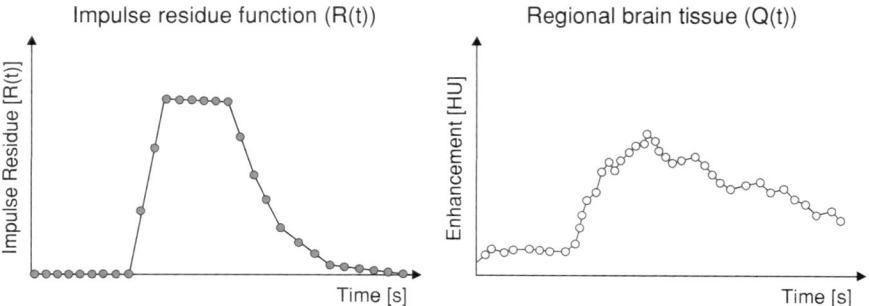

Fig. 2.4 *On the left* the hypothetical shape of the Impulse residue function R(t) obtained after the deconvolution $C_A(t)$ and $Q(t)$ from Eq. 2.3. *On the right* a hypothetical regional brain tissue, Q(t) (*open circles*), a contrast-enhancement curve obtained from CT scanning

assumed that a linear relationship exists between the enhancement in HU numbers and the concentration of the contrast material within an artery or brain tissue region, and that contrast material and blood have the same hemodynamic properties [14].

The contrast material is injected as a bolus of a very short duration. Theoretically, a CT scanner should allow us to observe an enhancement curve with an initial flat plateau followed by a continuous decrease toward the zero baseline (Fig. 2.4 left). This is the so-called Impulse residue function (R(t)).

R(t) describes the fraction of the contrast medium remaining in the tissue as a function of time, due to a unit input impulse of the contrast medium [15]. The duration of the plateau corresponds to the time interval during which all the injected contrast material remains in the capillary network [14]. After this time interval, the contrasted blood begins to leave brain vascularity, and the value of R(t) decreases. When R(t) is known, we can use it to compute the MTT according to given formula:

$$
\text{MTT} = \frac{\int\limits_{0}^{\infty} R(t)\mathrm{d}t}{R_{\max}}
\tag{2.2}
$$

However, R(t) cannot be directly determined by CT scanning because it is difficult to identify the specific arterial inlet(s) of a brain region [14]. To overcome this problem, Meier and Zierler proposed the following formula [12]:

$$
Q(t) = \text{CBF} \cdot [C_A(t) \otimes R(t)]
\tag{2.3}
$$

where $Q(t)$ is the tissue enhancement curve, $C_A(t)$ is the arterial enhancement curve, and $\otimes$ is a convolution operator. On the right side of Fig. 2.4, a hypothetical regional brain tissue (Q(t)) contrast-enhancement curve obtained by CT scanning is presented ($C_A(t)$ is similar in shape) (Fig. 2.5).

According to [16], the volume of blood passing through brain vascularity (CBV) can be estimated as

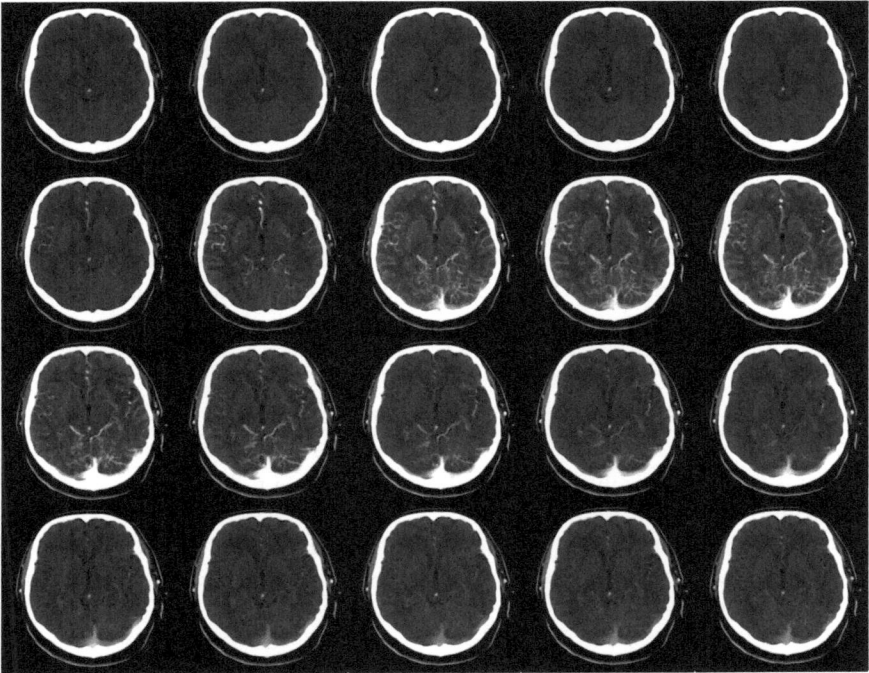

Fig. 2.5 An example set of 20 axial slices (the whole set consisted of 40). The slices are in order row by row from *left to right*. As can be seen while time passes the hyper-intense regions appear enhancing the vascularity of the brain with contrast material that arrived to them

$$\mathrm{CBV} = \frac{\int\limits_{0}^{\infty} Q(t)\mathrm{d}t}{\int\limits_{0}^{\infty} C_A(t)\mathrm{d}t} \tag{2.4}$$

The models (2.1)–(2.4) can be applied successfully only if the blood–brain barrier is intact and there are no recirculations of contrast material [16]. In cases in which the blood–brain barrier is compromised, $Q(t)$ would be the summation of the enhancement due to the contrast material in both the intravascular and extravascular spaces, and CBV would be overestimated. To eliminate the effect of recirculation, the procedure proposed in [14] can be applied. Finally, in order to determinate the CBF value, the following formula has to be computed:

$$\mathrm{CBF} = \frac{\mathrm{CBV}}{\mathrm{MTT}} = \frac{R_{\max} \cdot \int\limits_{0}^{\infty} Q(t)\mathrm{d}t}{\int\limits_{0}^{\infty} R(t)\mathrm{d}t \cdot \int\limits_{0}^{\infty} C_A(t)\mathrm{d}t} \tag{2.5}$$

In order to designate R(t) with the Meier–Zierler model, the Q(t) and $C_A(t)$ values in each sample of TDC must be known. Q(t) can be read directly from a CT scan. In order to measure $C_A(t)$, the common practice is to choose the right artery (or several arteries) in particular the axial slice. This can be done manually [17] or with the help of automatic methods [18]. To compute R(t) using (2.3) the impulse residuum function has to be obtained with the deconvolution (the inverse operation to a convolution). A singular-value-decomposition-based deconvolution technique is often reported as a way to solve this problem [15, 16, 19].

In some cases $C_A(t)$ curves are additionally fitted to the gamma function (the gamma—variate function, [18, 20]). It is done to denoise and eliminate tracer recirculation:

$$Q_\gamma(t) = K \cdot (t - t_0)^\alpha \cdot e^{\frac{-(t-t_0)}{\beta}} \tag{2.6}$$

where t is the time after injection, K is the constant scale factor, α, β, are γ-variety parameters.

Because TTP is the amount of time in which maximal blood flow is reached, the values of pixels in the TTP map can be easily computed pixel-by-pixel by analyzing the deconvolved curves.

2.3.2 Image Acquisition and Post Processing

In a CTP examination, the mass of contrast that remains in the capillary network is measured with a CT scanner. To generate a single set of perfusion maps (CBF, CBV, TPP, and MTT) CTP protocol acquires a series of CT slices in one axial position. A set of pixels that have same image coordinates are used to generate the time density curve (TDC$-Q(t)$). The deconvolution of (2.3) if performed pixel-by-pixel for all TDC curves. All of the examinations last about 40 s and generate 40 slices for each examined axial position. An example set of CT slices from the CTP examination is shown in Fig. 2.5.

In Fig. 2.6, we have presented three perfusion maps generated from the CT time series from Fig. 2.5 by Siemens Syngo Neuro Perfusion CT software. Each perfusion map visualizes a value of a single perfusion parameter and because of that it might be interpreted as a monochrome image. For an easier interpretation by a radiologist they are often additionally colored with a proper lookup table.

Generally, it is emphasized that CTP can provide quantitative data of brain perfusion parameters, which is important in medical data evaluation [19] and can provide valuable diagnostic information. However, the reliability of CTP data with regard to its quantitativeness remains to be established and validated [19]. It has been suggested that the reliability of CTP data depends on the quality of source images, temporal resolution, deconvolution algorithms, the vascular-pixel elimination (VPE) method, and arterial input functions. What is more, perfusion map

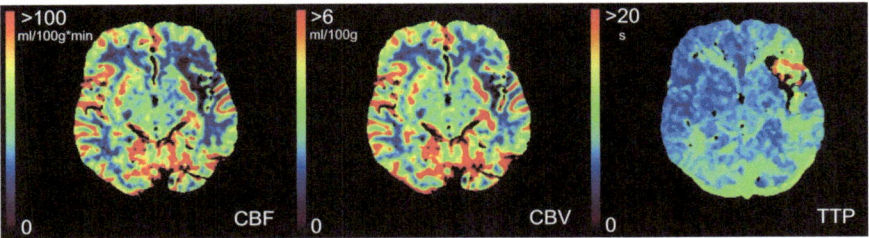

Fig. 2.6 CBF, CBV, and TTP perfusion maps generated from the CT time series from Fig. 2.5. Because CTP maps are grayscale images they are colored with a lookup table that is on the *left* of each figure, for easier interpretation. According to radiologists' description of the CTP maps presented, CBF and CBV are slightly decreased (TPP increased) on the *left* on the level of the *top* sides of the lateral ventricle frontally (the *left* side of the image is on the *right* side of a perfusion image)

generation protocol is not standardized and packages from different vendors might produce different quantity values on CTP maps from the same input data. For example, the perfusion dataset we used in this book for the evaluation of methods (Chap. 3) was generated with Syngo Neuro Perfusion CT by Siemens. We decided to do so because we have not found premises that a particular software is worse or better (more clinically usable) than another.

The assessment of cerebral ischemia by means of perfusion parameters derived from perfusion CT provides valuable information for the prediction of tissue outcome [20]. Also, according to [9, 21–23] a quantitative analyses of the severity of ischemic lesions might be implemented into the diagnostic management of stroke patients.

2.3.3 Prognostic Significance of Cerebral CTP

A great deal of medical research has been done in order to determine a correlation between the values of perfusion parameters and long- and short-term prognoses for examined brain tissues. Despite some minor differences, the authors determined the average value of CBF for health brain tissues as:

$$\overline{CBF_A} \approx 55 \frac{ml}{100\,g \cdot min} \tag{2.7}$$

and average CBV as

$$\overline{CBV_A} \approx 2.5 \frac{ml}{100\,g} \tag{2.8}$$

Table 2.1 Average relative values of perfusion parameters (CBF and CBV) and their interpretation according to the literature

rCBF decrease	rCBV decrease	Interpretation
0.60−0.70		Tissues can be salvaged [24, 27–29]
0.20−0.30		Tissues will eventually become infarcted [24, 27–29]
0.62 ± 0.17	0.78 ± 0.18	Tissues can be salvaged [21]
0.34 ± 0.20	0.43 ± 0.22	Tissues will eventually become infarcted [21]

[24]. The dysfunction of neural cells begins when a CBF value drops below $20\frac{ml}{100\,g\cdot min}$ [9, 10, 25]. Continuous drops of perfusion in range of $10 \sim 20\frac{ml}{100\,g\cdot min}$ may affect with cell death in many minutes to hours [9]. CBF of less than $10\frac{ml}{100\,g\cdot min}$ cannot be tolerated beyond a few minutes before infarction occurs causing permanent brain cell damage [9, 10, 25]. Because of some factors [26] the true CBF and CBV values in individual cases may be underestimated in a manner that is difficult to predict. As the result of this some authors prefer to use relative values of CBF and CBV (appropriately rCBF and rCBV—see Table 2.1). The authors in [26] state that a relative comparison of cerebral blood flow within the corresponding areas of both hemispheres of the brain is possible without any limitations because the error of measurement is the same for both high and low CBF values.

It is possible to detect the perfusion deficit area by CTP before noncontrast CT reveals early ischemic changes [30, 31]. The authors in [23] found that the perfused CBV, as imaged by the CTP, reflect the approximate minimum final infarct size in this clinical setting. As cerebral perfusion pressure falls, precapillary resistance vessels dilate (resulting in increased CBV) to maintain the CBF. Once maximum vasodilatation has been reached, autoregulation fails and the CBF begins to fall. As perfusion pressure continues to fall, there is disruption of cellular metabolism, vascular collapse, and the development of irreversible ischemia happens. In an acute ischemic stroke, collapse of vessels at low CBV is likely to occur only after prolonged, severe reductions in CBF, and continued collapse would be associated with a high probability of producing infarction. An increase in CBV reflects the collateral pathway or autoregulation and a decrease in CBV indicates an unfavorable state [32]. A decrease in CBF is a highly sensitive as well as a specific finding in predicting an infarction [27].

In conclusion, both CBF and CBV have prognostic values in the evaluation of the ischemic evolution [33–39]. In many cases, simultaneous analysis of both CBF and CBV perfusion parameters enables an accurate analysis of the ischemia visualized brain tissues and predicts its further changes permitting not only a qualitative (like CT angiography does) but also a quantitative evaluation of the degree of severity of the perfusion disturbance, which results from the particular type of occlusion and collateral blood. The multimodal CT evaluation (CT, CTP, and CTA) improves the detection rate and the prediction of the final size of the infarction in comparison with the unenhanced CT, CT angiography, and perfusion CT alone [40].

2.4 Computed Tomography Angiography

During the past decade CT angiography has become a standard noninvasive imaging modality for the depiction of vascular anatomy and pathology [41]. CTA is primarily performed for assessing the heart, arteries, or veins. After a contrast medium has been injected, the CT scanner acquires the data when the enhancement in the vessel reaches a predetermined operator selected level. The vessels that the contrast medium has already reached are visualized in CT scans as hyperintensive (brighter) areas. Enhancing the vessel position helps to further segment the circulatory system.

A complete interpretation of CTA includes a review of the transverse CT sections and, in selected cases, multiplanar/curved reformations, volume renderings, maximum-intensity projections, and other images produced during post processing [42].

In Fig. 2.7 example three-dimensional reconstructions of carotid artery CTA with vascular structures enhanced by a contrast agent are presented.

In Chap. 3, we will discuss different approaches for computer-based enhancing and segmentation postprocessing methods for vascular structures that are visualized with three-dimensional CTA images. This includes vessel-enhancing filtering, region growing-based algorithms, and deformable contour-based approaches [43–46].

2.5 Cognitive Methods in Computer Semantic Image Analysis

Cognitive analysis of medical images was made possible by advanced methods of identifying image semantics, which were created thanks to the development of a field called cognitive informatics within modern computer science. Cognitive informatics is a field that combines topics from both cognitive science and information theory, based on both the mechanisms of computer information processing and imitating processes occurring in human brain.

Cognitive informatics thus covers not only the aspects of using mathematical theories to describe and analyze data or information presented in a distributed form, but also engineering fields as well as informatics, cognitive sciences, neuropsychology, cybernetics, computer engineering, knowledge engineering, and computational engineering.

All research problems coming up in the area of cognitive informatics are aimed at understanding the rules followed by human intelligence and cognitive processes taking place in a person's brain. Understanding how the above processes operate allows their transfer and use for solving engineering problems.

Major applications of cognitive informatics methods include the development of the new generation of information systems (i.e., cognitive information systems),

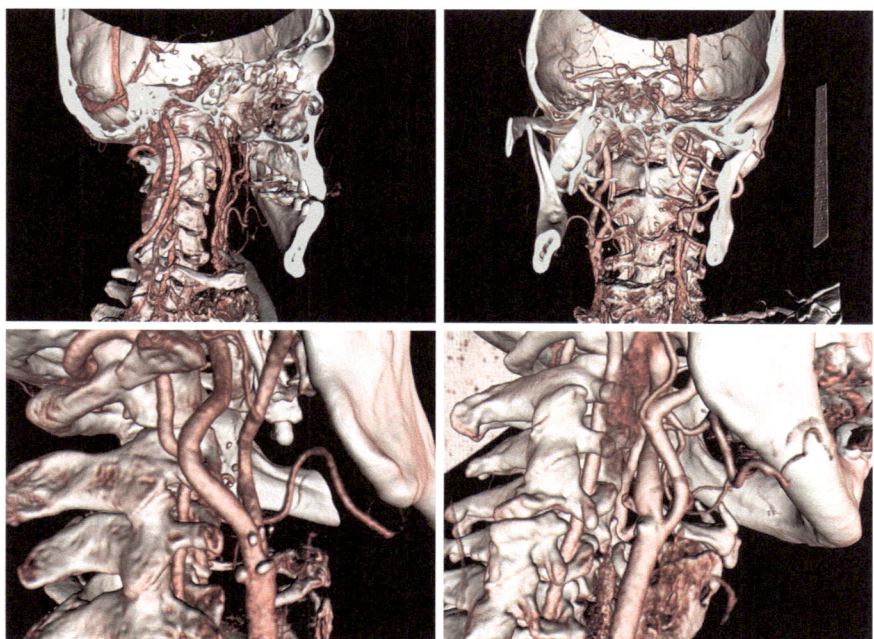

Fig. 2.7 An example three-dimensional reconstruction of a carotid artery CTA with vascular structures enhanced by a contrast agent

the design of cognitive robots, and attempts at the computer analysis of human impressions and sensations, as well as the design of an artificial brain that can perceive, receive, and analyze sensations and impressions. Multiple similar applications also include methods of cognitively analyzing image patterns (including the medical images we are considering) to understand their contents and meaning (semantics).

Similar problems can be solved thanks to the attempt to apply theoretical models of processes occurring in the human brain, associated with activities such as information acquisition, memory modeling, information extraction, or semantic interpretation and information understanding.

In cognitive informatics fields there are many different models allowing for the operation of basic cognitive processes to be identified. These models describe the operation of associational memories, identify methods of learning and perceiving, and also define mechanisms for understanding the world around us. These models are detailed in [52]. The most important of them include the model of information representation in the human brain, the cognitive informatics model built based on the structure of the natural human brain, the natural intelligence model, and the cognitive memory model [52]. However, to allow such biological models solve difficult problems with the use of computers, possible models of cognitive computers were also constructed and enhancements were made to models of cognitive machines based on cognitive memory models and models of visual perception, which in our case also enables the development of algorithms oriented toward cognitively analyzing medical images.

2.5.1 Cognitive Resonance Model

Semantic (meaning-based) analysis and computer understanding of medical images are made possible by implementing cognitive resonance processes [47–49]. A computer system that conducts this analysis by reference to features characteristic for the specific type of images holds in its base the indispensable knowledge, which allows certain expectations to be generated during the interpretation it carries out. These expectations are generated automatically using the expert knowledge bases collected in the system. Apart from the generated expectations, the information system also carries out an analysis aimed at defining and indicating the appropriate, actual characteristic features of the analyzed data. As a result of combining these significant features describing the analyzed data with expectations generated based on the knowledge held in the system and relating to the semantic contents of the pattern, cognitive resonance occurs [50–52].

Cognitive resonance becomes the cornerstone of the process of understanding the image datasets undergoing analysis. Resonance processes run as described below. The stream of expectations generated by the recognizing system and the stream of features characteristic for the specific dataset are compared, as a result of which certain pairs of expectations and features indicated for the analyzed patters can increase in importance and others, conversely, decrease in importance. By producing cognitive resonance, this comparison leads to confirming one of the possible hypotheses about the meaning of the pattern, or, on the contrary, demonstrates that the inconsistency of features and expectations is so significant that the hypothesis becomes untrue. The first case means that the analysis process was successful and the semantics of the examined image can be determined, the second means that the attempt to automatically understand the data failed.

In computer systems designed for cognitively analyzing images, cognitive resonance is based on mathematical linguistic methods [50, 51]. The structure of the analyzed image is compared to the structure of data constituting a certain pattern during the recognition process. The comparison is enabled by the strings of the derivation rules of a formal grammar which enable these or similar patterns to be generated unambiguously.

These rules, referred to as productions, are defined in a specially introduced grammar, which in turn defines a certain formal language. Data thus recognized is assigned to the class to which the pattern representing it belongs. In this case, cognitive analysis is based on a syntactic approach which uses additional techniques of processing and analyzing the examined image pattern to determine the semantics of the image. These additional techniques comprise the following operations:

- input image preprocessing;
- analyzing examined object features;
- image coding with picture primitives defined by the introduced formal language.

The completion of such stages makes it possible to re-represent the data in the form of hierarchical structures of a semantic tree and to take subsequent steps of deriving this representation from the initial symbol of the grammar [50, 51].

In a decisive majority of cases, a system carrying out a cognitive analysis while preprocessing image data must segment and identify picture primitives and also determine the relations between them.

The classification proper then consists in recognizing whether the specific obtained linguistic representation of input data belongs to the language generated by the defined formal grammar. Such grammars may come from the classes of sequential, tree, and graph grammars and they are used for recognition during a syntactic analysis conducted by the system [47, 50].

In data analysis processes run by cognitive information systems, a certain significant feature characteristic for these very systems is noted. Processes of semantic image analysis do not have to end at the stage of classifying the analyzed images and recognizing them as belonging to one of the defined classes: they are conducted further, until the image meaning is recognized. This is why cognitive image analysis systems now carry out a stage of automatically understanding the meaning of the image, completed using artificial intelligence technologies, which not only simply recognize but also extract significant semantic information. Only this information allows for the meaning of the image to be interpreted, in other words, supports the full understanding of the image pattern.

Research conducted in this field has led to significant progress in recent years. A number of classes of cognitive vision systems have been proposed for the semantic interpretation of images, including learning-capable E-UBIAS systems described in [49, 52]. The ability of cognitive systems to learn is a very desirable feature. Systems with such capabilities can extend their knowledge base which grows along with the number of semantically interpreted images and which is used to generate system expectations. In such systems, the learning process occurs in five stages.

In the first stage, the semantic information that can be of significance in further analysis process is extracted from sets of possible solutions, so if some information is useless in the current data analysis process, it is treated as superfluous for that process and will be omitted from it. After this stage, the features characteristic for the solution obtained at the first stage of the analysis process are identified. Identifying such features can cause a change in the solution obtained at the first stage, e.g., because the set of expectations or the expert knowledge base is broadened, and thus new patterns are defined.

The next stage focuses on indicating significant changes in the area of characteristic features leading to optimizing the solution formulated, as a result of which the set of characteristic features is redefined in the system.

The last stage of system learning is that of looking for solutions based on a new set of characteristic features and a new expert knowledge base, which at this stage takes the shape of a set of new patterns defined in the cognitive system.

Supplementing data analysis with stages at which the system learns new solutions means that the cognitive resonance must be repeated in the data analysis and image classification process, and if the learning process is multiplied, then cognitive resonance must be repeated more than once.

After the stage at which cognitive systems learn, the analysis and understanding process based on cognitive resonance is repeated, but unlike the traditional analysis process, it now makes use of new (extended) sets of analyzed data and a new base of expert knowledge. It is these very elements that become the primary foundation of cognitive data analysis processes in new systems for image pattern analysis and understanding enhanced with aspects of cognitive system learning.

2.5.2 Semantic Analysis in Cognitive Systems

Methods modeled on cognitive/decision-making processes, particularly those consisting in the description, analysis, and interpretation of the meaning contained in analyzed image datasets play a major role in semantic analysis algorithms. Such processes are inseparably connected with techniques of cognitive analysis, during which a significant role is played by semantic analysis stages. Semantic analysis is thus the key to the correct operation of cognitive data analysis systems. When this analysis is conducted, several different processes occur: interpretation, description, analysis, and semantic reasoning. The main stages in the semantic analysis of images focus on:

- data preprocessing;
- creating the linguistic representation of images, including:
  - recognizing picture primitives;
  - identifying relations between picture primitives;
  - defining relations between objects in the image;
- syntactic pattern analysis;
- pattern classification;
- cognitive resonance;
- determining the semantics of patterns and understanding image data.

Most of the above semantic analysis stages deal with the data understanding process as such, because beginning with the syntactic analysis conducted using the formal grammar defined in the system, tasks are executed to identify the features of the analyzed data with particular focus on its semantics, i.e., the meaning carried by such features.

To properly carry out the computerized process of understanding images, it is necessary to implement feedback techniques during which the features of analyzed images are compared to expectations generated by the system based on the knowledge it has. Such comparisons are performed using cognitive resonance processes which are crucial for the analysis conducted, i.e., they show the consistency of features and expectations, and the process of data understanding itself, during which the meaning of the analyzed images is identified.

Semantic analysis plays a significant role because it identifies the semantics in the areas within which patterns are interpreted. The proper identification of image semantics is done using the formal grammar, defined in the system, and the set of derivation rules associated with this grammar, which set defines a certain language for describing images and their semantic features. Analysis processes are applied to the features of medical images, which can help interpret diagnostic images [52]. For various classes of medical images, these features may be as follows:

- shape ratios identifying various lesions;
- morphometric values identifying the size, length, and width of the lesion;
- the number of lesions observed (frequently more than one);
- the number of repetitions of the given situation, lesion, pathology;
- the lesion location.

Identifying such lesions allows for a semantic record to be created, which record describes the examined diagnostic image and may also be used at further stages of prognosticating the planned therapy of the diagnosed patient.

2.5.3 Linguistic-Based Cognitive Interpretation of Images

An important aspect of the automatic image understanding method is a very close connection between our methodology and mathematical linguistics, especially a linguistic description of images [52]. There are two important reasons for the selection of linguistic techniques of image description as the fundamental tool for understanding images.

The first one derives from the fact that in the case of understanding we have no limited number of classes or templates known a priori. In fact when we try to understand absolutely an unknown image, the possible number of potential classes goes to infinity. So we must use a tool that offers us possibilities to describe a potentially infinite number of categories. Moreover, the tool under consideration must be constructed from a finite number of elements only, because computers cannot operate using an infinite number of components. This means that it is necessary to have a tool that generates descriptions of classes rather than to point to classes described a priori. For this reason the only suitable tool is a language that can generate an infinite number of sentences on the basis of a finite number of component words in vocabulary and rules in the grammar.

The second reason for using a linguistic method for automatic image understanding is connected with the fact that in the linguistic approach to after image processing, we obtain a description of the image content without the use of any

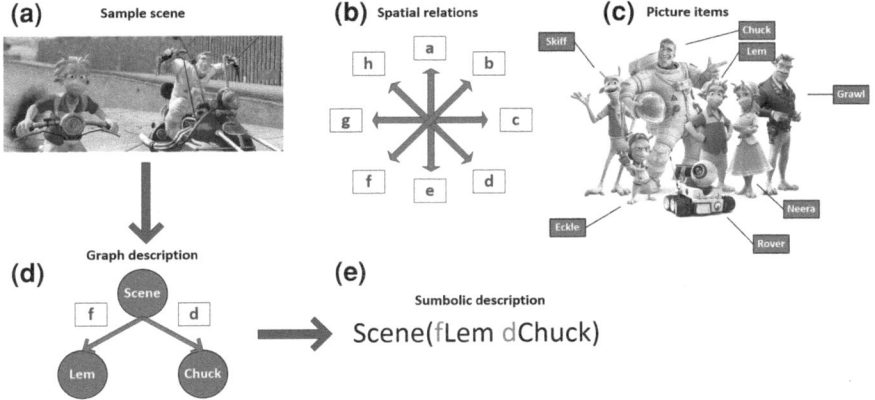

Fig. 2.8 Planet 51 heroes sample scene for syntactic description. **a** Analyzed scene,
b–c Elements of used vocabulary, **d** Symbolic representation of the scene before describing it
in terms of graph-grammar, **e** Conversion of a graph diagram of the image into its symbolic
description

classification known a priori due to the fact that even the criteria of the classification
are constructed and developed during the automatic reasoning process. This is
possible because of a very strong generalization mechanism included into the
grammar parsing process. Owing to formal and powerful technologies for the
automatic parsing of all linguistic formulas, describing actual images, we can recommend mathematical linguistic methods as the most powerful technology for any
pattern generalization. The only problem is connected with a correct adjustment of
the terms and methods of formal grammars and languages to the application in the
field of images.

When we try to build a language for the description of images we must start
with fundamental definitions of elements belonging to the suitable formal grammar. Let us assume that we must build a grammar for the description of a class of
scenes similar to the image shown in Fig. 2.8.

An analysis of such a scene shows that we have some classes of graphic objects
('primitives'), which can be built into the grammar as substantives (nouns). We
also have some classes of relations between objects, which can be treated as the
verbs of our grammar. So, the vocabulary of grammar for the images under
consideration can be shown as in Fig. 2.8b–c.

Using the proposed vocabulary, we can replace the scene with an equivalent
scheme for the grammar, as shown in Fig. 2.8d. On the basis of such a symbolic
description of the image under consideration we can also use symbolic notations
for elements of vocabulary; for every image they obtain a representation in terms
of terminal symbols belonging to the definition of the grammar used (see
Fig. 2.8e). After a final description of the image, using the elements of a selected
image description language, we must implement the cognitive resonance concept.
It is, of course, the most difficult part in the whole task. During cognitive

resonance we must generate a hypothesis about the semantic meaning of the image under consideration, and we must have an effective algorithm for its online verification. Both mentioned activities are performed by the parser of the grammar used. Hypothesis generation is connected with the use of the selected grammar rules (mappings included into the formal description of the grammar). In the case of medical support systems, the hypothesis generation process depends very much on the medical problem. Verification of the hypothesis is performed by the incessant comparison of selected features of the image with expectations taken from the source of knowledge (mostly it is a medical doctor's experience based on his or her previous visual expertise).

The main idea of cognitive resonance is based on an iterative performance of the following steps. Let us assume that a semantic linguistic description of an image is done in the usual form of a string of terminal symbols, denoted for example in a pattern in the form of text "*Natural user interface techniques in the cognitive analysis of brain and carotid artery images*":

"🕯︎🕯︎🕯︎🕯︎🕯︎🕯︎   🕯︎🕯︎🕯︎-🕯︎   🕯︎🕯︎🕯︎🕯︎-🕯︎-🕯︎🕯︎🕯︎🕯︎-🕯︎   🕯︎🕯︎-🕯︎🕯︎🕯︎-🕯︎🕯︎🕯︎🕯︎🕯︎-🕯︎   🕯︎🕯︎   🕯︎🕯︎🕯︎-🕯︎🕯︎🕯︎🕯︎
🕯︎🕯︎🕯︎-   🕯︎🕯︎🕯︎🕯︎🕯︎🕯︎🕯︎🕯︎🕯︎   🕯︎-🕯︎   🕯︎🕯︎🕯︎🕯︎🕯︎🕯︎   🕯︎🕯︎🕯︎🕯︎   🕯︎🕯︎🕯︎🕯︎🕯︎🕯︎🕯︎🕯︎🕯︎   🕯︎🕯︎🕯︎🕯︎🕯︎-🕯︎🕯︎   🕯︎🕯︎🕯︎🕯︎-🕯︎
🕯︎-🕯︎"

We are using *Wingdings2* font symbols as a signal to show that a man does not need to understand symbols produced by the linguistic processor, it is enough if the parser can manage them.

Now the parsing process begins. Let us assume that the working hypothesis about the meaning of this image leads to the assumption that the image must include at least one pattern (e.g. "*heart*"):

"🕯︎-🕯︎-🕯︎🕯︎🕯︎🕯︎"

The parser starts the search process through all the strings of the terminal symbols describing (in terms of the used language) important semantic features of the analyzed image.

The search process fails, which means that the strength of the first working hypothesis decreases. Another working hypothesis leads to the assumption that the image must include at least one pattern ("the *brain*"):

"🕯︎🕯︎🕯︎🕯︎🕯︎🕯︎"

This pattern can be found in the analyzed string:

"🕯︎🕯︎🕯︎🕯︎🕯︎🕯︎   🕯︎🕯︎🕯︎-🕯︎   🕯︎🕯︎🕯︎🕯︎-🕯︎-🕯︎🕯︎🕯︎🕯︎-🕯︎   🕯︎🕯︎-🕯︎🕯︎🕯︎-🕯︎🕯︎🕯︎🕯︎🕯︎-🕯︎   🕯︎🕯︎   🕯︎🕯︎🕯︎-🕯︎🕯︎🕯︎🕯︎
🕯︎🕯︎🕯︎-   🕯︎🕯︎🕯︎🕯︎🕯︎🕯︎🕯︎🕯︎🕯︎   🕯︎-🕯︎   🕯︎🕯︎🕯︎🕯︎🕯︎🕯︎   🕯︎🕯︎🕯︎🕯︎   🕯︎🕯︎🕯︎🕯︎🕯︎🕯︎🕯︎🕯︎🕯︎   🕯︎🕯︎🕯︎🕯︎🕯︎-🕯︎🕯︎   🕯︎🕯︎🕯︎🕯︎-🕯︎
🕯︎-🕯︎"

which means that our second hypothesis can now be considered more probable. Yet we are still not quite sure whether the hypothesis is true or not because for its full validation it is necessary to test also other assumptions taken from this hypothesis and from all other hypotheses.

References

1. DICOM (2013) strategic document, version revised in 2013-10-23. http://medical.nema.org
2. Digital Imaging and Communications in Medicine (DICOM, PS 3.5-2011) In: Part 5: data structures and encoding, National Electrical Manufacturers Association, 2011. http://medical.nema.org
3. Kopp AF, Klingenbeck-Regn K, Heuschmid M, Küttner A, Ohnesorge B, Flohr T, Schaller S, Claussen CD (2000) Multislice computed tomography: basic principles and clinical applications. Electromedica 68(2):95–105
4. Celenk C, Celenk P (2012), Bone density measurement using computed tomography. In: Saba L (ed) Computed tomography—clinical applications. ISBN: 978-953-307-378-1, doi: 10.5772/22884 (InTech). http://www.intechopen.com/books/computed-tomography-clinical-applications/bone-density-measurement-using-computed-tomography
5. Hachaj T, Ogiela MR (2012) Visualization of perfusion abnormalities with GPU-based volume rendering. Comput Graph-UK 36(3):163–169. doi:10.1016/j.cag.2012.01.002
6. Hachaj T, Ogiela MR (2012). Framework for cognitive analysis of dynamic perfusion computed tomography with visualization of large volumetric data. J Electron Imaging 21(4): 043017, doi: 10.1117/1.JEI.21.4.043017
7. Hachaj T (2014) Real time exploration and management of large medical volumetric datasets on small mobile devices—Evaluation of remote volume rendering approach. Int J Inf Manage 34:336–343. doi:10.1016/j.ijinfomgt.2013.11.005
8. Hachaj T, Ogiela MR (2010). Augmented reality interface for visualization of volumetric medical data. Adv Intell Soft Comput 84:271–277, (Springer, Berlin Heidelberg)
9. Latchaw RE, Yonas H, Hunter GJ, Yuh WTC, Ueda T, Sorensen AG, Sunshine JL, Biller J, Wechsler L, Higashida R, Hademenos G (2003) Guidelines and recommendations for perfusion imaging in cerebral ischemia. Stroke 34:1084–1104
10. Hoeffner EG, Case I, Jain R, Gujar SK, Shah GV, Deveikis JP, Carlos RC, Thompson BG, Harrigan MR, Mukherji SK (2004) Cerebral perfusion CT: technique and clinical applications. Radiology 231(3):632–644
11. Wintermarka M, Thirana JP, Maedera P, Schnydera P, Meuli R (2001) Simultaneous measurement of regional cerebral blood flow by perfusion ct and stable xenon CT: a validation study. Am J Neuroradiol 22:905–914
12. Meier P, Zierler KL (1954) On the theory of the indicator-dilution method for measurement of blood flow and volume. J Appl Physiol 6(12):731–744
13. Roberts GW, Larson KB (1973) The interpretation of mean transit time measurements for multi-phase tissue systems. J Theor Biol 39(2):447–475
14. Cenic A, Nabavi DG, Craen RA, Gelb AW, Lee TY (1999) Dynamic CT measurement of cerebral blood flow: a validation study. AJNR Am J Neuroradiol 20(1):63–73
15. Koh TS, Tan CKM, Cheong LHD, Limc CCT (2006) Cerebral perfusion mapping using a robust and efficient method for deconvolution analysis of dynamic contrast-enhanced images. NeuroImage 32(2):643–653
16. Axel L (1980) Cerebral blood flow determination by rapid-sequence computed tomography: a theoretical analysis. Radiology 137(3):679–686

17. Wittsack HJ, Wohlschläger AM, Ritzl EK, Kleiser R, Cohnena M, Seitz RJ, Mödder U (2008) CT-perfusion imaging of the human brain: advanced deconvolution analysis using circulant singular value decomposition. Comput Med Imaging Graph 32(1):67–77
18. Hirata M, Sugawara Y, Murase K, Miki H, Mochizuki T (2005) Evaluation of optimal scan duration and end time in cerebral CT perfusion study. Radiat Med 23(5):351–363
19. Sasaki M, Kudo K, Oikawa H (2006) CT perfusion for acute stroke: current concepts on technical aspects and clinical applications. Int Congr Ser 1290:30–36
20. Koh TS, Hou Z (2002) A numerical method for estimating blood flow by dynamic functional imaging. Med Eng Phys 24(2):151–158
21. Koenig M, Kraus M, Theek C, Klotz E, Gehlen W, Heuser L (2001) Quantitative assessment of the ischemic brain by means of perfusion-related parameters derived from perfusion CT. Stroke 32(2):431–437
22. Eastwood JD, Lev MH, Wintermark M, Fitzek C, Barboriak DP, Delong DM, Lee TY, Azhari T, Herzau M, Chilukuri VR, Provenzale JM (2003) Correlation of early dynamic CT perfusion imaging with whole-brain MR diffusion and perfusion imaging in acute hemispheric stroke. AJNR Am J Neuroradiol 24(9):1869–1875
23. Lev MH, Segal AZ, Farkas J, Hossain ST, Putman C, Hunter GJ, Budzik R, Harris GJ, Buonanno FS, Ezzeddine MA, Chang Y, Koroshetz WJ, Gonzalez RG, Schwamm LH (2001) Utility of perfusion-weighted CT imaging in acute middle cerebral artery stroke treated with intra-arterial thrombolysis: prediction of final infarct volume and clinical outcome. Stroke 32(9):2021–2028
24. Eastwood JD, Lev MH, Azhari T, Lee TY, Barboriak DP, Delong DM, Fitzek C, Herzau M, Wintermark M, Meuli R, Brazier D, Provenzale JM (2002) CT perfusion scanning with deconvolution analysis: pilot study in patients with acute middle cerebral artery stroke. Radiology 222(1):227–236
25. Aksoy FG, Michael HL (2000) Dynamic contrast-enhanced brain perfusion imaging: technique and clinical applications. Semin Ultrasound CT MR 21(6):462–477
26. Koenig M, Klotz E, Heuser L (1998) Perfusion CT in acute stroke: characterization of cerebral ischemia using parameter images of cerebral blood flow and their therapeutic relevance, Clinical experiences. Electromedica 66:61–67
27. Mayer TE, Hamann GF, Baranczyk J, Rosengarten B, Klotz E, Wiesmann M, Missler U, Schulte-Altedorneburg G, Brueckmann HJ (2000) Dynamic CT perfusion imaging of acute stroke. AJNR Am J Neuroradiol 21(8):1441–1449
28. Wintermark M, Reichhart M, Thiran JP, Maeder P, Chalaron M, Schnyder P, Bogousslavsky J, Meuli R (2002) Prognosis accuracy of cerebral blood flow measurement by perfusion computed tomography, at the time of emergency room admission, in acute stroke patients. Ann Neurol 51(4):417–432
29. Klotz E, König M (1999) Perfusion measurements of the brain: using dynamic CT for the quantitative assessment of cerebral ischemia in acute stroke. Eur J Radiol 30(3):170–184
30. Reichenbach JR, Röther J, Jonetz-Mentzel L, Herzau M, Fiala A, Weiller C, Kaiser WA (1999) Acute stroke evaluated by time-to-peak mapping during initial and early follow-up perfusion CT studies. AJNR Am J Neuroradiol 20(10):1842–1850
31. Guan X, Yu X, Liu X, Long J, Dai J (2003) CT perfusion imaging and CT subtraction angiography in the diagnosis of ischemic cerebrovascular disease within 24 hours. Chin Med J 116(3):368–372
32. Higashida RT, Furlan AJ, Roberts H, Tomsick T, Connors B, Barr J, Dillon W, Warach S, Broderick J, Tilley B, Sacks D (2003) Technology assessment committee of the american society of interventional and therapeutic neuroradiology; technology assessment committee of the society of interventional radiology, trial design and reporting standards for intra-arterial cerebral thrombolysis for acute ischemic stroke. Stroke 34(8):109–137
33. Hachaj T (2012) Pattern Classification Methods for Analysis and Visualization of Brain Perfusion CT Maps. Comput Intell Paradig Adv Pattern Classif 386:145–170

34. Hachaj T, Ogiela MR (2010) Automatic detection and lesion description in cerebral blood flow and cerebral blood volume perfusion maps. J Signal Process Syst Signal Image Video Technol 61(3):317–328. doi:10.1007/s11265-010-0454-0

35. Hachaj T, Ogiela MR (2011) Intelligent information system for interpretation of dynamic perfusion brain maps. Lect Notes Artif Intell 6591:406–415

36. Hachaj T, Ogiela MR (2011) CAD system for automatic analysis of CT perfusion maps. Opto-Electron Rev 19(1):95–103. doi:10.2478/s11772-010-0071-2

37. Hachaj T, Ogiela MR (2011) A system for detecting and describing pathological changes using dynamic perfusion computer tomography brain maps. Comput Biol Med 41(6):402–410. doi:10.1016/j.compbiomed.2011.04.002

38. Hachaj T, Ogiela MR (2011) Augmented reality approaches in intelligent health technologies and brain lesion detection. Lect Notes Comput Sci 6908:135–148

39. Hachaj T, Ogiela MR (2013) Application of neural networks in detection of abnormal brain perfusion regions. Neurocomputing 122:33–42. doi:10.1016/j.neucom.2013.04.030

40. Kloska SP, Nabavi DG, Gaus C, Nam EM, Klotz E, Ringelstein EB, Heindel W (2004) Acute stroke assessment with CT: do we need multimodal evaluation? Radiology 233(1):79–86

41. Yu T, Zhu X, Tang L, Wang D, Saad N (2007) Review of CT angiography of Aorta. Radiol Clin North Am 45(3):461–483

42. American College of Radiology (ACR), American Society of Neuroradiology (ASNR)(2010) ACR-ASNR practice guideline for the performance and interpretation of cervicocerebral computed tomography angiography (CTA). [online publication]. Reston (VA), American College of Radiology (ACR), p 7

43. Hachaj T, Ogiela MR (2012) Segmentation and visualization of tubular structures in computed tomography angiography. Lect Notes Artif Intell 7198:495–503

44. Hachaj T, Ogiela MR (2012) Evaluation of carotid artery segmentation with centerline detection and active contours without edges algorithm. Lect Notes Comput Sci 7465:469–479

45. Ogiela MR, Hachaj T (2012). The automatic two-step vessel lumen segmentation algorithm for carotid bifurcation analysis during perfusion examination. In: Watada J, Watanabe T, PhillipsWren G (eds) Intelligent decision technologies (IDT'2012), vol 2. Smart innovation systems and technologies, vol 16, pp 485–493

46. Ogiela MR, Hachaj T (2013) Automatic segmentation of the carotid artery bifurcation region with a region-growing approach. J Electron Imaging 22(3): 033029, doi: 10.1117/1.JEI.22.3.033029

47. Ogiela L (2008) Cognitive systems for medical pattern understanding and diagnosis. Lect Notes Artif Intell 5177:394–400

48. Ogiela L (2008) Syntactic approach to cognitive interpretation of medical patterns. Lect Notes Artif Intell 5314:456–462

49. Ogiela L (2009) UBIAS systems for the cognitive interpretation and analysis of medical images. Opto-Electron Rev 17(2):166–179

50. Ogiela L (2010) Cognitive informatics in automatic pattern understanding and cognitive information systems. Stud Comput Intell 323: 209–226 (Springer, Berlin Heidelberg)

51. Ogiela L, Ogiela MR (2009). Cognitive techniques in visual data interpretation. Stud Comput Intell 228 (Springer, Berlin Heidelberg)

52. Ogiela L, Ogiela MR (2012) Advances in cognitive information systems. Cognit Syst Monogr 17 (Springer: Berlin Heidelberg)

Chapter 3
Computer Analysis of Brain Perfusion and Neck Angiography Images

This chapter will be devoted to image processing, analyzing and recognizing algorithms for brain computed tomography perfusion (CTP) and neck angiography images (CTA). Both of those are popular medical imaging methods that are often used beside standard computed tomography (CT) in acute stroke imaging [1, 2]. Imaging of the carotid arteries is important for the evaluation of patients with an ischemic stroke or a Transient Ischemic Attack (TIA). You can learn more about the role of those types of examinations in Chap. 2 of this book.

At first we will discuss the automatic method for the detection and recognition of potential lesions in brain perfusion that can be localized with the help of CTP maps. The proposed automatic diagnostic schema includes the detection (D) of asymmetries in the brain perfusion between the hemispheres, measurement (M) of the parameters important from a medial point of view and a final diagnosis of the description (D) of the abnormalities displayed with a so-called prognostic map for the lesion evolution in the brain tissues. The abbreviation of the schema name, DMD, came from the first letters of those tasks. We will also present an evaluation of the proposed methodology.

The second part of this chapter contains different approaches for enhancing and segmenting vascular structures that are visualized with three-dimensional computed tomography angiography images. That includes vessel enhancing filtering, region growing-based algorithms and deformable contour-based approaches. We will discuss and evaluate the nearly automatic (it requires minimal initial configuration from the operator) framework that enables the segmentation of the single vessel lumen. We will present the results of this framework evaluation on the CTA images of the carotid artery bifurcation region.

3.1 An Analysis of Brain CTP Maps

In this section, we will present our image processing, analysis, and potential lesion detection framework called the DMD system for CTP brain maps. It is based on our earlier works [3–5].

M. R. Ogiela and T. Hachaj, *Natural User Interfaces in Medical Image Analysis*,
Advances in Computer Vision and Pattern Recognition,
DOI: 10.1007/978-3-319-07800-7_3,
© Springer International Publishing Switzerland 2015

3.1.1 Methodology

In Chap. 1 we have presented most of the image processing methods that were used in our image processing pipeline. Also, in Chap. 2, we have discussed the basis of brain CTP modality and its diagnostic relevance. However, we have not presented yet the state of the art of computer methods of automatic brain CTP analysis and some other specified image processing methods (like self-organized map-based image segmentation or CT scalping) that we utilized in our research. In this section, we will briefly describe those methods.

3.1.1.1 State of the Art Method of Automatic CTP Analysis

Strokes are the third-leading cause of death, after cardiovascular diseases and cancers [6]. CTP techniques combined with CTA provide a comprehensive non-invasive survey of the site of arterial occlusion and the resulting ischemia and infarction [7]. In clinical practice, CTP maps are interpreted in conjunction with nonenhanced CT and CTA images in patients with suspected strokes. Deconvo-lution-based dynamic CTP maps are more accurate than nonenhanced CT scans in the depiction of acute hemispheric strokes. Moreover, a CTP more accurately depicts the extent of the stroke; this advantage has implications on clinical deci-sion making.

The physicians who make a diagnosis as a result of CTP data may use various image processing procedures. One of the most notable methods, reported in [6, 8–10], relies on the CBF (cerebral blood flow) threshold of the ischemia and the preserved (penumbra) or the altered (infarct) autoregulatory processes. Thus, in this method, an ischemic cerebral area (penumbra plus infarct) was defined as including cerebral pixels with a CBF decrease of 34 % compared with the corresponding region in the cerebral hemisphere defined as healthy on the basis of clinical symptoms. Within this selected area, pixels with CBV (cerebral blood volume) values higher or lower than $2.5 \frac{ml}{100\,g}$ were selected as indicative of penumbra and infarct, respectively. The resulting cerebral infarct and penumbra maps were combined and graphically dis-played as a prognostic map.

An algorithm for the analysis of the CTP proposed by us in [3, 4] is a fusion of image processing, pattern recognition and image analysis procedures. The image processing step consists of the lesion detection algorithm. The lesion detection algorithm detects potential pathologic tissues (regions of interests—ROI). After the image processing step two symmetric regions are detected in the left and right hemisphere. The image analysis procedure measures parameters important from a medical point of view in the detected ROIs. In the pattern recognition step algo-rithm, knowing the previous measurements determines what type of lesion was detected and in which hemisphere. In order to do it, it is necessary to use medical knowledge about average perfusion values (similarly to Wintermark's approach). In this chapter, [5] we modified the existing image processing schema for computed tomography perfusion by adding a neural network-based image processing procedure. The procedure uses Kohonen's self-organizing map (SOM) architecture. In the following chapters, we will focus on a detailed description and evaluation of our approach.

3.1.1.2 Application of SOM in Medicine

Self-orginizing map (SOM, also called the Kohonen Network) [11] is among the group of structures and algorithms of so-called artificial neural networks. SOM has special property of effectively creating spatially organized "internal representations" of various features of input signals and their abstractions [12]. Because a SOM can be trained with an unsupervised algorithm, it is typically applied to data in which specific classes or outcomes are not known a priori. In this case, the SOM can be used to understand the structure of the input data, and in particular, to identify "clusters" of input records that have similar characteristics [13]. In the case of the analysis of dynamic contrast-enhanced perfusion images (MRI—magnetic resonance imaging—time series) it has been shown that clustering data is a useful extension to conventional perfusion parameter maps [14, 15].

SOM shows its effectiveness not only in pattern recognition tasks but also in image processing, especially in feature extraction, image matching, compression and segmentation [16].

In research [17] a batch of SOMs is applied to the feature image process for the dynamic behavior of an aerated agitation vessel. When time series images preprocessed by particle image velocimetry are computed by the SOM, the generated map provides visible and intelligible information for the periodic behavior of the patterns of gas dispersion. It is also shown that the sigmoid transformation of data enhances the efficiency of generating a more comprehensible map. Furthermore, the SOM is demonstrated to be effective in extracting the feature of small displacements of the impeller shaft inside the vessel.

The usage of a SOM is also reported in unimodal medical image matching [18]. Given a pair of two-dimensional medical images of the same anatomical region and a set of interest points in one of the images, the proposed algorithm effectively detects the set of corresponding points in the second image, by exploiting the properties of the Kohonen SOMs and embedding them in a stochastic optimisation framework. The correspondences are established by determining the parameters of local transformations that map the interest points of the first image to their corresponding points in the second image. The parameters of each transformation are computed in an iterative way, using a modification of the competitive learning, as implemented by SOMs. The proposed algorithm was tested on medical imaging data from three different modalities (CT, MR and red-free retinal images) subject to known and unknown transformations.

In paper [19], the authors used a fully automated image segmentation method based on an algorithm that provides adaptive plasticity in function approximation problems: the deformable (feature) map (DM) algorithm. The DM approach reduces a class of similar function approximation problems to the explicit supervised one-shot training of a single data set. This is followed by a subsequent, appropriate similarity transformation, which is based on a self-organized deformation of the underlying multidimensional probability distributions.

In [20] an unsupervised MR image segmentation method based on a self-organizing feature map network is presented. The algorithm includes spatial constraints by using a Markov Random Field (MRF) model. The MRF term introduces the prior distribution with clique potentials, thus improving the segmentation results without having extra data samples in the training set or a complicated network structure. Also, in [21] a computer-assisted method is used to evaluate of brain tumor grade (malignancy state), which has been designed using a mixture of unsupervised artificial neural networks (ANN) and hierarchical multi resolution wavelet. First, the medical images are decomposed by multi resolution wavelets, which are subsequently and selectively reconstructed to form wavelet filtered images. These wavelet filtered images along with MRI images have been utilized as the features to unsupervised neural network—SOMs—to segment the tumor, edema, necrosis and normal tissue and grade the malignant state of the tumor. A novel segmentation algorithm based on the number of hits experienced by Best Matching Units (BMU) on SOM maps is proposed. The results show that the SOM performs well in differentiating the tumor, edema, necrosis and normal tissue pattern vectors on the ADC images.

3.1.1.3 CTP Map Processing with SOM

Very often a crucial part that has to be performed before image analysis is the filtering of raw data in order to remove (mostly high or low frequency) noises and artefacts. The same applies to CTP maps where there are high-frequency artefacts. Because of algorithm [5] mime, the analysis procedure of a physician, we have made the assumption that a radiologist does not use all of the scale of the possible perfusion values that might be present in a map. It is sometimes more convenient to display preselected ranges of perfusion values in a single color to make regions of severe ischemia more conspicuous [22] and concentrate only on sufficiently large, homogenous abnormalities (visually apparent regional abnormalities [22]). Knowing that we concluded [5] that the physicians clusterise CTP values to a number of classes that differ in the perfusion parameter value, our solution utilises a SOM with a one-dimensional input vector (perfusion value) and 3×3 map grid size as shown in Fig. 3.1. The network is initialised "linearly" [23] and trained with the "batch training" method [23]. After the training is completed the original perfusion values are replaced by one of the nine closest values from the SOM map. In our research, we used a Matlab implementation of SOM [24].

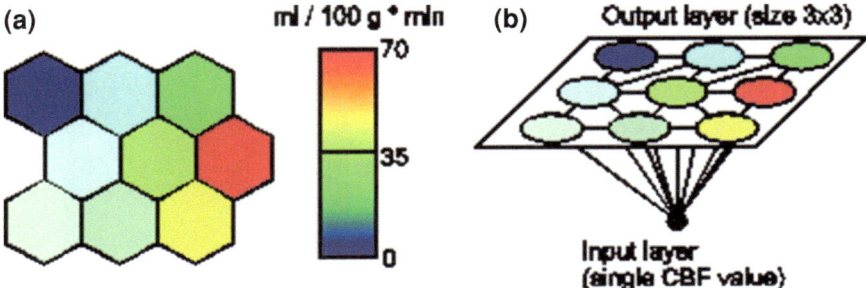

Fig. 3.1 The SOM architecture that was used for the CTP image clustering. **a** shows an example of a trained SOM for a cerebral blood flow (CBF) map, the neurons are colored according to a given look-up table. In **b** the used SOM vector architecture is presented: a single input in the first layer and a 3 × 3 neuron grid in the output layer

3.1.1.4 Scalping of CT Images

CT Scalping is a procedure of removing non-brain tissues from computed tomography data. A CT scalp might be useful for many various processes, image analysis and pattern recognition algorithms that require direct access to pixels that represent the brain. Scalping can be realised by a relatively simple image processing algorithm:

Scalping algorithm of a CT axial slice

A. Create a binary mask of bones by thresholding a CT image with a threshold in the range of the value of the bones. Fill the holes inside the obtained mask.
B. Create a binary mask of brain by thresholding a CT image with a threshold in the range of the value of the brain.
C. Take a common part of a binary mask of a brain from B and the bones from A. The resulting common part is a binary mask of a scalp.
D. Take only those tissues that are marked by a binary mask of a scalp.

An example of the above procedure can be seen in Fig. 3.2.

3.1.2 Asymmetry Detection and Measurement

An asymmetry detection algorithm plays a crucial role in the whole diagnostic algorithm. The proper detection of asymmetries (the position of potential perfusion lesions) significantly affects the rest of data processing. If a detection algorithm

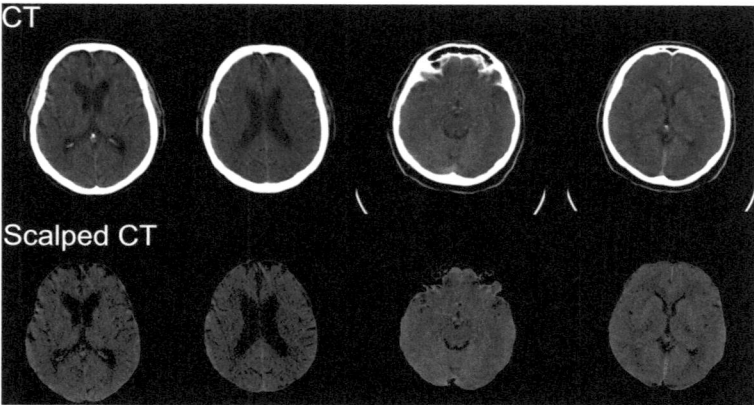

Fig. 3.2 In the first row there are four example CT images, in the second row, the same images after performing the scalping procedure as described in the text

finds asymmetries in the wrong place (or does not detect them at all) the proper diagnosis in further processing steps is nearly impossible. The algorithm for detecting asymmetries (potential abnormalities) in the cerebral blood flow (CBF) and the cerebral blood volume (CBV) maps is identical, and looks as follows:

A CTP map's asymmetry detection algorithm

1. In the first step, the system operator needs to manually indicate the line that separates the left and right hemisphere (later, we will call this line a symmetry axis of the CTP or just a symmetry axis).
2. In the second step, a reduction in the number of values in the perfusion map and median filtration with a window, sized 15×15, is performed—Fig. 3.3b. Due to this processing step regions with a homogenous perfusion value are obtained. This step is crucial for further processing because perfusion value reduction eliminates artefacts and fluctuations that disturb image processing while median filtration smooths the analysed regions and eliminates artefacts introduced by a CTP map generation algorithm. We have proposed two methods that can be used to perform this value reduction. The first is a simple linear filtration:

$$I(x, y) := \text{Floor}\left(I(x, y)/15\right) * 15$$

where I is an image being processed and x, y are image pixel indices.

The second filtration model is the SOM-based cauterization that was already discussed.

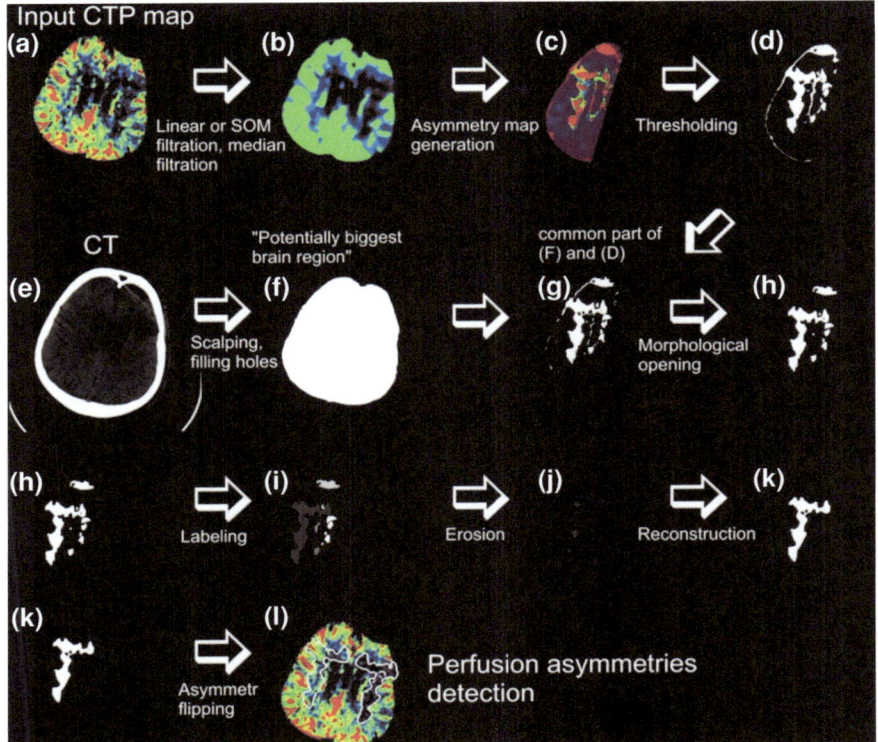

Fig. 3.3 The image processing pipeline of the CTP map's asymmetry detection algorithm. The description of this method is presented in the text

3. Generation of "potential biggest brain region"—Fig. 3.3e, f. "Potential biggest brain region" is a binary mask that can be generated from a scalped CT image. Pixels that represent tissues that do not belong to the brain have bits set to 0, and the rest of them have bits set to 1. The scalped image might be obtained from any CT image from the CTP time series.

4. Asymmetry map generation—in this step an algorithm compares the symmetric regions of the left and right hemispheres that lay on the corresponding sides of the symmetry axis—Fig. 3.3c. The comparison algorithm goes as follow:

A. For each pixel $I(x, y)$ which is on the left of the symmetry axis and the symmetric pixel $I_S(x, y)$ on the right check the following condition:

- If $I(x, y) > 0$ and $I_S(x, y) = 0$ or $I(x, y) = 0$ and $I_S(x, y) > 0$ then one of those pixels belongs to the brain region (because it has a nonzero perfusion) while the second one might be the background (a non-brain region) or might be a part of the brain with a very low perfusion. It is important to notice that even a perfusion map of a healthy patient can often be asymmetric.

If $I(x, y) > 0$ and $I_S(x, y) > 0$ both pixels belong to the brain.

- If $I(x, y) > I_S(x, y)$ Asymmetry$(x, y) := \frac{I(x,y)}{I_S(x,y)}$
- Else: Asymmetry$(x, y) := \frac{I_S(x,y)}{I(x,y)}$

  If $I(x, y)$ or $I_S(x, y)$ equals zero, the value 1 is used instead in the above quotient.

- If $I(x, y) = 0$ and $I_S(x, y) = 0$ that pixel belong to the background and it will not be analysed (the value 0 will also appear in the asymmetry map). Because values on the CTP map are always non-negative there will be no other conditions.

B. The asymmetry map is then thresholded, in order to leave only those pixels, for which perfusion asymmetry is "high enough"—Fig. 3.3d. Only the pixels that have values greater than t come to the next step of processing. In the case of linear filtration t = 6, when a SOM is used:

$$t = 0.6 \cdot \frac{\max(\text{SOM\_Vectors})}{\#\text{SOM\_Vectors}}$$

where SOM_Vectors are all neurons from the output layer of the SOM.

C. A common part of the thresholded asymmetry map and the "potential biggest brain region" mask is taken—Fig. 3.3g. During this step all pixels which do not belong to the brain are eliminated from further processing.

D. Morphological opening of the asymmetry map—with a circular element with a radius equal to 3—Fig. 3.3h. Quite often in this step of processing, an asymmetry map might have narrow regions in the border of the brain tissues that were generated during processing. The presence of those nonzero pixels is caused by the asymmetry of the CTP map, but they are irrelevant in further processing. In this step this border is removed together with the narrow links between the solid asymmetric perfusion regions.

E. Labeling of the asymmetry map, erosion and reconstruction—these three steps are used to filter only those perfusion asymmetric regions that have sufficient size to be potential perfusion lesions. The image is labeled—Fig. 3.3i and then eroded with a semi-circular structural element of a radius equal to 10—Fig. 3.3j. If at least one pixel from a particular region has survived erosion, the whole region is rewritten in the reconstruction step to the final asymmetry image—Fig. 3.3k.

F. The asymmetry map is flipped according to the symmetry axis to both hemispheres—Fig. 3.3l. At this stage we do not yet know in which hemisphere potential perfusion abnormalities reside. Knowing the size and position of those regions we can perform the measurements of the perfusion parameters in the detected ROIs. The average value of CBF and CBV in the left and right hemisphere can be computed: $\overline{CBF}_L$—the average CBF in the left asymmetric region, $\overline{CBF}_R$—the average CBF value in the right asymmetric region, $\overline{CBV}_L$—

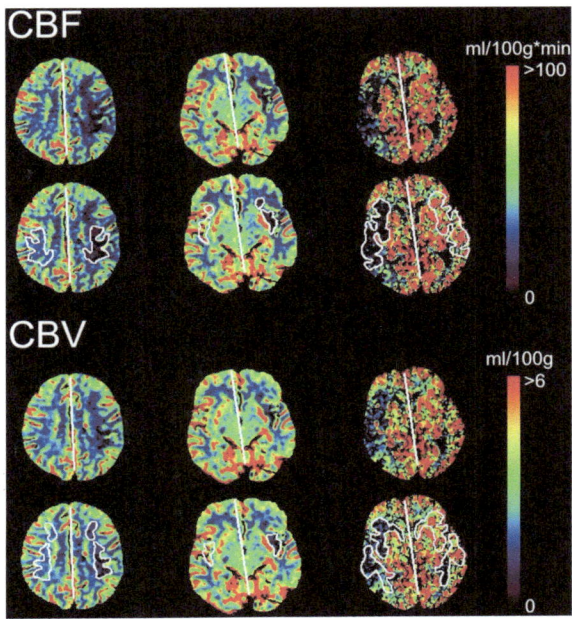

Fig. 3.4 This figure present three CBF maps (*first row*) and three CBV maps (*third row*). It should be remembered that the left side of the perfusion map is the right side of a patient's brain (CTP maps are mirrored). The maps in each column were generated from the same CTP time series. In the *second row* there are CBF maps from the *first row* with the perfusion abnormalities detected by our DMD algorithm. In the *fourth row* there are CBV maps from the *third row* with the perfusion abnormalities marked by the proposed method. The images from the *first* and *second column* are an axial slice of the same patient. In those maps the CBF and CBV are slightly decreased at the *left* on the level of the *top sides* of the lateral ventricle, frontally, and parietally. In the maps in the *third column* the CBF and CBV are decreased in the region of the right middle cerebral artery. In all cases a brain stroke was diagnosed

the average CBV value in the left asymmetric region and the average $\overline{CBV}_R$ in right asymmetric region.

In Fig. 3.4 we have presented example results of our asymmetry detection algorithm on a set of CBF and CBV perfusion maps.

3.1.3 Generation of Prognostic Maps

In the last step of data processing in a DMD algorithm the final diagnosis is generated. The automatic diagnosis is based on the CTP data evaluation method that was discussed in Chap. 2. The CBF and CBV have prognostic values in the evaluation of the ischemic evolution [25]. A simultaneous analysis of both the

CBF and CBV perfusion parameters may enable the analysis of the visualised ischemia of brain tissues and predict its further changes permitting not only a qualitative (like a CT angiography) but also a quantitative evaluation of the degree of the severity of the perfusion disturbance which results from the particular type of occlusion and collateral blood. At first, our algorithm determines in which hemisphere of the brain tissues are present and what is the type of the potential lesions (ischemic or hemorrhagic). It is done by comparing the average value of the perfusion parameters that should be measured in a healthy patient's brain with the results that were obtained in the step described in Sect. 3.1.2. In order to find the potential localization of an abnormality, the following procedure can be executed:

If the following condition is satisfied:

$$\left| \overline{CBF_L} - \overline{CBF_A} \right| > \left| \overline{CBF_R} - \overline{CBF_A} \right| \tag{3.1}$$

where:

$\overline{CBF_A}$—the average perfusion value in a healthy brain (according to literature reviewed in Chap. 2 it equals $55 \cdot \frac{ml}{100\,g \cdot min}$), we are observing a perfusion abnormality in the left hemisphere. It is due to the fact that the module of the difference between the healthy value of perfusion and that observed in left hemisphere is greater than the module of the difference between a healthy and observed values in the right hemisphere. In the opposite case, the abnormality resides in the right hemisphere.

This type of change in the left or right hemisphere can be determined by examining the following condition:

If $\overline{CBF_L} < \overline{CBF_A}$ (or $\overline{CBF_R} < \overline{CBF_A}$ if we are analysing the right hemisphere) then we are dealing with ischemia (the observed CBF is smaller than the healthy value of this parameter). In the opposite case, the region of abnormality is hemorrhagic.

The procedure that was used to evaluate the CBV maps is very similar:
Condition:

$$\left| \overline{CBV_L} - \overline{CBV_A} \right| > \left| \overline{CBV_R} - \overline{CBV_A} \right| \tag{3.2}$$

checks if the CBV abnormality is localised in the left hemisphere ($\overline{CBV_A}$ is the average value of the healthy perfusion, that according to according to literature reviewed in Chap. 2 equals $2.5 \cdot \frac{ml}{100\,g}$.

If $\overline{CBV_L} < \overline{CBV_A}$ then we are dealing ischemia with an (in opposite case a hemorrhage). The same reasoning can apply to the right hemisphere.

When we have already localised positions and types of perfusion aberrations, we can create so-called prognostic maps that show the potential ischemia evolution in brain tissues. Based on materials from Chap. 2 the algorithm is as follows:

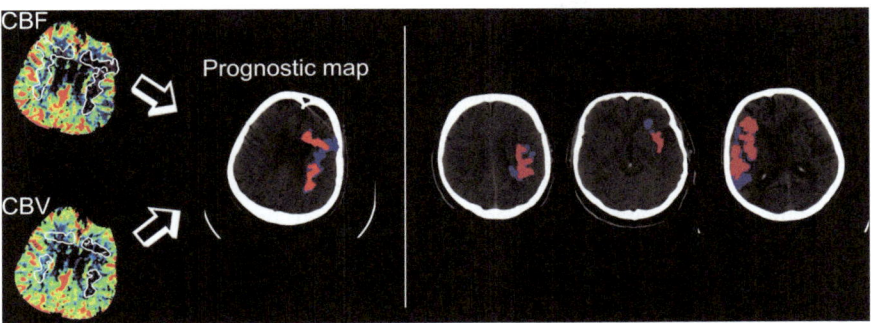

Fig. 3.5   An example of visualized prognoses for brain tissues. CBF and CBV are processed with an image processing algorithm in order to find asymmetries. After determining the abnormality positions both maps are simultaneously analyzed in order to generate prognostic maps. In the *left* part of the figure, the perfusion map from Fig. 3.3 is being processed. In the *right* part of this figure, the prognostic maps for perfusion maps from Fig. 3.4 are presented. *Red* regions are tissues that probably become infarcted, *blue regions*—an auto regulation mechanism might occur in the ischemic region

An algorithm for the generation of prognostic maps

For each pixel that belongs to a CBF map and a corresponding pixel in a CBV map, if the pixel contains a perfusion abnormality:

A. Particular tissues can be salvaged if abnormalities are present in the CBF and CBV asymmetry map and the values of the rCBF did not drop beyond 0.48.

B. Tissues that will eventually become infarcted if tissues are present in the CBF and CBV asymmetry map and the values of the rCBF did drop beyond 0.48.

C. Tissues that have an auto regulation mechanism in the ischemic region if CBF is decreased and CBV is correct or increased.

rCBF and rCBV parameters are computed as a division of the perfusion value in the analyzed pixel by the perfusion value in the symmetric pixel that resides in the opposite hemisphere. The example of visualized prognoses for brain tissues are presented in Fig. 3.5. Potential lesions should be compared with the corresponding CT image in order to check its presence there as part of the foregoing diagnostic protocol [26].

3.1.4 Dataset

In order to validate our approach we have gathered a test set consisting of 75 pairs of CTP images (one CBF and one CBV in each) from 30 patients (both men and women) suspected of ischemia / stroke. For each of these pairs we also have one CT image that is one of a series of images that was acquired during a perfusion examination. The maps were previously diagnosed by an expert. An expert described the position and type of pathologies that were visualised on the CTP maps. We also have the final patient diagnosis. 42 CTP maps were described as normal (no perfusion abnormalities), 33 maps showed syndromes of ischemic strokes of various severities. Patient scanning was done with a Siemens Somatom Sensation 10 CT scanner. CTP maps were generated with Syngo Neuro Perfusion CT software.

3.1.5 Evaluation

We have evaluated our DMD approach on the dataset that was described in the previous section. The results we present here have already been published [5] however, because of their importance to the presented methodology evaluation we decided to mention them in our book. The results obtained from the automatic method were compared with experts' descriptions and diagnoses. If the algorithm's diagnosis differed from the reference description we considered that case as an 'error'. Error situations are as follows:

- Detection of perfusion abnormality in a map that did not consist of any asymmetry that is a danger to a patient's health.
- Lack of perfusion abnormality detection in a map that is consistent with that kind of abnormality.
- Detection of excessive abnormalities besides those that were described.
- Detection of abnormalities in a different position or with a different type than those that were reported in the reference set.

Tests results presented in Table 3.1 were summed up according to terminology [27, 28]:

- TP—correctly predicted Positive samples (presence/position of lesions matched the radiologist's description).
- FP—incorrectly predicted Negative samples (Negative samples predicted as positives).
- TN—correctly predicted Negative samples (perfusion maps did not show lesions).
- FN—incorrectly predicted Positive samples (Positive samples predicted as negatives).

Table 3.1 Results of the DMD image processing algorithm's validation on our test dataset

Test result	Preprocessing type		
	Linear	SOM	Differences
TP	24	24	3
FP	8	4	3
TN	34	38	7
FN	9	9	3

Each row sums up the result of a particular type (TP, FP, TN, or FN). In the columns there are the results aggregated depending on the value reduction methods (Linear or SOM). The last column shows the differences between the validation results parameters between the Linear and the SOM method. For example, TP value 3 means that 3 cases that are very wrongly classified as Negative (N) with linear preprocessing are correctly classified as Positive with SOM preprocessing. FN value 3 means that 3 cases that were correctly classified as Positive (P) with linear preprocessing are wrongly classified as Negative with SOM preprocessing. In our case overall TP and FN values between Linear and SOM preprocessing do not change

Table 3.2 The FPR, FNR and TERR for the proposed algorithm with Linear and SOM preprocessing

Test result	Preprocessing type	
	Linear (%)	SOM (%)
FPR	19.0	9.5
FNR	27.3	27.3
ACC	77.3	82.7
TERR	22.7	17.3

We have compared the results of our DMD algorithm recognition using both types of perfusion value reduction methods, that is linear and SOM processing (see Sect. 3.1.1). The obtained results are presented in Table 3.1

We have also carried out a statistical analysis of the results using popular indicators, that is the total error rate (TERR) which measures the percentage of error of methodology, we have computed the false positive rate (FPR—how many healthy perfusion maps were classified as abnormal) and the false negative rate (FNR—how many abnormal perfusion maps were classified as healthy). The validation results elaborated according to this methodology are presented in Table 3.2.

$$ACC = \frac{TP + TN}{TP + TN + FP + FN} \tag{3.3}$$

$$TERR = 1 - ACC \tag{3.4}$$

$$FPR = \frac{FP}{TN + FP} \tag{3.5}$$

Table 3.3 Detailed medical descriptions of cases when our image processing algorithms return TP and FN results

	Diagnosis	Linear		SOM	
		TP	FN	TP	FN
1	Ischemia on the left between the frontal and parietal lobe	4	0	4	0
2	Ischemia on the left between the frontal, parietal and temporal lobe	4	0	4	0
3	Fractional ischemic changes in the left lateral ventricles	0	2	0	2
4	Fractional ischemic changes in the left middle cerebral artery region	1	0	1	0
5	Ischemic changes in the right middle cerebral artery region	2	0	2	0
6	Ischemic changes in the right middle cerebral artery region	1	1	2	0
7	Ischemia in the region of the right frontal lobe	0	2	2	0
8	Ischemic lesion on the left between the parietal and temporal lobe	2	0	2	0
9	Fractional ischemia in the right middle cerebral artery region	2	0	2	0
10	Ischemia on the left between the frontal and parietal lobe	2	0	2	0
11	Fractional ischemic changes in the right frontal lobe	1	1	0	2
12	Ischemia in the left middle cerebral artery region	1	1	1	1
13	Fractional changes in the right side of the occipital lobe	2	0	0	2
14	Fractional changes in the left side of the occipital lobe	0	2	0	2
15	Ischemia in the right middle cerebral artery region	2	0	2	0
	Σ	24	9	24	9

$$\text{FNR} = \frac{\text{FN}}{\text{TP} + \text{FN}} \qquad (3.6)$$

We could not carry out a Receiver Operating Characteristic (ROC) curve analysis of our dataset because the DMD method is not a typical binary classifier although the algorithm for asymmetry detection has a threshold parameter that has a crucial role in the segmentation process (see Sect. 3.1.2 stage 4-B of an algorithm pipeline). The role of this parameter is to filter pixels with perfusion values that do not relatively differ too much between the hemispheres. If an algorithm does not detect improper perfusion regions or it places them in the wrong position it is interpreted as FN. When a threshold parameter increases the FP indicator decreases while FN and TN become higher. If a threshold parameter decreases TP will not increase significantly because the algorithm will be classifying irrelevant small asymmetries in healthy patients data as lesions. That will cause an increase in the FP indicator. Because of that the characteristic for the ROC curve, trading sensitivity for specificity (and vice versa), cannot be observed.

What is important is the fact that the FP in the SOM processing is two times smaller than in the Linear processing, the FP and FN sets of the SOM preprocessing are not a subset of the FP and FN sets of linear preprocessing and vice versa. To make this situation clearer we created Table 3.3 in which we provided detailed medical descriptions of cases when our image processing algorithms return TP and FN results. The results prove that both types of preprocessing methods have the ability to detect perfusion asymmetries that are not visible to the other algorithm.

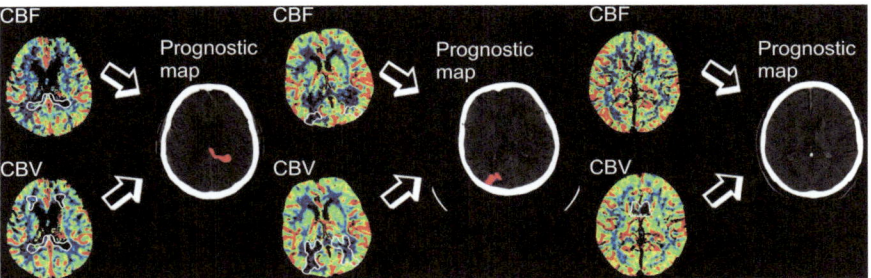

Fig. 3.6 In these pictures, we present example abnormality detection and automatic diagnosis results carried out by our DMD method. From *left* to *right* they are: the FP error of our method—the asymmetry without medical relevance is detected near the symmetry axis of the CBF and CBV map, the wrong image processing results affects the final diagnosis in the prognostic map. In the middle is the TP detection of an asymmetry in the parietal lobe near the borders of the brain and background. On the *right* there is another FP error—an asymmetry without medical relevance is detected near the symmetry axis of the CBV map

Both algorithms have made FP errors—the SOM made only one identical FP error as the linear processing, however, it is generated in three different ones.

The example results of abnormality detection and prognostic maps are shown in Fig. 3.6. Left and right pictures show the most common cause of the FP error in Linear and SOM processing that is the detection of asymmetry without medical relevance near the symmetry axis of the CBF and/or CBV map. The difference in the FP and FN sets between both types of preprocessing is caused by the different nature of the preprocessing [5]. While linear preprocessing arbitrarily reduces the number of different perfusion values it might sometimes prevent including asymmetries with low perfusion difference in the final detection. On the other hand, the SOM does not have a predefined range of values for classes. That fact might prevent both FP and FN detections caused by an arbitrary value reduction.

As we mentioned before, the image processing algorithm determines the success or failure of further image analysis and prognostic map generation. It seems obvious that when asymmetries are detected in the wrong places, not detected at all or detected in a healthy brain an algorithm will fail to provide a correct diagnosis. This was also confirmed by our evaluation. We have determined whether an image analysis and recognition algorithm is capable of finding a potential lesion position and type in already processed perfusion maps (when symmetrical perfusion asymmetric regions are found in both hemispheres). There is no point in carrying out tests on images without any visible perfusion abnormalities (TN and FN), because that data will not generate a diagnosis other than "lack of visible changes"—all of these cases were excluded for our validation set. Now we have only two possible situations:

- TP—correctly predicted Positive samples (presence/position of lesion matched radiologist description).

Table 3.4 The results of the validation of lesion identification algorithm

Test result	Preprocessing type	
	Linear	SOM
TP	24	24
FP	8	4

- FP—incorrectly predicted Negative samples (Negative samples predicted as positives).

The results of the validation of a lesion identification algorithm are summed up in Table 3.4.

As can be seen all correctly localized abnormalities in the image processing step with Linear or SOM-based preprocessing were correctly interpreted by an algorithm for potential lesion type identification and positioning. Summing up, our experiment showed that SOM-based processing increases the ACC of the DMD algorithm by 5.4 % compared to the Linear value reduction. The SOM approach reduced the false positive rate by nearly 10 %. This means that more maps visualizing healthy blood flow will be properly diagnosed by our algorithm. The false negative rate remained unchanged (still the same number of CTP maps that show abnormalities are classified as healthy). The reduction of the FPR has lowered the chance that our automatic procedure will classify healthy patients as ones with diseases. The overall accuracy of our method is 82.7 % (taking into account the image processing, the analysis and the lesion type recognition results), which represents quite satisfying results for this kind of automatic solution.

3.2 An Analysis of the Carotid Artery CTA

Vascular diseases are among the most important public health problems in developed countries [29]. Given the size and complexity of modern angiographic acquisitions, segmentation is a key step towards the accurate visualization, diagnosis, and quantification of vascular pathologies. Often even the same type of blood vessels might differ much not only in shape but they can also contain abnormalities like calcifications or stenosis. Also, the image of a particular vascular structure depends on the acquisition technique (for example, X-ray, computed tomography angiography, magnetic resonance angiography (MRA), and ultrasound (which we also utilized in our previous research [30, 31] etc.). Depending on the technique and its parameters an image might have a different resolution, dimensionality, and contain noise and artifacts. Those biological and technical factors make vascular segmentation a challenging task.

Computed tomography angiography is an effective diagnostic tool in acute stroke detection [1] and is often used to estimate the degree of carotid artery stenosis during an ischemic stroke event or a Transient Ischemic Attack (TIA)

[32]. The examination of carotid arteries is an important step in the course of assessing the risk of a cerebral stroke [33]. The analysis is based on locating and assessing the severity of the stenosis of blood vessels. In the following sections, we will present various computer methods that can be helpful during vascularity structure filtering and segmentation.

3.2.1 Methodology: State of the Art in Vessel Lumen Segmentation

In recent years, many 3D vessel lumen segmentation techniques have been proposed. The systematic overview of different schemas can be found in paper [29]. In this section, we will only summarize selected approaches that were applied to the CTA. We divided the algorithms into groups by the type of principal image processing method that drives the segmentation.

3.2.1.1 Mathematical Morphology

In their article [34], the authors propose an automatic algorithm for coronary artery segmentation from a 3D-CT scan. This method is based on mathematical morphology techniques (blur gray-level hit-or-miss transformations, some of them being extended in this article). It is also guided by anatomical knowledge, using discrete geometric tools to fit on the artery shape independently from any perturbation of the data. In [35], the authors have developed a new technique for the detection of arteries from CTA images by the use of a morphological operation. In this technique an N-Quoit filter is applied to identify the arteries in CTA images. N-Quoit is a type of morphological filter. It is sensitive to the distribution of pixels in a circular formation. A practical method for patient-specific modeling of the aortic arch and the entire carotid vasculature from computed tomography angiography scans for morphologic analysis and for interventional procedure simulation was presented in [36]. The method starts with the automatic watershed-based segmentation of the aorta and the construction of an a priori intensity probability distribution function for arteries. The carotid arteries are then segmented with a graph min-cut method based on a new edge weighting function that adaptively couples voxel intensity, intensity prior, and local vesselness shape prior. Finally, the same graphcut optimization framework is used to interactively remove a few unwanted vein segments and to fill in minor vessel discontinuities caused by intensity variations. Also, the article [37] presents vessel segmentation and filtering techniques, relying on mathematical morphology. The proposed methodology contains three steps: vessel detection (it utilizes the hessian of an image), directional field correction, and vessel reconnection.

3.2.1.2 Snakes and Level-Set Methods

In study [38], a hybrid semi-supervised pixel-based classification algorithm is proposed for the automatic segmentation of intracranial aneurysms in CTA images. The algorithm was designed to discriminate image pixels as belonging to one of two classes: blood vessel and brain parenchyma. Its accuracy in vessel and aneurysm detection was compared with two other reliable methods that have already been applied in vessel segmentation applications: the frequency histogram of connected elements (FHCE), and the gradient vector flow snake. Paper [39] describes an evaluation framework that allows for a standardized and objective quantitative comparison of carotid artery lumen segmentation and stenosis grading algorithms. What is more, the authors present eight different algorithms that perform automated segmentation of the vessel lumen with a precision that is comparable to manual annotation. The majority of the presented algorithms are two-step procedures. In the first step, the centerline inside vessels to be segmented between the seed endpoints is computed. In the second step, the centerline is utilized to find the vessel walls. Also, the algorithm [40] involves two parts: a user defines a start- and endpoint upon which a lumen path is automatically defined, and which is used for the initialization and the automatic segmentation of the vessel lumen on the computed tomographic angiography images. Both parts are based on the detection of vessel-like structures by analyzing intensity, edge, and ridge information. The extracted lumen path is used to initialize a level set method for the segmentation of the vessel lumen. Level set segmentation can be regarded as the evolution of a surface toward the boundaries of the lumen based on a speed function. The segmentation method [41] is implemented in the level set framework, more specifically Geodesic Active Surfaces, in which a surface is evolved to capture the aneurysmal wall via an energy minimization approach. The energy term is composed of three different image features, namely; intensity, gradient magnitude, and intensity variance. The method requires minimal user interaction, i.e., a single seed point inside the aneurysm needs to be placed, based on which image intensity statistics of the aneurysm are derived and used in defining the energy term. In [2], the authors propose and validate a semi-automatic method for the lumen segmentation of the carotid bifurcation in the computed tomography angiography. First, the central vessel axis is obtained using path tracking between three user-defined points. Second, starting from this path, the segmentation is automatically obtained using a level set. The cost and speed functions for path tracking and segmentation make use of intensity and homogeneity slice-based image features. The authors in [42] present a level-setbased method to segment and quantify stenosed internal carotid arteries (ICAs) in 3D contrast-enhanced computed tomography angiography. The proposed model is an extension of Active contours without the edges algorithm [43].

3.2.1.3 Region Growing

In the algorithm [44], a small local cube is segmented to detect a vessel segment, and the following local cube(s) is determined based on the segmentation result. This procedure is repeated until the segmentation is completed. By confining the segmentation inside each local cube, a robust result can be obtained even in a tubular structure of steadily changing intensity. For segmentation, a locally adaptive and competitive region growing scheme is adopted to obtain well-defined vessel boundaries. In paper [45], the authors propose a series of methods and techniques that separate and segment the portal vein and the hepatic vein from CT images, and extract the centerlines of both vessel trees. Segmentation of the trees is a four-step iterative process. It involves a traditional region growing method, a skeletonization algorithm, an adaptive directional region growing method, and a reconnection step. The algorithm [46] recursively tracks branches and detects bifurcations by analyzing the binary connected components on the surface of a sphere that moves along the vessels. Local segmentation within the sphere is performed using a clustering algorithm based on both geometric and intensity information. It minimizes a combination of the intra-class intensity variances and of the inertia moment of the 'vessel' class, which emphasizes the cylindrical structures.

3.2.1.4 Model-Based Segmentation and Image Registration

In [47] the authors introduce a new joint segmentation and registration approach for the quantification of the aortic arch morphology that combines 3D model-based segmentation with elastic image registration. With this combination, the approach benefits from the robustness of model-based segmentation and the accuracy of elastic registration. The approach can cope with a large spectrum of vessel shapes and particularly with pathological shapes that deviate significantly from the underlying model used for segmentation. A model-based approach to interactive segmentation of abdominal aortic aneurysms from CTA data is presented in [48]. After the manual delineation of the aneurysm sac in the first slice, the method automatically detects the contour in subsequent slices, using the result from the previous slice as a reference. If an obtained contour is not sufficiently accurate, the user can intervene and provide an additional manual reference contour.

3.2.2 Vessel Enhancement Filtering

Very often a simple thresholding of the volume Hounsfield Unit (HU) values is not sufficient to detect tissues of interest. Because of that additional image processing is required. With the vessel enhancement filtering, it is not necessary to indicate any particular vascular region to be segmented but rather the range of filter parameters in which the tissues of interests consist. One possible solution to designing this type of filter is to utilize the second order structure of an image (Hessian). In this approach [49] the authors obtained the vessel enhancement as a filtering process that searches for geometrical structures, which can be regarded as tubular. In order to do so a local behavior of the image I has to be examined. A common approach for this type of analysis is to consider its Taylor expansion in the neighborhood of a point x_0:

$$I(x_0 + \delta x_0, s) \approx I(x_0 + \Delta x) + \delta x_0^T \nabla_{0,s} + \delta x_0^T H_{0,s} \delta x_0 \qquad (3.7)$$

where $\nabla_{0,s}$ is a gradient vector, $H_{0,s}$ is a hessian matrix (3.8) and s is a scale parameter. A scale parameter is introduced because vessels may appear in different sizes and it is important to introduce a measurement which varies within a certain range.

$$H = \begin{pmatrix} \frac{\partial^2 I}{\partial x^2} & \frac{\partial^2 I}{\partial x \partial y} & \frac{\partial^2 I}{\partial x \partial z} \\ \frac{\partial^2 I}{\partial y \partial x} & \frac{\partial^2 I}{\partial y^2} & \frac{\partial^2 I}{\partial y \partial z} \\ \frac{\partial^2 I}{\partial z \partial x} & \frac{\partial^2 I}{\partial z \partial y} & \frac{\partial^2 I}{\partial z^2} \end{pmatrix} \qquad (3.8)$$

The elements of a hessian matrix approximate second order derivatives, therefore encoding the shape information—both a qualitative and quantitative description of how the normal to an isosurface changes [50]. Assuming that function I is continuous, Hessian matrix H is symmetric. The H matrix, as a real-valued and symmetric matrix, has real-valued eigenvalues.

Frangi et al. computes the differentiation of I as a convolution with derivatives of Gaussians:

$$\frac{\partial}{\partial x} I(x, s) = s^\gamma I(x) * \frac{\partial}{\partial x} G(x, s) \qquad (3.9)$$

where γ is a parameter that defines a family of normalized derivatives (for the rest of this section we will consider $\gamma = 2$), $*$ is a convolution operator and G is a n-dimensional Gaussian kernel (in our case, because we are dealing with volumetric data, n equals 3).

Analyzing the second order information (Hessian) has an intuitive justification in the context of vessel detection [49]. The second derivative of a Gaussian kernel at scale s generates a probe kernel that measures the contrast between the regions inside and outside the range $(-s, s)$ in the direction of the derivative. In order to perform such an analysis Frangi extracts the eigenvalues of (3.9).

The idea behind the eigenvalue analysis of the hessian is to extract the principal directions in which the local second order structure of the image can be decomposed. Let as assume that eigenvalues will be ordered from the smallest to the largest magnitude ($|\lambda_1| \leq |\lambda_2| \leq |\lambda_3|$). For each pixel of a 3D image Frangi's filter generates a vesselness measure defined as:

$$v(s) = \begin{cases} 0 & \text{if } \lambda_1 > 0 \text{ or } \lambda_2 > 0 \\ \left(1 - e^{\left(-\frac{R_A^2}{2\cdot\alpha^2}\right)}\right) \cdot \left(-e^{\left(-\frac{R_B^2}{2\cdot\beta^2}\right)}\right) \cdot \left(1 - e^{\left(-\frac{S^2}{2\cdot c^2}\right)}\right) \end{cases} \tag{3.10}$$

where

$$R_A = \frac{|\lambda_2|}{|\lambda_3|} \tag{3.11}$$

R_A ratio is essential for distinguishing between plate-like and line-like structures.

$$R_B = \frac{|\lambda_1|}{\sqrt{|\lambda_2 \cdot \lambda_3|}} \tag{3.12}$$

R_B ratio accounts for the deviation from a blob-like structure but cannot distinguish between a line- and a plate-like pattern.

$$S = \sqrt{\sum_{i=1}^{3} \lambda_i^2} \tag{3.13}$$

S ratio is used to distinguish the background pixels from vessel structures (in MRA and CTA vessel structures are often brighter than the background especially after the injection of contrasting material).

α, β, and c are thresholds that control the sensitivity of the line filter for the measures, R_A, R_B and S. For the rest of this section in this case $\alpha = \beta = 0.5$ as suggested in [49] while c was chosen to have a relatively low value $c = 3$.

The vesselness measure in Eq. (3.10) is analyzed at different scales, s. The response of the line filter is maximal at a scale that approximately matches the size of the vessel to detect.

$$v_0(\gamma) = \max_{s_{min} \le s \le s_{max}} v_0(s, \gamma) \tag{3.14}$$

From an implementation point of view, in order to calculate (3.14) the following steps have to be taken:

Algorithm of Frangi's filtration

1. Initiate the table that contains result V_{es} with zeros.
2. For each considered scale s_i.

- Compute the convolution with a Gaussian kernel of volume I and store the result in temporary variable GI_i
- For each voxel the volume contains:

- Compute Hessian matrices of GI_i, compute the eigenvalue for each hessian matrix, compute (3.10) and store the results in temporary table V_{es1}
- Check each element of V_{es}, to determine if it has a smaller value than the corresponding element from V_{es1} replace that element from V_{es} by this corresponding element from V_{es1} (Eq. (3.14)).

It is important to realize that we do not obtain a segmentation of the vasculature. Only if an accurate model of the typical luminance in the perpendicular direction of the vessel is known, an estimate of the size of the vessel can be made based on the response of the filter over the scales. In the first column of Figs. 3.6 and 3.7 we have presented the results of Frangi's filtration with different threshold values of $v_0(\gamma)$ (v_{es}). As can be seen Frangi's filter is also sensitive to noises and scanning artifacts. Those noises are visible as a cloud of small short thick lines that occupy nearly the whole volume. What is more because Frangi's method operates under the constraints that there are no large continuous regions with a higher HU value than the contrasted tissues, the volume I should be additionally thresholded in order to remove regions that contain tissues whose densities are outside the range of interests.

In order to eliminate the problems mentioned, in the paper [51] we have proposed another filtration procedure that incorporates Frangi's method. The additional filter is a neighborhood analysis filter that, for each voxel of the image, generates the following response:

Algorithm of Neighborhood filtration

1. Initiate the table that will contain result N_{es} with zeros.
2. For each voxel the volume contains

- Check if the considered voxel $v_{i,j}$ has a value that is inside the considered range of interest

    - If above condition is true, count how many voxels in the one voxel neighborhood of $v_{i,j}$ have a value that is inside the considered range of interest. The response of the filter for $v_{i,j}$ is 1 + the number of neighborhood voxels whose values are inside the considered range of interest.
    - If above condition is false, the response of the filter for $v_{i,j}$ is 0.

Our vessel enchantment filter [51] incorporates Frangi's filtration and the Neighborhood filtration. The algorithm has two parameters: the threshold value of V_{es} (v_{es}) and the threshold value of N_e (n_e). If a particular value of V_{es} is greater than v_{es} and a particular value of N_e is greater than n_e the corresponding voxel of volume is added to the final results. In the opposite case that voxel is excluded (filtered) from the results.

We have implemented our filter in a Matlab environment. For the computation of the eigenvalues of the real symmetric 3×3 matrix we utilized the DSYEV routine from the Lapack library [52]. The test data consisted of four CTAs of carotid artery volumes scanned by Siemens Somatom Sensation 10 with a size of approximately 512^3 voxels.

In Figs. 3.7 and 3.8, we have presented the results of the vessel enhancing filtering with the proposed method along the a coronal and sagittal plane. Each column corresponds to from a different value of neighborhood filtering threshold, respectively: $n_e = 0$ (no neighborhood filtering), $n_e > 5$, $n_e > 15$, and $n_e > 25$. Each row corresponds to for a different threshold value of vesselness filter threshold, respectively $v_{es} = 0$ (no filtering), $v_e > 0$, $v_e > 0.2$, $v_e > 0.4$, $v_e > 0.6$, $v_e > 0.8$. When $v_e > 0.9$ the vesseleness filtration filters out all of the voxels from the volume. As can be seen, the neighborhood filter has the capability to find solid regions containing voxels in a given HU range but it cannot differentiate between tubular structures and surfaces. On the other hand, Frangi's filter eliminates surfaces but does not exclude short thick lines. The common part of the filtered regions combines the advantages of both filtering methods.

In Table 3.5 we presented the dependents of the percentage of remaining voxels from a proposed filtration process as a function of the vesselness coefficient and neighbor count threshold for the volume from Figs. 3.7 and 3.8. The 3D plot showing this dependence is presented in Fig. 3.9.

The numerical results confirm the visualizations we obtained. As can be seen neighborhood filtering is not sufficient to distinguish between vessels and other tubular structure. Even if the threshold value is high (approximately 15 or more), there are still many excessive voxels. The large number of excessive voxels can also be observed while carrying out Frangi's filtration alone. While both thresholding parameters n_e/v_{es} increase the number of remaining pictures decreases very quickly. The filtration is leaving only those voxels, which satisfy given conditions which leads to satisfactory results.

In Fig. 3.10, we have presented the results of the detection of tubular structures in all four CTA volume datasets in the coronal and sagittal view. The algorithm's parameters were chosen to be: $n_{es} > 0.4$ and $n_e > 15$. As can be seen nearly all thick-line artifacts were eliminated. The rest of them might be eliminated by increasing the parameter of the filtering thresholds, but it might also damage the continuity of correctly detected thick vessels. Because of that threshold values should be carefully tuned to each case separately.

A filtration method of this type cannot be used alone for the segmentation of blood vessels. It lacks the appropriate accuracy and might exclude some parts of the vascular system like leaving out additional tubular structures that are not tissues of interests. That is mainly because this method does not analyze the continuity of vascularity and does not have any prior knowledge about the segmented structure (for example, initial points inside the vessels of interests). This algorithm can, however, be successfully utilized as an initial step for other segmentation algorithms. It can also be used to enhance vascular structures in the data visualization process without the necessity to perform a complete segmentation of a particular part of the vascularization. With this approach the tissues of interest will be much more visible than when they were only colored with a transfer function in direct volume rendering [53–55].

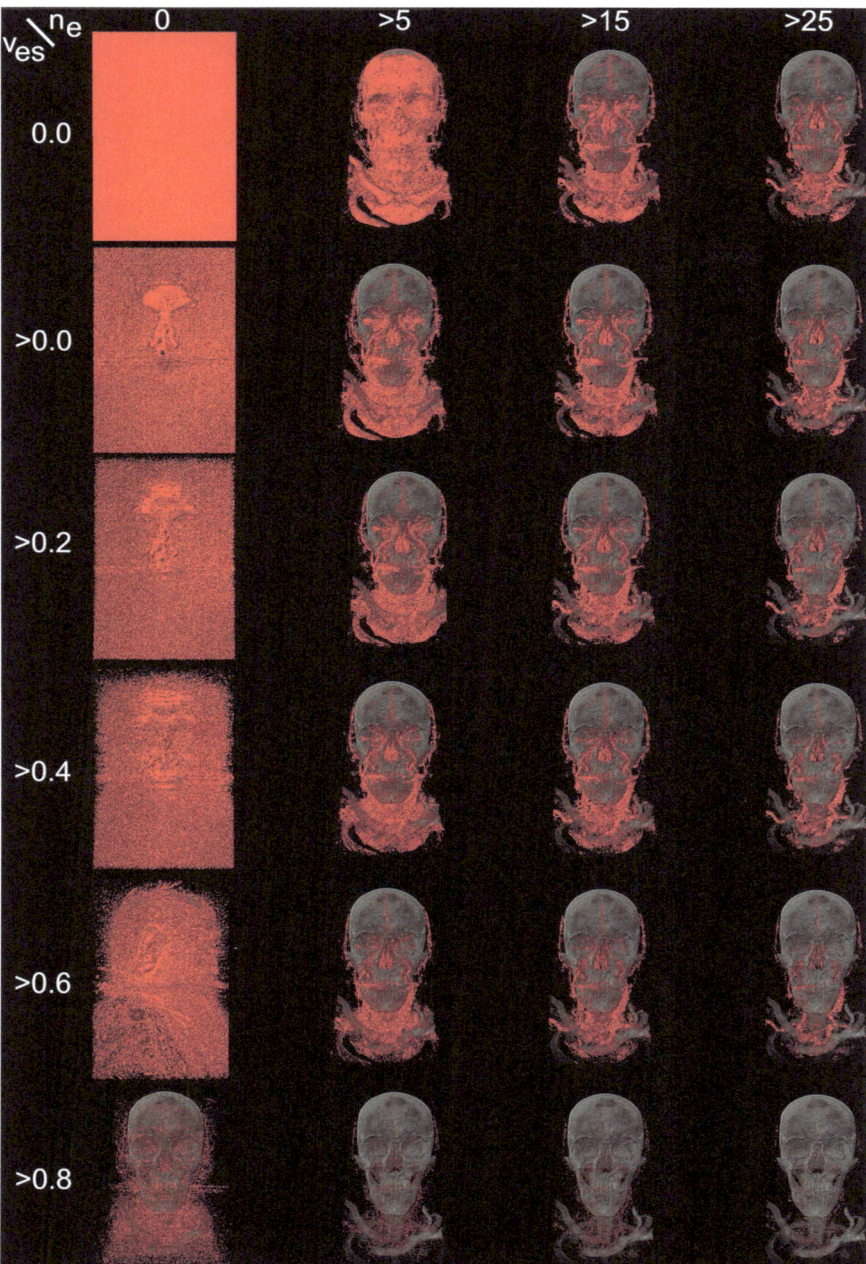

Fig. 3.7 Results of vessel enhancing filtering with the proposed method along a coronal plane. Each column corresponds to different values of the neighborhood filtering thresholds, each row corresponds to a different threshold value of a vesselness filter threshold

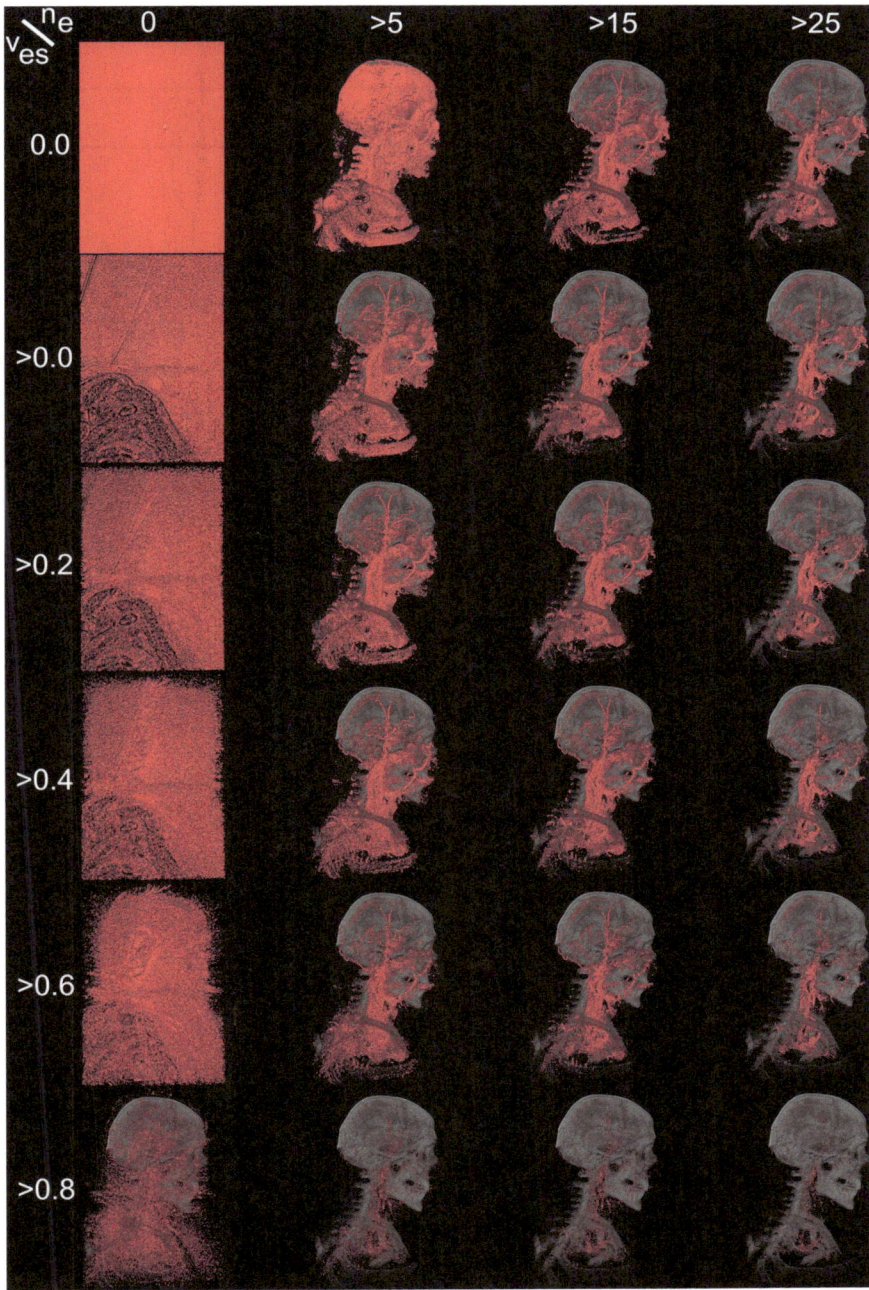

Fig. 3.8 Results of vessel enhancing filtering with the proposed method along a sagittal plane. Each column corresponds to a different value of a neighborhood filtering threshold, each row corresponds to a different threshold value for a vesselness filter threshold

Table 3.5 The dependants of the percentage of the remaining voxels from a proposed filtration process as a function of the vesselness coefficient and the neighbor count threshold for the volume from Figs. 3.6 and 3.7

$Ne \geq$ and $Ves \geq 0$ (%)		0.1 (%)	0.2 (%)	0.3 (%)	0.4 (%)	0.5 (%)	0.6 (%)	0.7 (%)	0.8 (%)	0.9 (%)	1 (%)
0	100	23	21	18	16	12	9	4	1	0	0
1	72	6	6	5	5	4	3	2	0	0	0
2	67	6	5	5	4	3	2	1	0	0	0
3	62	6	5	5	4	3	2	1	0	0	0
4	60	6	5	4	4	3	2	1	0	0	0
5	50	5	5	4	3	3	2	1	0	0	0
6	46	5	4	4	3	3	2	1	0	0	0
7	46	5	4	4	3	3	2	1	0	0	0
8	44	5	4	4	3	3	2	1	0	0	0
9	43	5	4	4	3	3	2	1	0	0	0
10	43	5	4	4	3	3	2	1	0	0	0
11	42	4	4	4	3	3	2	1	0	0	0
12	42	4	4	3	3	2	2	1	0	0	0
13	42	4	4	3	3	2	2	1	0	0	0
14	41	4	4	3	3	2	2	1	0	0	0
15	36	4	4	3	3	2	2	1	0	0	0
16	36	4	3	3	2	2	2	1	0	0	0
17	36	4	3	3	2	2	1	1	0	0	0
18	35	4	3	3	2	2	1	1	0	0	0
19	34	3	3	3	2	2	1	1	0	0	0
20	33	3	3	2	2	2	1	1	0	0	0
21	32	3	3	2	2	2	1	1	0	0	0
22	32	3	2	2	2	2	1	1	0	0	0
23	24	2	2	2	2	1	1	1	0	0	0
24	16	1	1	1	1	1	1	0	0	0	0
25	4	1	1	1	1	1	1	0	0	0	0
26	1	0	0	0	0	0	0	0	0	0	0

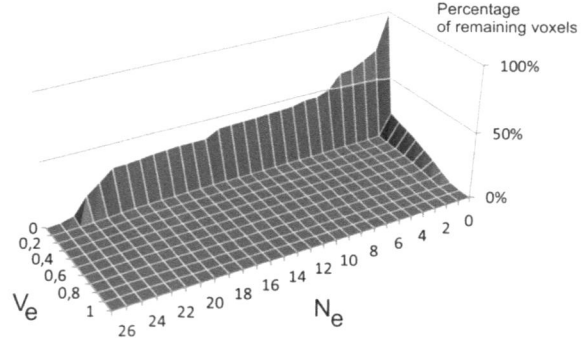

Fig. 3.9 The 3D plot showing the dependence of the percentage of the remaining voxels from a proposed filtration process as a function of the vesselness coefficient and the neighbor count threshold from Table 3.5

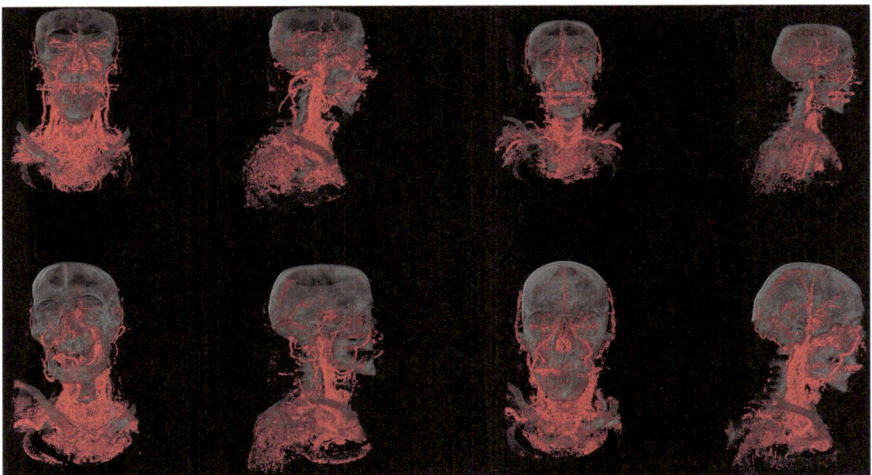

Fig. 3.10 Results of the detection of tubular structures in four CTA volume datasets in the coronal and sagittal view of four different CTA volumes. The algorithm parameters were chosen to be $n_{es} > 0.4$ and $n_e > 15$

3.2.3 The Region Growing Approach

A very interesting approach for blood vessel segmentation can be carried out by applying the region growing approach. We have proposed such an algorithm in [56]. This intensity-based segmentation was initially tailored for extracting the carotid artery bifurcation region, but it can also be an effective framework for segmenting larger arterial structures and in this paragraph, we will discuss this particular application. Our method is based on the assumption that the blood that runs along the vessel lumens has similar HU value. That means that starting from some single predefined initial voxel with a proper propagation algorithm it should be possible to segment large amounts of connected vascularity.

The proposed algorithm consisted of two elements: a region growing procedure and homogeneity criteria. The role of a region growing procedure is to analyze the surroundings of each voxel that was already "visited" by an algorithm starting from the initial voxel (or more than one initial voxel). If any of the voxels from the surroundings satisfies the homogeneity criteria that neighboring voxel will also be "visited" by the algorithm. Each initial and "visited" voxel together form the final segmentation. Before applying our algorithm the input volume data is thresholded in order to exclude tissues with densities beyond the values of interest of the segmentation process.

The homogeneity criteria we propose are based on similar assumptions as the Neighborhood filtration method form in Sect. 3.2.2. We decided to use it because the volume might contain some voxels with densities similar to those of the arterial tissues but which are not part of the arteries. In order to exclude them from the segmentation results, only voxels that are surrounded by sufficient numbers of voxels of similar HU are included in the homogeneity criteria, which is described as follows [56]:

Region growing

1. Initialize the set X with starting voxel x_0

$$X := \{x_0\}$$

2. Initialize the result set (the segmented data) as an empty set
   $Y := \emptyset$
3. Perform a filtration of volumetric data leaving only voxels with HU values in the range $[i_0 - 40, i_0 + 200]$, where i_0 is a value of x_0.
4. While $X \neq \emptyset$

   a. Remove any one element x_i from the set X

   $$X := X - \{x_i\}$$

   b. Add element x_i to the set Y
      $Y := Y \cup \{x_i\}$
   c. Examine each point x_j of the surroundingsX_i ofx_i, if the homogeneity criteria are satisfied add that point to set X (surroundings are a $3 \times 3 \times 3$ voxel cube)
      $X := X \cup x_j$ where $x_j \in X_i$ and X_i is the surrounding of x_i with a radius 1 (26 voxels).
      End While

5. Perform the 3D morphological closing with a cubical structural element sized $3 \times 3 \times 3$ voxels.

End region growing

Homogeneity criteria
The homogeneity criteria for a voxel x_j are satisfied if and only if:
The absolute value of the difference of the HU values between a voxel x_i and x_j is smaller or equal to 20.
AND
In the surroundings of a voxel x_j with a radius of 1 (26 voxels) there are more than 9 voxels x_k for which the absolute value of the difference of the HU values of the voxel x_j and x_k is smaller or equal to 20.

$$x_j \in X \Leftrightarrow |i_i - i_j| \leq 20 \wedge \#\{x_k : |i_j - i_k| \leq 20\} > 9$$

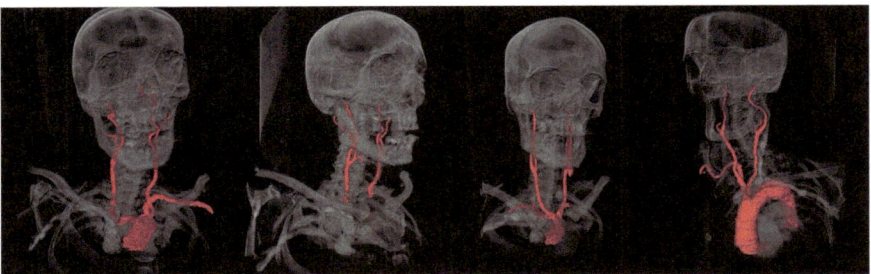

Fig. 3.11 Example results of a region growing segmentation procedure applied to four different CTA images. The segmented data are marked as *red* regions. Concerning each of the volumes, the segmentation procedure was completed twice: once when the initial voxels were situated several millimeters below the *left* carotid artery bifurcation region and the second time when the initial voxels were situated several millimeters below the right carotid artery bifurcation region. The segmentations were then combined in order to create the sum of the segmented regions. As can be seen two initial voxels are sufficient to segment large, continuous parts of the vasculature

where i_i, i_j, i_k is the HU value of x_i, x_j, x_k respectively.

End Homogeneity criteria

The threshold values introduced in point (3) of a Region growing algorithm, the size of the surroundings of a homogeneity criterion, the HU range in a homogeneity criterion and the number of voxels with similar densities were derived empirically by us. In Fig. 3.11 we have shown example results of a region growing segmentation procedure applied to four different CTA images. The proposed method has very important features:

- It requires only one initial point to start the segmentation procedure.
- The size of the segmented region might be easily expanded by adding more starting voxels.
- It is possible to influence the size of the final segmentation region by optimizing the threshold of the neighboring criteria (both the HU range and the neighbors count) to fit a particular problem.
- The principles of the algorithm can be described easily what makes its parameters easy to interpret and intuitively change.
- The algorithm does not require postprocessing procedures like smoothing the obtained segmentation because the local smoothness is obtained by the homogeneity criterion that prevents isolated voxels from being added to the final solution.

The main drawback of the region growing approach with homogeneity criteria such as ours is its sensitivity to the nonlinear shifts of the HU values in the region of interest. This algorithm is invulnerable to the linear shifts of the HU, but the nonlinear shifts in the HU range of the tissues to be segmented might disturb the propagation of the segmentation. What is more homogeneity criteria do not allow very narrow vessel structures to be segmented. Also, if the tolerance value of the homogeneity criterion is increased, it may lead to an incorrect segmentation area growth (for example, due to the included adjacent arteries that are separated by a layer of tissues of a HU value similar to the considered arteries in the result voxel set). Also, our criterion does not take into consideration the shape of the tissues to be segmented which border should be a tubular structure. This explicit information about the shape of an object will be utilized in the next possible solution of a vessel lumen segmentation which is the deformable contours approach.

3.2.4 The Deformable Contours Approach

One of the most popular image segmentation procedure called a snake was introduced in paper [57]. A snake is an energy-minimizing spline guided by external constraint forces and influenced by image forces that pull it toward features such as lines and edges. Snakes are active contour models: they lock onto nearby edges, localizing them accurately. In classical active models an edge detector depending on the gradient of image I is used to stop the evolving curve on the boundary of the desired object [43]. Let Ω be a bounded open subset of R^2.

$C(s), s \in [0, 1] \rightarrow R$ is the parameterized curve that represents the boundary of the segmented region in Ω. An active contour algorithm is designed to solve the following optimization problem:

$$\inf_s(E(s)) = \inf_s \left(\alpha \cdot \int_0^1 |C'(s)|^2 ds + \beta \cdot \int_0^1 |C''(s)|^2 ds + \lambda \cdot \int_0^1 Q(C(s)) ds \right)$$

(3.15)

where:

α is the elasticity parameter, β is the rigidity parameter of a so-called internal force, and λ is the scaling parameter of a so-called external force. All three are positive numbers.

$Q(C) = -|\nabla P(C(s))|^2$ and $P = G_{\sigma 0} * I$ is the initial image I convolved with a Gaussian filter with variance σ_0.

A snake that minimizes E(s) must satisfy the following Euler-Lagrange equation [58, 59]:

$$\alpha \cdot C''(s) - \beta \cdot C''''(s) - \nabla Q(C(s)) = 0 \qquad (3.16)$$

$C(0)$, $C'(0)$, $C(1)$ and $C'(1)$ being given.

To find the solution of (3.16), the snake is made dynamic by treating C as a function of time t and s. The partial derivative of C with respect to t is:

$$\begin{cases} \dfrac{\partial C(s,t)}{\partial t} = \alpha \cdot C''(s,t) - \beta \cdot C''''(s,t) + F(C(s,t)) \\ C(0,s) = C_0(s) \\ C(t,0) = C_0(0) \\ C(t,1) = C_0(1) \\ C'(t,0) = C_0'(0) \\ C'(t,1) = C_0'(1) \end{cases} \qquad (3.17)$$

where:

$F(C(s,t)) = -\nabla Q(C(s,t))$ is an external force.

Depending on the external force F used, many variations of snake algorithms have been proposed.

3.2.4.1 Balloon Snake

To make the snake find its way, an initial guess of the contour has to be provided manually. This has many consequences on the evolution of the curve (or surface) [58]:

- If the curve is not close enough to an edge, it is not attracted to it.
- If the curve is not subjected to any counterbalancing forces, it tends to shrink on itself.

Knowing that the authors of [58] introduced an internal pressure by considering the evolving curve as a balloon which is inflated. The internal pressure force prevents the curve from being 'trapped' by spurious isolated edge points, and makes the final result much less sensitive to the initial conditions. The initial contour can be located far from the boundary to be segmented because the equation contains an additional constant force to inflate the growth of the contour:

$$F = k_1 \bar{n}(C(s)) - k \frac{\nabla P(C(s))}{|\nabla P(C(s))|} \qquad (3.18)$$

where $\bar{n}(s)$ is the unit vector normal to the curve at the point $C(s)$ and k_1 is the amplitude of the force. Parameter k is the external force weight.

3.2.4.2 Distance Snake

In a deformation strategy called the distance snake [58] the external force field on the image is constructed as the negative of the external energy gradient, which is the distance from each point to its closest edge points in the image:

$$F = -\nabla d(C(s)) \qquad (3.19)$$

where d is a function that computes the smallest normalized Euclidean distance from C to an edge point, which is identified using a thresholded gradient.

The proposed external energy allows the external force to be strong everywhere in the image, thus the distance snake has a large capture range [58]. The distance between the actual position of the counter and the boundary is not limited in space provided that there are no additional edges along the way.

3.2.4.3 Gradient Vector Flow

The most important problems we have to struggle with while dealing with snakes is the proper initialization of the starting shape and the poor convergence leading to boundary concavities. Paper [60] presents a new external force for active contours, intended to solve both of those problems. This external force, which we call the *gradient vector flow* (GVF), is computed as a diffusion of the gradient vectors of a gray-level or binary edge map derived from the image. It differs fundamentally from traditional snake external forces in that it cannot be written as the negative gradient of a potential function. To obtain the corresponding dynamic snake equation, the potential force in (3.16) $-\nabla Q(C(s))$ is replaced with a static external force $V(x, y)$, yielding:

$$\frac{\partial C(s, t)}{\partial t} = \alpha \cdot C''(s, t) - \beta \cdot C''''(s, t) + V \qquad (3.20)$$

We define the gradient vector flow field to be the vector field $V(x, y) = [u(x, y), v(x, y)]$ that minimizes the energy functional:

$$\varepsilon = \int \int \mu(u_x^2 + u_y^2 + v_x^2 + v_y^2) + |\nabla f|^2 |V - \nabla f|^2 \mathrm{d}x\mathrm{d}y \qquad (3.21)$$

where $f(x, y)$ is the so-called edge map derived from image I having the property that it is larger near the image edges. The parameter μ is a regularization parameter governing the trade-off between the first-term and the second-term in the integrand. The analytic equation of the solution as well as the numerical implementation of the GVF can be found in paper [60].

3.2.4.4 Active Contours Without Edges

Another minimization of an energy-based segmentation model is the active contours without edges (ACWE) algorithm [61]. The basic idea of the model is similar to previous snakes, however, there are some noticeable differences. The boundary of the object C is the minimizer of the fitting energy:

$$\inf_{c_1,c_2,C} (F_1(C,c_1) + F_2(C,c_2)) \approx 0 \approx F_1(C,c_1) + F_2(C,c_2) \tag{3.22}$$

$$F_1(C,c_1) + F_2(C,c_2) = \int_{\text{inside}(C)} |I(x,y) - c_1|^2 dxdy + \int_{\text{outside}(C)} |I(x,y) - c_2|^2 dxdy$$

$$\tag{3.23}$$

where:

C—parameterized curve (we will skip argument "s" in the rest of this chapter).

$I(x, y)$ is the pixel intensity value of the image to be segmented with coordinates x, y.

c_1 is the average value of pixel intensity inside the region with boundary C.

c_2 is the average value of pixel intensity outside the region with boundary C.

Equation (3.23) may also contain regularization terms [43] and obtains the form:

$$F(c_1, c_2, C) = \mu \cdot \text{Length}(C) + v \cdot \text{Area}(\text{inside}(C))$$
$$+ \lambda_1 \int_{\text{inside}(C)} |I(x,y) - c_1|^2 dxdy \tag{3.24}$$
$$+ \lambda_2 \int_{\text{outside}(C)} |I(x,y) - c_2|^2 dxdy.$$

The first-term depends on the length of the curve, the second on the area inside it. Parameters μ, v, λ_1 and λ_2 ($\mu, v \geq 0$, $\lambda_1, \lambda_2 > 0$) are constants.

This particular case of the minimal partition problem can be formulated and solved using the level set method, for example [62]. That algorithm enables the following fronts to propagate with a curvature-dependent speed. The speed may be an arbitrary function of the curvature, and the front can also be passively advected by an underlying flow. It supports automatic changes of the topology such as merging and breaking, and the calculations are made on a fixed rectangular grid.

A given curve C is represented by a zero level set of a scalar Lipschitz continuous function $\phi : \Omega \to R$ such that:

$$\begin{cases} C = \partial\omega = \{(x,y) \in \Omega : \phi(x,y) = 0\} \\ \text{inside}(C) = \omega = \{(x,y) \in \Omega : \phi(x,y) > 0\} \\ \text{outside}(C) = \Omega\backslash\omega = \{(x,y) \in \Omega : \phi(x,y) < 0\} \end{cases} \tag{3.25}$$

The energy from (3.24) might be rewritten as:

$$F(c_1, c_2, \phi) = \mu \int_\Omega \delta(\phi(x, y))|\nabla \phi(x, y)|dxdy$$
$$+ v \int_\Omega H(\phi(x, y))dxdy$$
$$+ \lambda_1 \int_\Omega |I(x, y) - c_1|^2 H(\phi(x, y))dxdy$$
$$+ \lambda_2 \int_\Omega |I(x, y) - c_2|^2 (1 - H(\phi(x, y)))dxdy \qquad (3.26)$$

where H is the Heaviside function and $\delta_0(z)$ is a Dirac measure:

$$H(z) = \begin{cases} 1 & \text{if} \quad z \geq 0 \\ 0 & \text{if} \quad z < 0 \end{cases} \qquad (3.27)$$

$$\delta_0(z) = \frac{\mathrm{d}}{\mathrm{d}z} H(z) \qquad (3.28)$$

In the numerical solution, the nonzero value of δ_0 is defined within the range $(z - \varepsilon, z + \varepsilon)$, where $\varepsilon > 0$ is a small value. In the rest of this article, we assume that $v = 0$ and we do not consider the area regularization term in our calculations.

In order to minimize $F(c_1, c_2, \phi)$ with respect to ϕ, we have to solve the following equation for ϕ [63].

$$\frac{\partial \phi}{\partial t} = \delta(\phi)\left(\mu \cdot div\left(\frac{\nabla \phi}{|\nabla \phi|}\right) - \lambda_1(I - c_1)^2 + \lambda_2(I - c_2)^2\right) = 0 \quad \text{in } t \geq 0 \text{ and in } \Omega$$

$$\phi(0, x, y) = \phi_0(x, y) \quad \text{in } \Omega$$

$$\frac{\delta(\phi)}{|\nabla \phi|}\frac{\delta \phi}{\delta \overrightarrow{n}} = 0 \quad \text{in } \delta \Omega$$

$$(3.29)$$

where:
   $\bar{n}$ is the exterior normal of the boundary $\delta \Omega$
   $\frac{\delta \varphi}{\delta n}$ is the normal derivative of ϕ at the boundary.
   Of course, the parameters μ (the curve smoothing term), λ_1 and λ_2 affect results of the optimization procedure and have to be properly fitted to the particular task.

3.2.5 Segmentation of the Carotid Bifurcation Region

In this section, we will present our vessel structure segmentation framework that was introduced in our papers [64, 65]. The proposed algorithm consisted of two stages. In the first stage, an algorithm operator needs to indicate the two points that are at the ends of the tissue to be segmented. An initial algorithm finds the centerline inside the vessel lumen. The path that was found starts and ends in the indicated voxels and is one voxel wide. All points that are included in this path are used in the second step of the algorithm as initial voxels for the various deformable contour algorithms. Our framework may utilize any type of snakes that we mentioned before.

The centerline detection algorithm detects the possible path between the start and end points (in a way similar to the typical region growing procedure). In the second step of the first algorithm, it performs the thinning of the previously obtained path. The generated path between the start and end points becomes 1 voxel wide but retains the same length as the path from the first step.

In the algorithm's description we will use the following designations:

Frozen points—points already visited. Each visited point beside its coordinates has additional information about the number of iterations, in which it was visited.

Narrow band$_i$—points visited in the ith step.

Start point—the starting point of the path.

End point—the end point of the path.

Delta value—the maximum accepted difference between adjacent points.

$S(x_j)$—Surroundings of point x_j with a radius of 1 (26 voxels).

$V(x_j)$—The value of voxel HU in point x_j.

Path length—the length of the path (in voxels).

Delta value—the maximum accepted difference between two voxel densities. If the difference is greater than the Delta value, the considered voxel is not included in the path.

The first step of the algorithm is the convolution of a three-dimensional image with the Gaussian kernel in order to remove noise and scanning artifacts from the volume. After this, resulting volume is thresholded in order to remove voxels with HU values that are not in the range of interest:

[min(V(Start point), V(End point))—40, max(V(Start point), V(End point)) + 200]

The parameters −40 and 200 are the same as in Sect. 3.2.3.

Path finding algorithm, step I – detecting the path between *Start point* and *End point*

```
Delta value:=-1
While (End point ∉Frozen points)
        Delta value:=Delta value+1
        i:=0
        Narrow band₀:={Start point}
        Frozen point:={(Start point, i)}
        While ( #Narrow bandᵢ>0 ∧ End point ∉Frozen points)
                i:=i+1
                ∀xⱼ ∈Narrow bandᵢ₋₁
                ∀yₖ∈S(xⱼ)

                if(|V(xⱼ)- V(yₖ)|<Delta value)
                            Narrow bandᵢ:= Narrow bandᵢ∪yₖ
                            Frozen point:= Frozen pointᵢ∪(yₖ,i)
                Path length:=i
```

After the previous step we have the path that links the starting point with the end point. However, this path might be more than one pixel in width and it also might have excessive brunches in many directions. The task of the second step of the algorithm is to narrow the path to be one voxel wide and to remove those excessive branches. The second step of the path finding algorithm starts from the end of the path choosing descending indices of voxels from the frozen points list. In each iteration, only one point from the frozen point set is chosen. Thanks to this, the path generated in the second step has the same length as the previous path, but it is only one voxel wide.

Path finding algorithm, step II—thinning the path obtained in step I

Path:= $\emptyset$ – path from End point to Start point
Path:=Path$\cup$End point
k:=Path length -1
i:=0
x_i:=End point
While(Start point $\notin$ Path)
    X_{i+1}:=$(y_j$:$|V(y_j)-V(x_i)|$=min$|V(y_l)-V(x_i)|$, $(y_l,k)\in$Frozen   points,
$y_l\in S(x_i))$
        Path:= Path$\cup x_{i+1}$
        i:=i+1
        k:=k-1

3.2.6 Evaluation

In this section, we will present the evaluation results of our carotid bifurcation region segmentation algorithm described in Sect. 3.2.5. We have completed two experiments. In the first, we initially determined which of the snake models from Sect. 3.2.4 fit our problem best. In the second experiment, we found the optimal values of the ACWE parameters which are appropriate for our research problem.

3.2.6.1 Dataset

We have evaluated our framework on a set of 32 artery lumens: 16 from the Common Carotid Artery (CCA)—the Internal Carotid Artery (ICA) section and 16 from the CCA—the External Carotid Artery (ECA) section, acquired by a Siemens Somatom Sensation 10 CT scanner (see Table 3.6 for detailed information about the dataset). The evaluation procedure is similar to the one presented in [39]. The segmentation contains the CCA, starting at least 20 mm caudally from the bifurcation slice, the ICA, up to at least 40 mm cranially from the bifurcation slice, and the ECA, up to between 10 and 20 mm cranially from the bifurcation slice.

Table 3.6 CTA dataset that was used for the framework evaluation procedure

Patient Id	Right artery CTA description	Left artery CTA description	Diagnosis
1	A 40 % narrowing of the lumen in the first 6 mm of the right internal carotid artery above the bifurcation	A 30 % narrowing of the lumen in the first 6 mm of the left internal carotid artery above the bifurcation	Right hemisphere ischemic stroke
2	Small atherosclerotic stenosis	Small atherosclerosis stenosis	Right hemisphere ischemic stroke
3	No lesions	No lesions	Left hemisphere ischemic stroke
4	No lesions	No lesions	Left hemisphere ischemic stroke
5	No lesions	An atherosclerotic stenosis in the left carotid bifurcation region and in the internal carotid artery (a 2/3 narrowing of the lumen) with a visible poststenotic widening	Left hemisphere ischemic stroke
6	No lesions	No lesions	Left hemisphere ischemic stroke
7	No lesions	No lesions	Temporary visual and memory disturbances of an unknown etiology
8	No lesions	No lesions	A TIA of the right hemisphere

Each CTA volume was approximately 512^3 in size. The distance between the axial slices was 0.7 mm. First, we applied our Path finding algorithm to each of the examined volumes. In this method, the seed points have to be manually placed on both sides of the vessel to be segmented. We situated them in voxels inside the lumen where the HU value was the highest. These assumptions guarantee the repeatability of the procedure. Each point of the segmented path was used as a seed point for a snake algorithm from Sect. 3.2.4.

In addition to the volumetric data we also had results for the manual segmentation of the tissues of interest that were carried out by a radiologist (an expert). We treated that manual segmentation as reference data for further evaluation.

3.2.6.2 Experiment I: Testing the Snake Model

The role of the first experiment was to find the snake model that best fits our problem of segmentation of carotid arteries from the CTA images. In order to measure the quality of segmentation we used Dice's coefficient:

Table 3.7 Average and standard deviation values of Dice's coefficient for all of the considered snakes obtained for the segmented dataset

Method	Average	Standard deviation
Balloon	0.453	0.131
Distance	0.449	0.074
GVF	0.637	0.095
ACWE	0.745	0.092

Fig. 3.12 The bar plot of results from Table 3.7. We additionally marked the standard deviation as smaller *black bars*

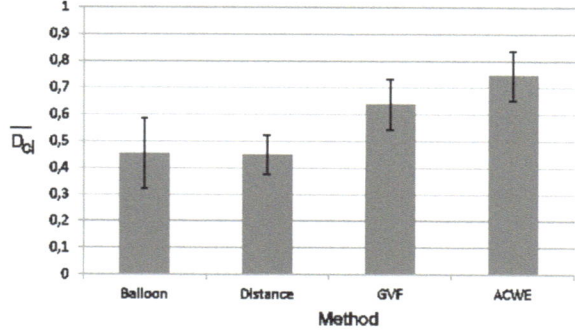

Fig. 3.13 An example segmentation result of the same carotid artery region carried out by different active contour algorithms. The *white arrows* mark the regions of interest that are discussed in the text

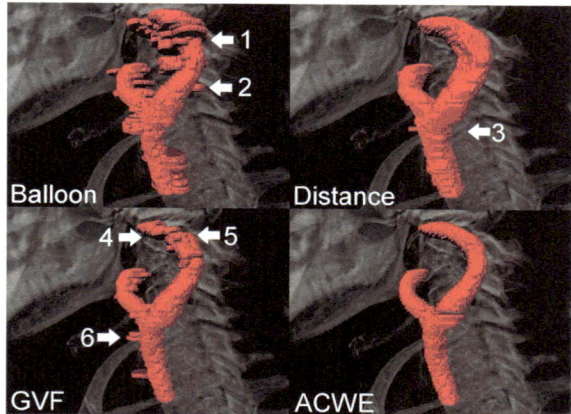

$$D_{ci} = \frac{2 \cdot |pv_r \cap pv_p|}{|pv_r| + |pv_p|} \tag{3.30}$$

where pv_r and pv_p are the reference artery tissue and an algorithmically determined one.

We performed the active contour segmentation of the test dataset with each of the snake algorithms separately. We used the same implementation of the Balloon, Distance and GVF snakes as the authors in [59] (done in a Matlab environment) with coefficients suggested by the authors of the snake library. For the ACWE, we

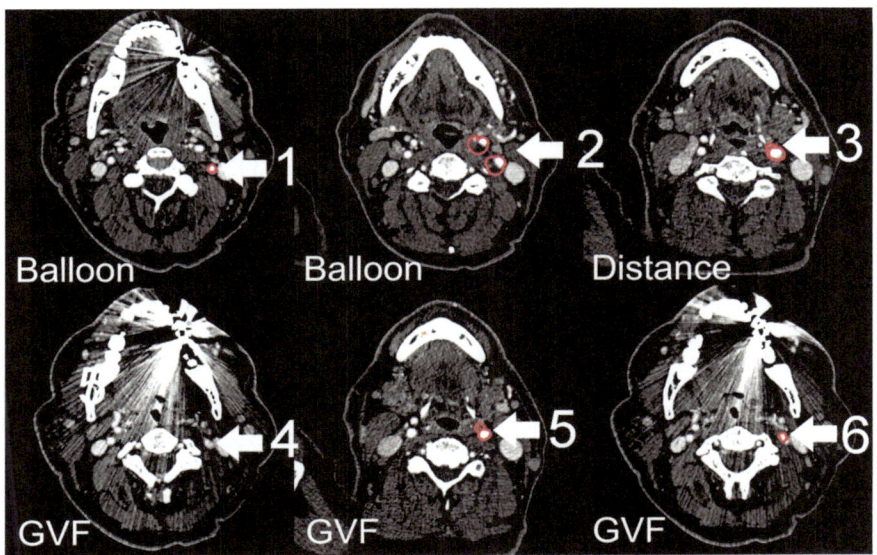

Fig. 3.14 A detailed view of the axial slices that were marked with *white arrow* in Fig. 3.13

used our implementation with $\lambda_1 = 1, \lambda_2 = 1, \mu = 0.5$. In the case of the Balloon and GVF snakes, CTA slices were additionally filtered with a Sobel edge detector and transformed into black-and-white images. We used the suggested parameters to initially compare the segmentation results of different snake models in order to exclude those whose deformation model cannot overcome the noise in the input images.

In order to guarantee the same statistical distribution between the results of the CCA–ICA and the CCA–ECA classes, the whole carotid bifurcation region was evaluated together. In Table 3.7 we have presented average and standard deviation values of Dice's coefficient for all of the considered snakes. The bar plot in Fig. 3.12 visualizes the obtained results.

In Fig. 3.13, we present example segmentation results of the same carotid artery region done by different active contour algorithms. In Fig. 3.14, we present a detailed view of the axial slices that were marked with a white arrow in Fig. 3.13. As can be seen even though they are using the same initial points determined by the centerline detection algorithm, the results differ. The segmentations contains two types of errors: an overestimation of the lumen (the contours expand to the neighboring tissues that have similar HU values as the region of interest) or an underestimation of the region or even a collapse of a snake (the contracting force was not stabilized by the expanding force).

In the case of the Balloon snake, the common problem is an overestimation of the segmentation region by the excessive growth of the contours. This can be seen in Figs. 3.13-2 and 3.14-2. However, an algorithm with the same parameters might

Table 3.8 The average value of Dice's coefficient calculated from all of the segmentation results as the function of λ_1/λ_2 and μ, bolded values indicate the best segmentation results

λ_1/λ_2 μ	1	2	4	6	8	10	12	14	16	18	20
0.0	0.686	0.767	0.843	0.879	0.898	0.907	0.911	0.908	0.902	0.892	0.884
0.1	0.697	0.776	0.853	0.889	0.907	0.916	0.917	0.912	0.902	0.890	0.878
0.2	0.714	0.790	0.862	0.898	0.914	0.923	0.921	0.911	0.898	0.884	0.871
0.3	0.727	0.800	0.872	0.909	0.924	0.930	0.924	0.908	0.891	0.877	0.861
0.4	0.743	0.815	0.885	0.918	0.932	0.935	0.924	0.906	0.888	0.871	0.853
0.5	0.745	0.816	0.889	0.921	0.938	**0.939**	0.919	0.900	0.881	0.864	0.848
0.6	0.753	0.820	0.891	0.923	**0.939**	0.936	0.913	0.893	0.872	0.854	0.836
0.7	0.763	0.826	0.898	0.925	0.936	0.928	0.903	0.883	0.863	0.843	0.825
0.8	0.771	0.833	0.903	0.929	0.937	0.922	0.897	0.877	0.855	0.835	0.819
0.9	0.779	0.838	0.905	0.933	0.938	0.918	0.890	0.869	0.847	0.829	0.813
1.0	0.784	0.844	0.911	0.935	0.938	0.912	0.888	0.863	0.842	0.821	0.804

also produce the correct (precise) segmentation results like those in Figs. 3.13-1 and 3.14-1. Because of the high value of the standard deviation of the Dice coefficient (nearly 30 % of the average value) we can conclude that the segmentation with the balloon model is quite unreliable.

Distance snake-based segmentation also contains overestimated regions (see Figs. 3.13-3 and 3.14-3), however, the standard deviation of Dice's coefficient has a smaller value which indicates that segmentation behaves in a more stable way. However, the average value of Dice's coefficient is quite small compared with the and ACWE, what makes this algorithm unsuitable for our problem.

The GVF snake segmentation also has a problem with the extensive growth of the segmented region like the one in Figs. 3.13-6 and 3.14-6 and with collapses, caused by the contracting force (Figs. 3.13-4 and 3.14-4). However, besides this problem, many parts of the lumen are correctly segmented (Fig. 3.13-5 and 3.14-5). This particular snake algorithm has the second highest average value of Dice's parameter.

The best segmentation results, while taking into account the criterion (3.30) was obtained with the ACWE-based segmentation (0.745 ± 0.092 and the standard deviation value equals about 12 % of the average value). Also, the visual effects of the segmentation carried out using the ACWE model were the most accurate. Moreover, the ACWE did not require any preprocessing of the CTA (like an additional edge detection).

Based on the results we have obtained, the correct decision was to choose ACWE as the most suitable algorithm for carotid artery bifurcation region segmentation and for further evaluations.

Table 3.9 The standard deviation of Dice's coefficient calculated from all of the segmentation results as the function of λ_1/λ_2 and μ, bolded values indicate the best segmentation results

λ_1/λ_2 μ	1	2	4	6	8	10	12	14	16	18	20
0.0	0.099	0.083	0.053	0.043	0.038	0.040	0.048	0.057	0.062	0.068	0.071
0.1	0.101	0.082	0.050	0.041	0.038	0.042	0.056	0.059	0.064	0.071	0.073
0.2	0.104	0.082	0.048	0.036	0.036	0.045	0.059	0.063	0.068	0.069	0.072
0.3	0.100	0.078	0.046	0.032	0.032	0.045	0.059	0.062	0.066	0.068	0.071
0.4	0.097	0.077	0.042	0.030	0.031	0.046	0.055	0.058	0.063	0.065	0.069
0.5	0.092	0.070	0.039	0.027	0.033	**0.049**	0.056	0.059	0.064	0.065	0.069
0.6	0.090	0.068	0.042	0.030	**0.038**	0.052	0.060	0.063	0.067	0.068	0.073
0.7	0.088	0.065	0.039	0.033	0.042	0.054	0.059	0.063	0.064	0.067	0.072
0.8	0.086	0.062	0.036	0.030	0.045	0.054	0.059	0.060	0.063	0.067	0.070
0.9	0.079	0.063	0.035	0.033	0.045	0.056	0.061	0.063	0.066	0.069	0.071
1.0	0.076	0.058	0.035	0.033	0.049	0.056	0.060	0.063	0.068	0.071	0.074

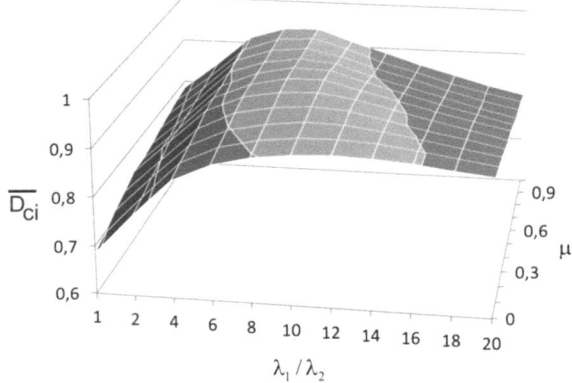

Fig. 3.15 The plot of average value of Dice's coefficient calculated from all segmentation results as the function of λ_1/λ_2 and μ basing on data from Table 3.8

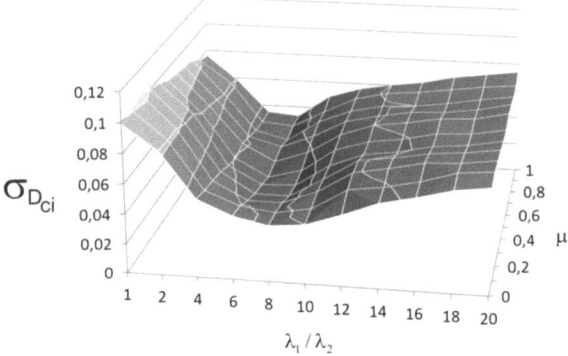

Fig. 3.16 The plot of the standard deviation value of Dice's coefficient calculated from all segmentation results as the function of λ_1/λ_2 and μ basing on data from Table 3.9

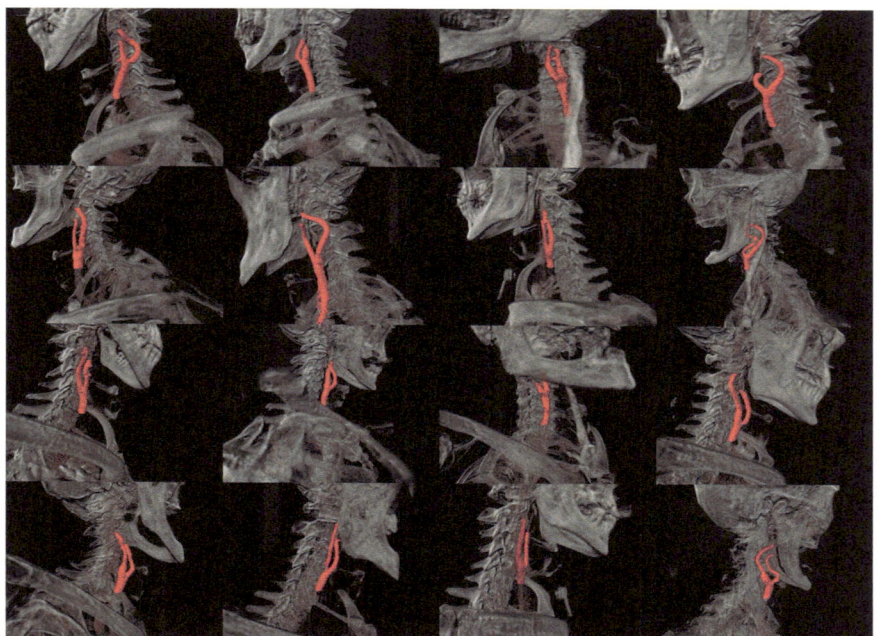

Fig. 3.17 Segmentation results of all volumes from dataset for ACWE parameters $s_1 = \left(\frac{\lambda_1}{\lambda_2} = 8, \mu = 0.6 \right)$

3.2.6.3 Experiment II: Finding the Optimal Values of the ACWE Parameters

The aim of the second experiment was to evaluate the optimal values of the ACWE parameters for carotid artery segmentation. We took into account two parameters: λ_1/λ_2 a ratio in the range of $[1, 20]$ and μ in the range $[0, 1]$. For all combinations of those two parameters we performed a segmentation using our framework on the same dataset as before. An average value and the standard deviation of Dice's coefficient were used to evaluate the results. In Tables 3.8 and 3.9, we present the average value and the standard deviation, respectively, of Dice's coefficient calculated from all of the segmentation results as the function of λ_1/λ_2 and μ.

In Figs. 3.15 and 3.16 we present a three-dimensional plot of the results from Tables 3.8 and 3.9, respectively. As can be seen, the average of Dice's coefficient has a maximal value in two cases: when $s_1 = \left(\frac{\lambda_1}{\lambda_2} = 8, \mu = 0.6 \right)$ and when $s_2 = \left(\frac{\lambda_1}{\lambda_2} = 10, \mu = 0.5 \right)$. The standard deviations for both of those solutions are at

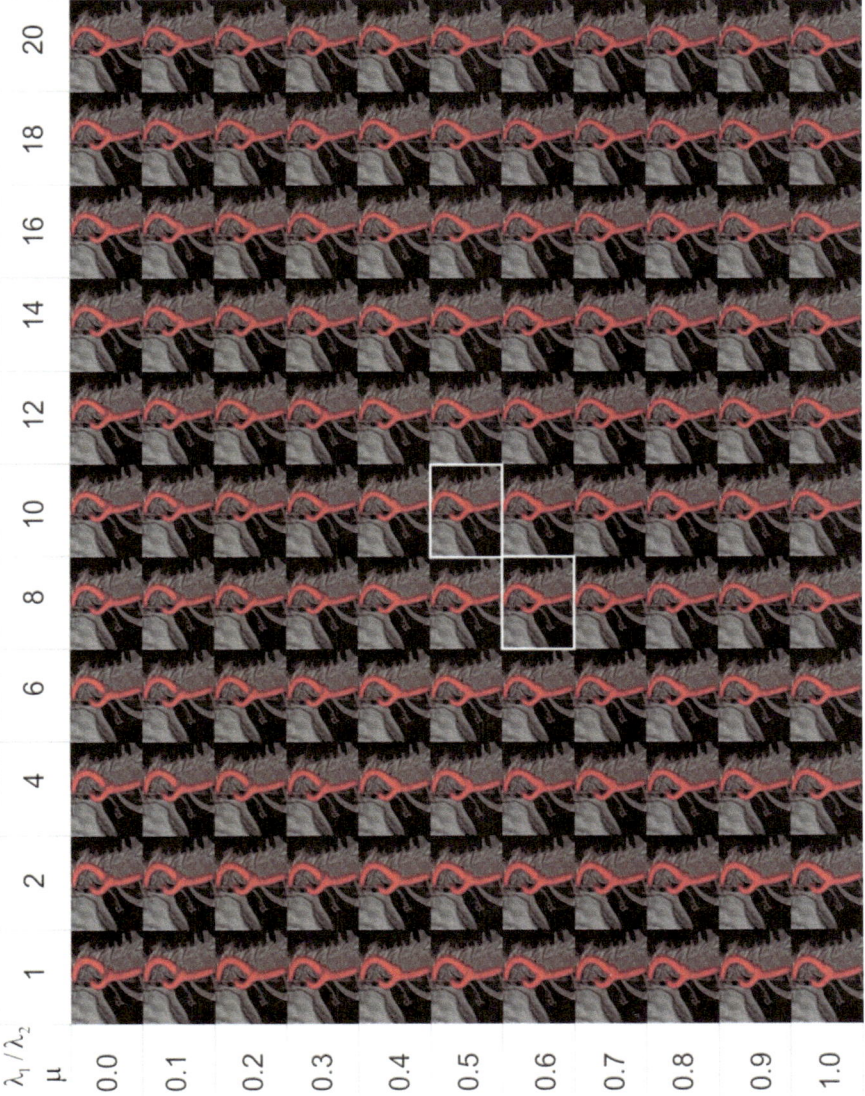

Fig. 3.18 A visualization of an evaluation of ACWE parameters of one example CCA–ICA and CCA–ECA region taken from our dataset

a relatively low level (about 5 % of the average value). That suggests that for those parameters Dice's coefficient values in our dataset do not differ much (the method provides stable results, meaning that the average number of correctly and incorrectly segmented voxels is similar between the cases). The shape of the plot in

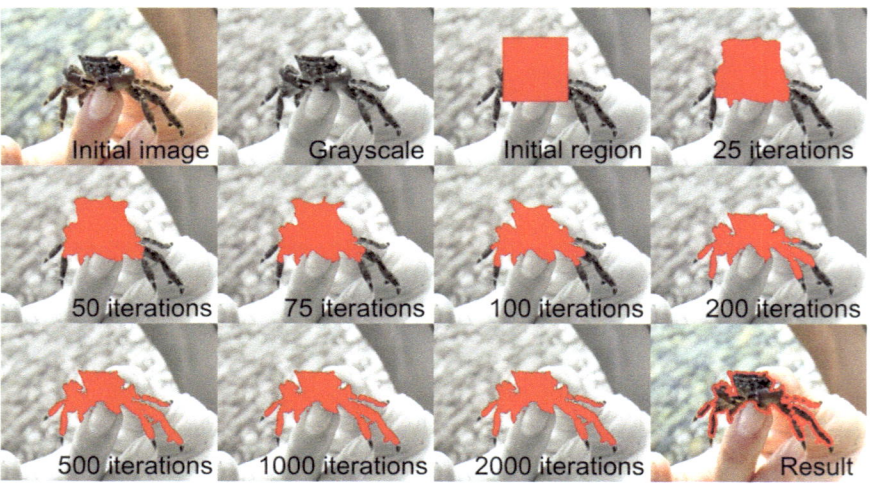

Fig. 3.19 Example performance results of the ACWE algorithm. After the initial image is loaded it is converted to a *grayscale*. Then a region which is restricted by initial contours is set. There are no visible differences in contour shapes after evolving them with more than 500 iterations of ACWE. In the *bottom-right corner* of this figure, edges of the final region are imposed onto the initial image. Algorithm parameters were: $\mu = 0.05$, $\lambda_1 = 1$, $\lambda_2 = 1$

Fig. 3.16 also suggests that for those two selected parameter sets the standard deviation has the smallest value in comparison with other examined parameters.

In Fig. 3.17, we present segmentation results of all volumes from the dataset for ACWE parameters $s_1 = \left(\frac{\lambda_1}{\lambda_2} = 8, \mu = 0.6 \right)$. The segmented carotid artery regions are marked with red color. As can be seen also the visualization of results shows the smoothness of final solutions. An algorithm manages to detects vessels walls properly, both in cases when particular cases do not show any pathological changes and also when a narrowing of lumen was present.

In Fig. 3.18, we present a visualization of the evaluation of ACWE parameters of one example CCA–ICA and CCA–ECA region taken from our dataset. With white brackets we have marked the solutions for which the highest average value of Dice's coefficient was obtained. As can be seen the results for different parameters do not differ much, however when λ_1/λ_2 and μ value is low, more segmentation errors are visible: both contours of arterial structures expand too much including into segmented region tissues with a similar HU as the initial region but not forming a part of a vessel lumen and some part of the vasculature is not segmented properly because the contours have collapsed. The segmentation errors become less visible while λ_1/λ_2 and μ are increasing, and for high boundary values of those parameters they are hardly visible in the visualization without a precise examination of particular axial slices.

The proposed vessel lumen segmentation framework proved to be an efficient algorithm, and the quality of the final solution measured with Dice's coefficient is respectively high for this type of systems. Of course this type of approach has some drawbacks we have to remember about. The first is that the deformable contour framework may produce inconsistently segmented regions, as shown in Fig. 3.13. This is caused by noise that may be present in this particular CTA data, which causes the initial segmentation region to be split into smaller separate planes. The second one is the relatively long execution time of the segmentation procedure, especially the path finding algorithm. That is because that proposed procedure may be difficult to parallelize on a massive SIMD (single instruction multiple data) architecture (like GPU processors). This is caused by the fact that the algorithm is highly sequential (not parallel). It is difficult to predict how the region growing procedure will evolve in each step.

3.3 Implementations

In this section, we will present an implementation of the ACWE algorithm [43, 61]. Our implementation is an adaptation to C# of a Matlab code written by Shawn Lankton (www.shawnlankton.com). Figure 3.19 shows example performance results of the presented ACWE algorithm.

```
/**
 *  Image - input grayscale image
 *  init_mask - initial region, which contours will be evolved
 *  0 is a background, 1 marks a region
 *  max_its - maximal number of iterations of algorithm
 *  mu, lambda1, lambda2 - see (4.24)
 *  output - region segmented by ACWE algorithm, 0 is
 *  a background, 1 marks a region
 *  Example call:
 *  //image array is already initialized
 *  //initialization of a region inside contours, here it is
 *  //square with center defined by coordinates centerX
 *  //and centerY
 *  int centerX = 140;
 *  int centerY = 87;
 *  double [][]initReg = new double[array.Length][];
 *  for (int a = 0; a < array.Length; a++)
 *  {
 *      initReg[a] = new double[array[0].Length];
 *  }
```

```
    *   for (int xx = -45; xx <= 45; xx++)
    *        for (int yy = -45; yy <= 45; yy++)
    *        {
    *               initReg[centerX + xx][centerY + yy] = 1;
    *        }
    *   short[][] returnSeg = ACWESegementation(array, initReg, 2000,
    *   0.05, 1, 1);
    */


        public static short[][] ACWESegementation(double[][] Image,
            double[][] init_mask, int max_its,
            double mu, double lambda1, double lambda2)
{
    double[][] phi = get_signed_distance_function(init_mask);
    //Main loop
    int its = 0;
    while (its < max_its)
    {
            int n = phi.Length;
            int m = phi[0].Length;
            int count = 0;
            //Computes length of contour
            for (int a = 0; a < n; a++)
                    for (int b = 0; b < m; b++)
                    //Get the curve's narrow band
                            if (phi[a][b] <= 1.2 && phi[a][b] >=
                            -1.2)
                                    count++;
            int[][] curvHelp = new int[count][];
            for (int a = 0; a < curvHelp.Length; a++)
                    curvHelp[a] = new int[2];
int ii = 0;
for (int a = 0; a < n; a++)
        for (int b = 0; b < m; b++)
                //Get the curve's narrow band
                if (phi[a][b] <= 1.2 && phi[a][b] >=
                -1.2)
                {
                        curvHelp[ii][0] = a;
                        curvHelp[ii][1] = b;
                        ii++;
                }
double sumupts = 0;
double lupts = 0;
double sumvpts = 0;
double lvpts = 0;
```

```
for (int a = 0; a < n; a++)
      for (int b = 0; b < m; b++)
      {
              //Interior points
              if (phi[a][b] <= 0)
              {
                      sumupts = sumupts + Image[a][b];
                      lupts = lupts + 1;
              }
              //Exterior points
              else
              {
                      sumvpts = sumvpts + Image[a][b];
                      lvpts = lvpts + 1;
              }
         }
  //Find interior and exterior mean
  double uT = sumupts / (lupts + eps);
double vT = sumvpts / (lvpts + eps);

  //Force from image information
double[] FT = new double[count];
double maxABSF = -1; ;

//See (4.26)-(4.29)
for (int a = 0; a < count; a++)
{
      FT[a] = (lambda1
      * (Image[curvHelp[a][0]][curvHelp[a][1]] - uT)
      * (Image[curvHelp[a][0]][curvHelp[a][1]]
      - uT))
      - (lambda2
      * (Image[curvHelp[a][0]][curvHelp[a][1]] - vT)
      * (Image[curvHelp[a][0]][curvHelp[a][1]]
      - vT));
      if (Math.Abs(FT[a]) > maxABSF)
            maxABSF = Math.Abs(FT[a]);
}
```

```
//Force from curvature penalty
if (count > 0)
{
        //Force from curvature penalty
        double[]curvatureT
        = get_curvature(phi,curvHelp);
        double[] dphidtT = new double[count];
        //Gradient descent to minimize energy
        double maxDphidt = double.MinValue;
        for (int a = 0; a < count; a++)
{
        dphidtT[a] = (FT[a] / maxABSF)
        + (mu *  curvatureT[a]);
        if (dphidtT[a] > maxDphidt)
                maxDphidt = dphidtT[a];
}

//Maintain the CFL condition
double dtT = 0.45 / (maxDphidt + eps);
//Evolve the curve
for (int a = 0; a < count; a++)
{
        phi[curvHelp[a][0]][curvHelp[a][1]] =
         phi[curvHelp[a][0]][curvHelp[a][1]]
        + dtT * dphidtT[a];
}
        //Keep signed distance function smooth
                phi = reinitialize_sussman(phi, 0.5);
                its++;
        }
else
        its = max_its + 1;
}

//Generate output region mask from signed distance function
   short[][] seg = new short[phi.Length][];
for (int a = 0; a < seg.Length; a++)
{
        seg[a] = new short[phi[0].Length];
        for (int b = 0; b < seg[a].Length; b++)
        //positive values are outside region restricted
          //by curves and negative inside
```

```
                    if (phi[a][b] <= 0)
                            seg[a][b] = 1;
        }
        return seg;
}

/**
 * "Small" epsilon value
 */
private static double eps = 0.000001;

/**
 * Helper function of ACWESegementation
 * Compute curvature along signed distance function
 */
private   static   double[]  get_curvature(double[][]  phi,   int[][]
curvHelp)
{
    int dimy = phi.Length;
    int dimx = phi[0].Length;
    int n = curvHelp.Length;
    int m = curvHelp[0].Length;
    double[] curvature = new double[n];
    for (int a = 0; a < n; a++)
    {
            int yy = curvHelp[a][0];
            int xx = curvHelp[a][1];
            double phi_x = phi[yy - 1][xx] - phi[yy + 1][xx];
            double phi_y = phi[yy][xx - 1] - phi[yy][xx + 1];
            double phi_xx = phi[yy - 1][xx] - 2 * phi[yy][xx]
            + phi[yy + 1][xx];
            double phi_yy = phi[yy][xx - 1] - 2 * phi[yy][xx]
            + phi[yy][xx + 1];
```

```
        double phi_xy = -0.25 * phi[yy - 1][xx - 1]
        - 0.25 * phi[yy + 1][xx + 1]
        + 0.25 * phi[yy + 1][xx - 1] + 0.25
        * phi[yy - 1][xx + 1];

        double phi_x2 = phi_x * phi_x;
        double phi_y2 = phi_y * phi_y;
        //Compute curvature (Kappa)
        curvature[a] = ((phi_x2 * phi_yy + phi_y2
        * phi_xx - 2 * phi_x * phi_y * phi_xy) /
        Math.Pow((phi_x2 + phi_y2 + eps), 3.0 / 2.0))
        * Math.Pow((phi_x2 + phi_y2), (1.0 / 2.0)));
    }
return curvature;
}
/**
 * Helper function of ACWESegementation
 * Level set re-initialization by the sussman method
 * (see [66] and [67])
 */
private static double[][] reinitialize_sussman(double[][] D,
double dt)
{
    // forward/backward differences
        int n = D.Length;
    int m = D[0].Length;
    //backward
    double[][] a = new double[n][];
    for (int aa = 0; aa < n; aa++)
            a[aa] = new double[m];
    for (int aa=0; aa <n; aa++)
        {
                for (int bb=1; bb <m; bb++)
                        a[aa][bb] = D[aa][bb] - D[aa][bb-1];
                a[aa][0] = 0;
        }
        //forward
        double[][] b = new double[n][];
        for (int aa = 0; aa < n; aa++)
                b[aa] = new double[m];
        for (int aa=0; aa <n; aa++)
        {
                for (int bb=0; bb <m-1; bb++)
                        b[aa][bb] = D[aa][bb+1] - D[aa][bb];
                b[aa][m-1] = 0;
        }
```

```
          //backward
          double[][] c = new double[n][];
          for (int aa = 0; aa < n; aa++)
                  c[aa] = new double[m];

          for (int bb=0; bb <m; bb++)
          {
                  for (int aa=1; aa <n; aa++)
                          c[aa][bb] = D[aa][bb] - D[aa-1][bb];
                  c[0][bb] = 0;
          }
          //forward
          double[][] d = new double[n][];
          for (int aa = 0; aa < n; aa++)
                  d[aa] = new double[m];

          for (int bb=0; bb < m; bb++)
{
      for (int aa=0; aa<n-1; aa++)
              d[aa][bb] = D[aa+1][bb] - D[aa][bb];
      d[n-1][bb] = 0;
}

double[][] dDT = new double[n][];
for (int aa = 0; aa < n; aa++)
      dDT[aa] = new double[m];

double a_p = 0; double a_n = 0;
double b_p = 0; double b_n = 0;
double c_p = 0; double c_n = 0;
double d_p = 0; double d_n = 0;
```

```
for (int aa = 0; aa < n; aa++)
      for (int bb = 0; bb < m; bb++)
      {
            if (D[aa][bb] > 0)
            {
                  a_p = a[aa][bb];
                  if (a_p < 0)
                        a_p = 0;
                  b_n = b[aa][bb];
                  if (b_n > 0)
                        b_n = 0;

                  a_p = a[aa][bb];
                  if (a_p < 0)
                        a_p = 0;
                  b_n = b[aa][bb];
                  if (b_n > 0)
            b_n = 0;

      c_p = c[aa][bb];
      if (c_p < 0)
            c_p = 0;
      d_n = d[aa][bb];
      if (d_n > 0)
            d_n = 0;
      dDT[aa][bb] = Math.Sqrt(Math.Max(a_p
      * a_p, b_n * b_n)
      + Math.Max(c_p * c_p, d_n * d_n)) - 1;
}
if (D[aa][bb] < 0)
```

```
                    {
                        a_n = a[aa][bb];
                        if (a_n > 0)
                                a_n = 0;
                        b_p = b[aa][bb];
                        if (b_p < 0)
                        b_p = 0;
                        c_n = c[aa][bb];
                        if (c_n > 0)
                                c_n = 0;
                        d_p = d[aa][bb];
                        if (d_p < 0)
                                d_p = 0;
                        dDT[aa][bb] = Math.Sqrt(Math.Max(a_n
                        * a_n, b_p * b_p)
                        + Math.Max(c_n * c_n, d_p * d_p)) - 1;
                    }
}
double[][] S = get_sign_sussman(D);
        for (int aa = 0; aa < n; aa++)
                for (int bb = 0; bb < m; bb++)
                        D[aa][bb] = D[aa][bb] - (dt * S[aa][bb]
                        * dDT[aa][bb]);
        return D;
}


/**
 * Helper function of ACWESegementation
 * Compute sign for sussman re-initialization method
 */
private static double[][] get_sign_sussman(double[][] D)
{
        int n = D.Length;
        int m = D[0].Length;
        double[][] S = new double[n][];
        for (int a = 0; a < S.Length; a++)
                S[a] = new double[m];
```

```
        for (int a = 0; a < n; a++)
             for (int b = 0; b < m; b++)
                 {
                      S[a][b] = D[a][b] / Math.Sqrt((D[a][b]
                      * D[a][b]) + 1);
                 }
        return S;
}


/**
 * Helper function of ACWESegementation
 * Calculates the signed distance function
 */
private static double[][] get_signed_distance_function(
double[][] init_a)
{
    double[][] init_a2 = new double[init_a.Length][];
    for (int a = 0; a < init_a.Length; a++)
          init_a2[a] = new double[init_a[0].Length];
    //Change background with non-background pixels and vice versa
    for (int a = 0; a < init_a.Length; a++)
          for (int b = 0; b < init_a[0].Length; b++)
                init_a2[a][b] = 1 - init_a[a][b];
    double[][] i1 = shortestDist(init_a);
    double[][] i2 = shortestDist(init_a2);

    double[][] phi = new double[init_a.Length][];
    for (int a = 0; a < init_a.Length; a++)
          phi[a] = new double[init_a[0].Length];
    //phi will be having smallest absolute values
    //at curve's narrow band
    //positive values are outside region restricted by curves
    //and negative inside
    //it is reversed to (4.25) because it is more natural
    //to mark regions with 1 and have 0 as background
    for (int a = 0; a < phi.Length; a++)
          for (int b = 0; b < phi[a].Length; b++)
                phi[a][b] = i1[a][b] - i2[a][b] + init_a[a][b]
          - 0.5;
    return phi;
}


/**
 * Helper function of ACWESegementation
 * Computes the shortest distance between background point
 * and non-background point
```

```
 */
private static double[][] shortestDist(double[][] init_a)
{
     double[][] distArray = new double[init_a.Length][];
     for (int a = 0; a < init_a.Length; a++)
             distArray[a] = new double[init_a[0].Length];
     int pointsCount = 0;
     //Count non-background points
     for (int a=0; a < init_a.Length; a++)
             for (int b=0; b < init_a[0].Length; b++)
                     if (init_a[a][b] > 0)
                             pointsCount++;
     if (pointsCount == 0)
             return distArray;
     int[][] points = new int[pointsCount][];
     for (int a = 0; a < points.Length; a++)
     points[a] = new int[2];
int count = 0;
//Get coordinates of non-background points
for (int a=0; a < init_a.Length; a++)
        for (int b=0; b < init_a[0].Length; b++)
                if (init_a[a][b] > 0)
                {
                        points[count][0] = a;
                        points[count][1] = b;
                        count ++;
                }
double minDist = double.MaxValue;
double dist;
for (int a=0; a < init_a.Length; a++)
        for (int b=0; b < init_a[0].Length; b++)
```

```
        {
            minDist = double.MaxValue;
            //Computes the shortest distance
            //between background point and non-background
point
            if (init_a[a][b] == 0)
            {
                for (int aa = 0; aa < pointsCount;
aa++)
                {
                dist = Math.Sqrt(((a - points[aa][0])
                * (a - points[aa][0]))
                + ((b - points[aa][1])
                * (b - points[aa][1])));
                if (dist < minDist)
                        minDist = dist;
                }
            }
            else
                minDist = 0;
            distArray[a][b] = minDist;
        }
    return distArray;
}
```

References

1. Scharf J, Brockmann MA, Daffertshofer M, Diepers M, Neumaier-Probst E, Weiss C, Paschke T, Groden C (2006) Improvement of sensitivity and interrater reliability to detect acute stroke by dynamic perfusion computed tomography and computed tomography angiography. J Comput Assist Tomogr 30(1):105–110
2. Manniesing R, Schaap M, Rozie S, Hameeteman R, Vukadinovic D, van der Lugt A, Niessen W (2010) Robust CTA lumen segmentation of the atherosclerotic carotid artery bifurcation in a large patient population. Med Image Anal 14:759–769
3. Hachaj T, Ogiela MR (2011) CAD system for automatic analysis of CT perfusion maps. Opto-Electron Rev 19(1):95–103. doi:10.2478/s11772-010-0071-2
4. Hachaj T, Ogiela MR (2010) Automatic detection and lesion description in cerebral blood flow and cerebral blood volume perfusion maps. J Sig Proc Syst 61(3):317–328
5. Hachaj T, Ogiela MR (2013) Application of neural networks in detection of abnormal brain perfusion regions. Neurocomputing 122(25):33–42
6. Wintermark M et al (2002) Comparison of admission perfusion computed tomography and qualitative diffusion- and perfusion-weighted magnetic resonance imaging in acute stroke patients. Stroke 33:2025–2031
7. Wintermark M, Fischbein NJ, Smith WS, Ko NU, Quist M, Dillon WP (2005) Accuracy of dynamic perfusion CT with deconvolution in detecting acute hemispheric stroke. AJNR Am J Roentgenol 26(1):104–112

8. Wintermark M, Reichhart M, Thiran J-P, Maeder P, Schnyder P, Bogousslavsky J, Meuli R (2002) Prognostic accuracy of cerebral blood flow measurement by perfusion computed tomography, at the time of emergency room admission, in acute stroke patients. Ann Neurol 51:417–432

9. Tietke M, Riedel C (2008) Whole brain perfusion CT imaging and CT angiography with a 64-channel CT system. MedicaMundi 52/1(07):21–23

10. Ho CY, Hussain S, Alam T, Ahmad I, Wu IC, O'Neill DP (2013) Accuracy of CT cerebral perfusion in predicting infarct in the emergency department: lesion characterization on CT perfusion based on commercially available software. Emerg Radiol 20(3):203–212

11. Kohonen T (1998) The self-organizing map. Neurocomputing 21(1–3):1–6

12. Kohonen T (1990) The self-organizing map. Proc IEEE 78(9):1464–1480

13. Lawrence RD, Almasi GS, Rushmeier HE (1999) A scalable parallel algorithm for self-organizing maps with applications to sparse data mining problems. Data Min Knowl Disc 3:171–195

14. Lange O, Meyer-Baese A, Wismuller A, Hurdal M (2005) Analysis of dynamic cerebral contrast-enhanced perfusion MRI time-series based on unsupervised clustering methods. In: Proceedings of SPIE 5818, independent component analyses, wavelets, unsupervised smart sensors, and neural networks III, 26 (April 05, 2005). doi:10.1117/12.601005

15. Wismüller A, Lange O, Dersch DR, Hahn K, Leinsinger GL (2001) Analysis of dynamic perfusion MRI data by neural networks. In: ESANN'2001 Proceedings—European symposium on artificial neural networks Bruges (Belgium), pp 19–24. D-Facto public., ISBN 2-930307-01-3, 25–27 Apr 2001

16. Egmont-Petersena M, de Ridder D, Handels H (2002) Image processing with neural networks—a review. Pattern Recogn 35:2279–2301

17. Matsumoto H, Masumoto R, Kuroda C (2009) Feature extraction of time-series process images in an aerated agitation vessel using self organizing map. Neurocomputing 73:60–70

18. Markaki VE, Asvestas PA, Matsopoulos GK (2009) Application of Kohonen network for automatic point correspondence in 2D medical images. Comput Biol Med 39:630–645

19. Wismüller A, Vietze F, Behrends J, Meyer-Baese A, Reiser M, Ritter H (2004) Fully automated biomedical image segmentation by self-organized model adaptation. Neural Netw 17:1327–1344

20. Li Y, Chi Z (2005) MR brain image segmentation based on self-organizing map network. Int J Inf Technol 11(8):45–53. ISSN 0218-7957

21. Vijayakumar C, Damayanti G, Pant R, Sreedhar CM (2007) Segmentation and grading of brain tumors on apparent diffusion coefficient images using self-organizing maps. Comput Med Imaging Graph 31(7):473–484 Epub 2007 Jun 14

22. Eastwood JD et al (2002) CT perfusion scanning with deconvolution analysis: pilot study in patients with acute middle cerebral artery stroke. Radiology 222(1):227–236

23. Kohonen T (1995) Self-organizing maps, Springer series in information sciences, vol 30. Springer, New York

24. Vesanto J, Himberg J, Alhoniemi E, Parhankangas J (2000) SOM toolbox for Matlab 5. http://www.cis.hut.fi/somtoolbox/

25. Kumpulainen P, Mettänen M, Lauri M, Ihalainen H (2009) Relating halftone dot quality to paper surface topography. In: Engineering applications of neural networks, Communications in computer and information science, vol 43, pp 178–189

26. Srinivasan A, Goyal M, Azri FA, Lum C (2006) State-of-the-art imaging of acute stroke. Radiographics 26:75–95

27. Allchin D (2001) Error types. Perspect Sci 9:38–59

28. Lasko TA, Bhagwat JG, Zou KH, Ohno-Machado L (2005) The use of receiver operating characteristic curves in biomedical informatics. J Biomed Inform 38(5):404–415

29. Lesage D, Angelini ED, Bloch I, Funka-Lea G (2009) A review of 3D vessel lumen segmentation techniques: models, features and extraction schemes. Med Image Anal 13:819–845

30. Bodzioch S, Ogiela MR (2009) New approach to gallbladder ultrasonic images analysis and lesions recognition. Comput Med Imaging Graph 33:154–170
31. Ogiela MR, Bodzioch S (2011) Computer analysis of gallbladder ultrasonic images towards recognition of pathological lesions. Opto-Electron Rev 19(2):155–168
32. Josephson SA, Bryant SO, Mak HK, Johnston SC, Dillon WP, Smith WS (2004) Evaluation of carotid stenosis by CT angiography in the initial evaluation of stroke and TIA. Neurology 10;63(3):457–460
33. Steinman DA, Poepping TL, Tambasco M, Rankin RN, Holdsworth DW (2000) Flow patterns at the stenosed carotid bifurcation: effect of concentric versus eccentric stenosis. Ann Biomed Eng 28(4):415–423. doi:10.1114/1.279
34. Bouraoui B, Ronse C, Baruthiob J, Passat N, Germainc P (2010) 3D segmentation of coronary arteries based on advanced mathematical morphology techniques. Comput Med Imaging Graph 34:377–387
35. Itai Y, Yamamoto A, Kim H, Tan JK, Ishikawa S (2009) Automatic detection of blood vessels from CTA images employing morphological operation. Artif Life Robotics 13:428–433. doi:10.1007/s10015-008-0594-5
36. Freiman M, Joskowicz L, Broide N, Natanzon M, Nammer E, Shilon O, Weizman L, Sosna J (2012) Carotid vasculature modeling from patient CT angiography studies for interventional procedures simulation. Int J Comput Assist Radiol Surg 7(5):799–812
37. Dufour A, Tankyevych O, Naegel B, Talbot H, Ronse C, Baruthio J, Dokládal P, Passat N (2013) Filtering and segmentation of 3D angiographic data: Advances based on mathematical morphology. Med Image Anal 17:147–164
38. Kostopoulos S, Glotsos D, Kagadis GC, Daskalakis A, Spyridonos P, Kalatzis I, Karamessini M, Petsas T, Cavouras D, Nikiforidis G (2007) A hybrid pixel-based classification method for blood vessel segmentation and aneurysm detection on CTA. Comput Graph 31:493–500
39. Hameeteman K, Zuluaga MA, Freiman M, Joskowicz L, Cuisenaire O, Valencia LF, Gülsün MA, Krissian K, Mille J, Wong WCK, Orkisz M, Tek H, Hoyos MH, Benmansour F, Chung ACS, Rozie S, van Gils M, van den Borne L, Sosnam J, Berman P, Cohen N, Douek PC, Sánchez I, Aissat M, Schaap M, Metz CT, Krestin GP, van der Lugt A, Niessen WJ, van Walsum T (2011) Evaluation framework for carotid bifurcation lumen segmentation and stenosis grading. Med Image Anal 15:477–488
40. van Velsen EFS, Niessen WJ, de Weert TT, de Monyé C, van der Lugt A, Meijering E, Stokking R (2007) Evaluation of an improved technique for lumen path definition and lumen segmentation of atherosclerotic vessels in CT angiography. Eur Radiol 17(7):1738–1745
41. Firouzian A, Manniesing R, Flach ZH, Risselada R, van Kooten F, Sturkenboom MCJM, van der Lugt A, van Niessen WJ (2011) Intracranial aneurysm segmentation in 3D CT angiography: method and quantitative validation with and without prior noise filtering. Eur J Radiol 79:299–304
42. Scherl H, Hornegger J, Prümmer M, Lell M (2007) Semi-automatic level-set based segmentation and stenosis quantification of the internal carotid artery in 3D CTA data sets. Med Image Anal 11:21–34
43. Chan TF, Vese LA (2001) Active contours without edges. IEEE Trans Image Process 10(2):266–277
44. Yi J, Ra JB (2003) A locally adaptive region growing algorithm for vascular segmentation. Int J Imaging Syst Technol 13(4):208–214
45. Shang Q, Clements L, Galloway RL, Chapman WC, Dawant BM (2008) Adaptive directional region growing segmentation of the hepatic vasculature. In: Proceedings of SPIE 6914, medical imaging 2008: image processing, 69141F (March 11, 2008). doi:10.1117/12.769565
46. Carrillo FJ, Hoyos MH, Dávila EE, Orkisz M (2007) Recursive tracking of vascular tree axes in 3D medical images. Int J Comput Assist Radiol Surg 1(6):331–339
47. Biesdorf A, Rohr K, Feng D, von Tengg-Kobligk H, Rengier F, Böckler D, Kauczor H-U, Wörz S (2012) Segmentation and quantification of the aortic arch using joint 3D model-based segmentation and elastic image registration. Med Image Anal 16:1187–1201

48. de Bruijne M, van Ginneken B, Viergever MA, Niessen WJ (2004) Interactive segmentation of abdominal aortic aneurysms in CTA images. Med Image Anal 8:127–138

49. Frangi AF, Niessen WJ, Vincken KL, Viergever MA (1998) Multiscale vessel enhancement filtering. In: Medical image computing and computer-assisted intervention—MICCAI '98, pp 130–137

50. Hladuvka J, König A, Gröller E (2001) Exploiting eigenvalues of the Hessian matrix for volume decimation. In: The 9th international conference in central Europe on computer graphics, visualization, and computer vision (WSCG)

51. Hachaj T, Ogiela MR (2012) Segmentation and visualization of tubular structures in computed tomography angiography. In: Intelligent information and database systems. Lecture notes in computer science, vol 7198/2012, pp 495–503. doi:10.1007/978-3-642-28493-9_52

52. LAPACK—Linear Algebra PACKage. http://www.netlib.org/lapack/

53. Hachaj T, Ogiela MR (2012) Visualization of perfusion abnormalities with GPU-based volume rendering. Comput Graph UK 36(3):163–169. doi:10.1016/j.cag.2012.01.002

54. Hachaj T, Ogiela MR (2012) Framework for cognitive analysis of dynamic perfusion computed tomography with visualization of large volumetric data. J Electron Imaging 21(4), Article Number: 043017, doi:10.1117/1.JEI.21.4.043017

55. Hachaj T, Ogiela MR (2010) Augmented reality interface for visualization of volumetric medical data. Adv Int Soft Comput 84:271–277

56. Ogiela MR, Hachaj T (2013) Automatic segmentation of the carotid artery bifurcation region with a region-growing approach. J Electron Imaging 22(3):033029

57. Kass M, Witkin A, Terzopoulos D (1988) Snakes: active contour models. Int J Comput Vis 1(4):321–331

58. Hea L, Pengb Z, Everdingb B, Wangb X, Hanb CY, Weissc KL, Weeb WG (2008) A comparative study of deformable contour methods on medical image segmentation. Image Vis Comput 26(2):141–163

59. Xu C, Prince JL (1997) Gradient vector flow: a new external force for snakes. In: Proceedings of IEEE conference on computer vision and pattern recognition (CVPR), Los Alamitos, Computer Society Press, pp. 66–71

60. Xu C, Prince JL (1998) Snakes, shapes, and gradient vector flow. IEEE Trans Image Process 7(3):359–369

61. Chan T, Vese L (1999) An active contour model without edges, scale-space theories in computer vision. Lect Notes Comput Sci 1682:141–151

62. Osher S, Sethian JA (1988) Fronts propagating with curvature dependent speed: algorithms based on Hamilton-Jacobi formulation. J Comput Phys 79:12–49

63. Chan TF, Vese LA (2002) A Multiphase level set framework for image segmentation using the Mumford and Shah model. Int J Comput Vis 50(3):271–293

64. Ogiela MR, Hachaj T (2012) The automatic two–step vessel Lumen segmentation algorithm for carotid bifurcation analysis during perfusion examination. In: Intelligent decision technologies, smart innovation, systems and technologies, vol 16, Part 2, pp 485–493. doi:10.1007/978-3-642-29920-9_50

65. Hachaj T, Ogiela MR (2014) The application of centerline detection and deformable contours algorithms to segmenting the carotid lumen. J Electron Imaging 23(2):023006. doi:10.1117/1.JEI.23.2.023006

66. Sussman M, Smereka P, Osher S (1994) A level set approach for computing solutions to incompressible two-phase flow. J Comput Phys 114(1):146–159

67. Zhao HK, Chan T, Merriman B, Osher S (1996) Multiphase motion. J Comput Phys 127:179–195

Chapter 4
Brain and Neck Visualization Techniques

The creation of an algorithm for visualizing volumetric computed tomography (CT) images for real-time applications is a challenging task. That is because of the large size of the dataset (the volumes the authors are dealing with are about $512^3 \approx 10^8$ voxels) and the time constraints on the minimal frames per second (fps) number. Nowadays, it is impossible to render high-quality images of that size without using graphics processing unit (GPU) hardware support. In this chapter, we will present contemporary visualization algorithms that satisfy the need of the medical visualization of large datasets. We will concentrate on direct volume rendering algorithms because they have proven themselves to be computationally efficient and reliable (produce acceptable image quality) in common medical practice.

Before we present visualization algorithms, we will refresh the reader's knowledge of linear algebra and the GPU rendering pipeline , which is crucial for understanding these methods. The GPU programs are strongly dependent on graphic libraries that were used for their implementation. What is more, it is impossible to describe such programs without going into some detail. Because our implementation was developed in the XNA Framework [1–5] (managed libraries based on DirectX 9.0), whenever the pseudo-code notation is not sufficient in this chapter for the proper explanation, we will use elements of C# for CPU and of the high-level shader language (HLSL) for the GPU code. What is more, the use of a specified technology might be more interesting for readers who are not familiar with computer graphics programming and can be applied directly by those who want to check them in practice.

The XNA code can be easily migrated to MonoGame technology [6]. Mono-Game is an Open Source implementation of the Microsoft XNA 4 Framework that uses low-level OpenGL libraries. MonoGame allows XNA developers who primary used Xbox 360, Windows and Windows Phone to port application to the iOS, Android, Mac OS X, Linux, and Windows 8 Metro. What is very important is that the application source code remains the same, only some parts of the Content Pipeline have to be compiled separately. Because those technical details exceed the scope of this book, we recommend reading the official documentation of MonoGame [7].

M. R. Ogiela and T. Hachaj, *Natural User Interfaces in Medical Image Analysis*,
Advances in Computer Vision and Pattern Recognition,
DOI: 10.1007/978-3-319-07800-7_4,
© Springer International Publishing Switzerland 2015

4.1 Linear Algebra for 3D Modeling

In order to generate a 3D image (whether using GPU programming or not), we have to be familiar with elements of the linear algebra theory [8]. That is because we have to know how to display a three-dimensional object on a two-dimensional computer screen. We will only define and derive equations that are crucial for this task.

In the rest of this chapter, we will write equations in respect to a right-handed coordinate system (Fig. 4.1). That is because the XNA framework uses the right-handed coordinate system. OpenGl has the same orientation of axes. DirectX uses a left-handed system.

Let us assume that matrices use a row vector layout (a 3D $\overline{V_3} = [x, y, z]$ vector is a row matrix $M_{V1x3} = [x, y, z]$).

Let $\overline{V} = [x, y, z]$ be a three-dimensional vector.

Definitions

Vector length is a function $|| : R^n \rightarrow R$ defined as:

$$|\overline{V}| = \sqrt{x^2 + y^2 + z^2} \tag{4.1}$$

Vector norm is a function Normalization$() : R^n \rightarrow R^n$ defined as:

$$\text{Normalization}(\overline{V}) = \frac{[x, y, z]}{|\overline{V}|} = \left[\frac{x}{|\overline{V}|}, \frac{y}{|\overline{V}|}, \frac{z}{|\overline{V}|} \right] \tag{4.2}$$

After the normalization, the vector's length equals 1. $|\text{Normalization}(\overline{V})| = 1$
The dot product (scalar product) is the operator $R^n \circ R^n \rightarrow R$ defined as:

$$\overline{V_1} \circ \overline{V_2} = [x_1, y_1, z_1] \circ [x_2, y_2, z_2] = x_1 \cdot x_2 + y_1 \cdot y_2 + z_1 \cdot z_2 = |\overline{V_1}| \cdot |\overline{V_2}| \cdot \cos\theta \tag{4.3}$$

where θ is the angle between vectors $\overline{V_1}$ and $\overline{V_2}$ (Fig. 4.2).
The cross product (vector product) is the operator $R^n \circ R^n \rightarrow R^n$ defined as:

$$\begin{aligned} \overline{V_1} \times \overline{V_2} &= [x_1, y_1, z_1] \times [x_2, y_2, z_2] \\ &= [y_1 \cdot z_2 - z_1 \cdot y_2, z_1 \cdot x_2 - x_1 \cdot z_2, x_1 \cdot y_2 - y_1 \cdot x_2] \end{aligned} \tag{4.4}$$

Let us assume, for simplicity's sake, that A and B are square matrices with the same dimensions and λ is a scalar.

The matrix multiplication has the following properties:

- Is not commutative:

$$A \cdot B \neq B \cdot A \tag{4.5}$$

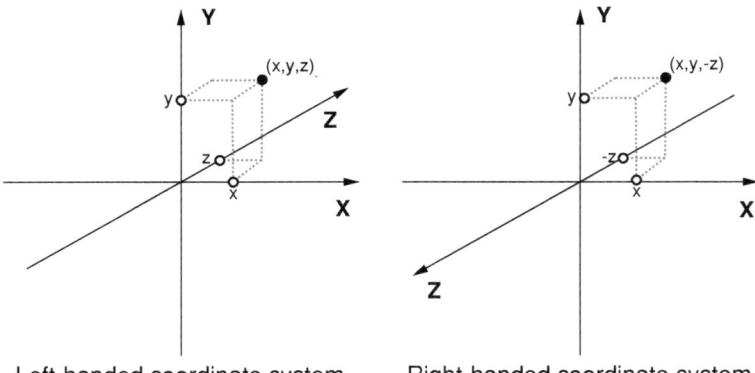

Fig. 4.1 Axis orientation in left- and right-handed coordinate systems

Fig. 4.2 Dot product and cross product

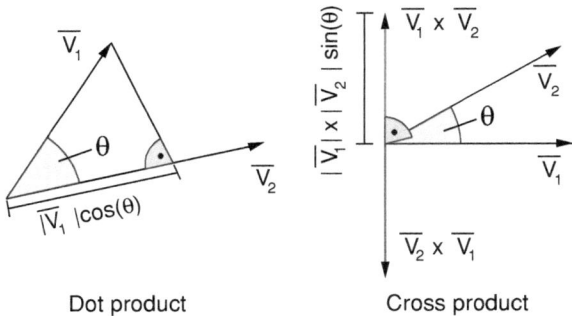

- Is Associative:

$$A \cdot (B \cdot C) = (A \cdot B) \cdot C \tag{4.6}$$

- Is distributive over matrix addition:

$$A \cdot (B + C) = A \cdot B + A \cdot C, (A + B) \cdot C = A \cdot C + B \cdot C \tag{4.7}$$

- The scalar multiplication is compatible with the matrix multiplication:

$$\lambda \cdot (A \cdot B) = (\lambda \cdot A) \cdot B = (A \cdot B) \cdot \lambda = A \cdot (B) \cdot \lambda \tag{4.8}$$

- Identity element (I):

$$A \cdot I = I \cdot A = A \tag{4.9}$$

- Inverse matrix

$$A \cdot A^{-1} = A^{-1} \cdot A \qquad (4.10)$$

A linear transformation between two vector spaces V and W is a map $T : V \to W$ such that the following is true:

1.

$$T(\overline{V}_1 + \overline{V}_2) = T(\overline{V}_1) + T(\overline{V}_2) \text{ for any vectors in } V \qquad (4.11)$$

2.

$$T(\alpha \cdot \overline{V}) = \alpha \cdot T(\overline{V}) \text{ for any scalar } \alpha \qquad (4.12)$$

In computer graphics practice, in order to project a three-dimensional point to a two-dimensional plane, three transformations are applied in the following order: world, view, and projection transformation. The role of the world transformation is to change the position and orientation of the point in the three-dimensional space (we will call that space the "world space"). The role of the view transformation is to transfer the world space into a view space that is relative to the observer's position ("camera position"). The projection transformation converts the viewing frustum into a cuboid shape. These transformations are represented by the appropriate transformation matrices.

4.1.1 World Matrix

The world matrix is represented by a 4×4 square matrix of the following form:

$$W = \begin{bmatrix} w_{11} & w_{12} & w_{13} & 0 \\ w_{21} & w_{22} & w_{23} & 0 \\ w_{31} & w_{32} & w_{33} & 0 \\ w_{41} & w_{42} & w_{43} & 1 \end{bmatrix} \qquad (4.13)$$

In order to transform the three-dimensional vector $\overline{V} = [x, y, z]$, we add the fourth-dimension to it with a value equal to 1 $\overline{V}_+ = [x, y, z, 1]$. We obtain transformation T of $\overline{V}$ by multiplying $\overline{V}_+$ by the appropriate matrix W_T which represents that linear transform.

$$T(\overline{V}) = \overline{V}_+ \cdot W_T \qquad (4.14)$$

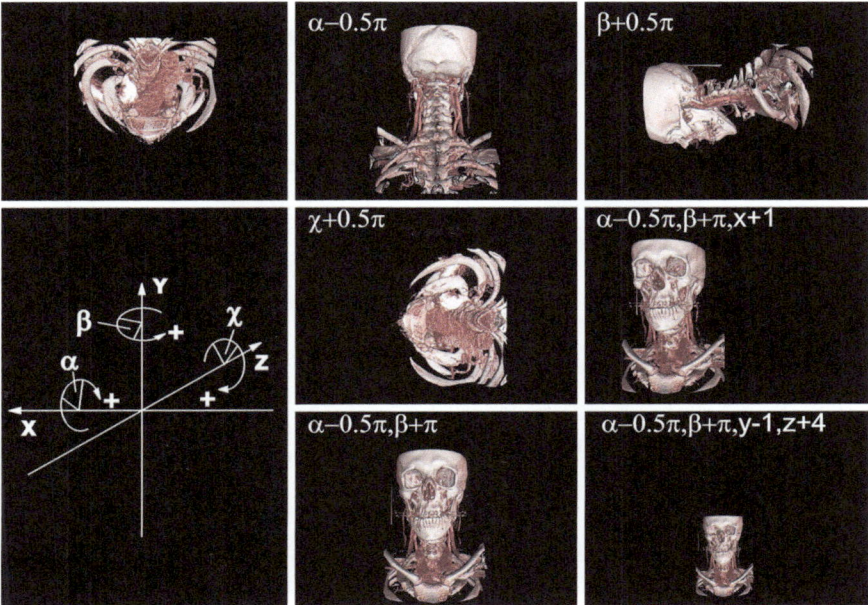

Fig. 4.3 Example visualization rotations and translations of points set in a three-dimensional space. The orientations of rotations are presented in the *bottom-left* corner of the picture

The result vector has four dimensions with the fourth element equal to 1. This fourth element is eventually skipped. The transformation was defined in this manner in order to represent the translation of the vector inside one matrix with another linear transformation.

In our case, the three most useful transformations are the rotation, translation, and scaling (see Fig. 4.3).

The matrices representing these transforms are defined as follows:

$$
X\text{-axis rotation } R_x = \begin{bmatrix} 1 & 0 & 0 & 0 \\ 0 & \cos(\alpha) & \sin(\alpha) & 0 \\ 0 & -\sin(\alpha) & \cos(\alpha) & 0 \\ 0 & 0 & 0 & 1 \end{bmatrix} \tag{4.15}
$$

$$
Y\text{-axis rotation } R_y = \begin{bmatrix} \cos(\beta) & 0 & -\sin(\beta) & 0 \\ 0 & 1 & 0 & 0 \\ \sin(\beta) & 0 & \cos(\beta) & 0 \\ 0 & 0 & 0 & 1 \end{bmatrix} \tag{4.16}
$$

$$\text{Z-axis rotation } R_z = \begin{bmatrix} \cos(\chi) & \sin(\chi) & 0 & 0 \\ -\sin(\chi) & \cos(\chi) & 0 & 0 \\ 0 & 0 & 1 & 0 \\ 0 & 0 & 0 & 1 \end{bmatrix} \qquad (4.17)$$

$$\text{Scaling } S = \begin{bmatrix} s_x & 0 & 0 & 0 \\ 0 & s_y & 0 & 0 \\ 0 & 0 & s_z & 0 \\ 0 & 0 & 0 & 1 \end{bmatrix} \qquad (4.18)$$

where s_x, s_y, s_z are amounts for scaling along the x, y, and z-axes.

$$\text{Translation } S = \begin{bmatrix} 1 & 0 & 0 & 0 \\ 0 & 1 & 0 & 0 \\ 0 & 0 & 1 & 0 \\ t_x & t_y & t_z & 1 \end{bmatrix} \qquad (4.19)$$

where t_x, t_y, t_z are amounts for translating by along the x, y, and z-axes.

4.1.2 View Matrix

The view space, sometimes called the camera space, is similar to the world space, but the in view space, the origin is at the viewer or camera, looking in the negative z-direction. Recall that we use a right-handed coordinate system, so z is negative into a scene.

The view matrix is also known as the camera matrix. It transforms the entire world space into a camera space. Similarly, the world matrix transform puts the object from the object space into the world space—Fig. 4.4.

In order to prepare the view matrix, let us assume that:

$P = (x_p, y_p, z_p)$ is the camera (observer) position.
$\overline{V_p} = [-x_p, -y_p, -z_p]$ is a vector which links the camera position to the beginning of the World Cartesian frame.
$T = (x_t, y_t, z_t)$ is the point at which the camera "is looking".
$\overline{V_u} = [x_u, y_u, z_u]$ is an up-vector of the camera.

The camera should be looking along the negative direction of the axis of which the first versor is:

$$\overline{V}_{h1} = \frac{[x_p - x_t, y_p - y_t, z_p - z_t]}{\left|[x_p - x_t, y_p - y_t, z_p - z_t]\right|} = \text{Normalization}(\overline{TP}) = [x_{h1}, y_{h1}, z_{h1}] \quad (4.20)$$

Fig. 4.4 The Cartesian
frame of the world space and
the camera frame

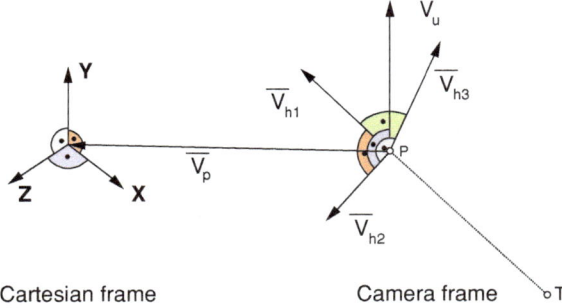

Cartesian frame   Camera frame

The next two versors are defined as:

$$\overline{V}_{h2} = \text{Normalization}\left(\overline{V}_u \times \overline{V}_{h1}\right) = [x_{h2}, y_{h2}, z_{h2}] \tag{4.21}$$

$$\overline{V}_{h3} = \overline{V}_{h1} \times \overline{V}_{h2} = [x_{h3}, y_{h3}, z_{h3}]. \tag{4.22}$$

To change the coordinates of point A from the Cartesian frame $(x_a, y_a, z_a)_C$ to
the Camera frame $(v_{1a}, v_{2a}, v_{3a})_H$, the following transform has to be executed:

$$[x_a, y_a, z_a, 1] \cdot V = [x_a, y_a, z_a, 1] \cdot \begin{bmatrix} e_{11} & e_{12} & e_{13} & 0 \\ e_{21} & e_{22} & e_{23} & 0 \\ e_{31} & e_{32} & e_{33} & 0 \\ e_{41} & e_{42} & e_{43} & 1 \end{bmatrix} = [v_{1a}, v_{2a}, v_{3a}, 1]. \tag{4.23}$$

In other words, the coordinates of each row of the transfer matrix V (view
matrix) consist in the linear combination coefficients of the Camera frame that
represent Cartesian frame versors. In addition, we can write vector $\overline{V}_p$ as a similar
linear combination.

$$\begin{cases} [1,0,0] = e_{11} \cdot \overline{V}_{h2} + e_{12} \cdot \overline{V}_{h3} + e_{13} \cdot \overline{V}_{h1} \\ [0,1,0] = e_{21} \cdot \overline{V}_{h2} + e_{22} \cdot \overline{V}_{h3} + e_{23} \cdot \overline{V}_{h1} \\ [0,0,1] = e_{31} \cdot \overline{V}_{h2} + e_{32} \cdot \overline{V}_{h3} + e_{33} \cdot \overline{V}_{h1} \\ [-x_p, -y_p, -z_p] = e_{41} \cdot \overline{V}_{h2} + e_{42} \cdot \overline{V}_{h3} + e_{43} \cdot \overline{V}_{h1} \end{cases} \tag{4.24}$$

These equations can be solved by Cramer's Rule [8]. The resulting V matrix
(the so-called "View" matrix) has the following components:

$$V = \begin{bmatrix} x_{h2} & x_{h3} & x_{h1} & 0 \\ y_{h2} & y_{h3} & y_{h1} & 0 \\ z_{h2} & z_{h3} & z_{h1} & 0 \\ -\overline{V}_{h2} \circ \overline{V}_p & -\overline{V}_{h3} \circ \overline{V}_p & -\overline{V}_{h1} \circ \overline{V}_p & 1 \end{bmatrix} \tag{4.25}$$

4.1.3 Projection Matrix

The projection space refers to the space after the projection transformation from the view space has been executed. After the projection transformation, the visible content has x- and y-coordinates ranging from -1 to 1, and a z-coordinate ranging from 0 to 1 (z-coordinates are then utilized in computer graphics as the so-called "z-buffer"). The position of the 3D point on the 2D plane is given by equation:

$$\overline{V}_{3D} = [x_{3D}, y_{3D}, z_{3D}]$$

$$\overline{V}_h = [x_{3D}, y_{3D}, z_{3D}, 1] \cdot (W \cdot V \cdot P) = [x_h, y_h, z_h, w_h] \tag{4.26}$$

$$\overline{V}_{2D} = [x_{2D}, y_{2D}, z_{2D}]$$
$$= \left[\frac{(x_h + 1) \cdot 0.5 \cdot \text{window\_width}}{w_h}, \frac{(-y_h + 1) \cdot 0.5 \cdot \text{window\_height}}{w_h}, \frac{z_h}{w_h} \right] \tag{4.27}$$

where window_width, window_height are dimensions of the viewport (the square part of the projection plane that is visible on the computer screen) and x_{2D}, y_{2D} are $\overline{V}_{3D}$ coordinates on the projection plane.

The reverse transform (the projection of a vector from the screen space into the object space) is given by equation:

$$\overline{V}_{h2} = \left[\frac{x_{2D}}{2 \cdot \text{window\_width} - 1}, \frac{-y_{2D}}{2 \cdot \text{window\_height} - 1}, z_{2D}, 1 \right] \cdot (W \cdot V \cdot P)^{-1}$$
$$= [x_{h2}, y_{h2}, z_{h2}, w_{h2}] \tag{4.28}$$

$$\overline{V}_{3D} = \left[\frac{x_{h2}}{w_{h2}}, \frac{y_{h2}}{w_{h2}}, \frac{z_{h2}}{w_{h2}} \right]. \tag{4.29}$$

The projection matrix is based on the near and far view distance (the distance range (z-coordinate) inside which points will be projected onto the screen plane), the camera viewing angle, and your screen resolution proportions—Fig. 4.5. Let us define:

α field of view, $\alpha \in (0, \pi)$

ar   aspect ratio (the proportional relationship between the width and the height of the projection screen), ar > 0

np, fp   near and far plane distance, $0 < \text{np} < \text{fp}$

Fig. 4.5 The graphic representation of the projection transform

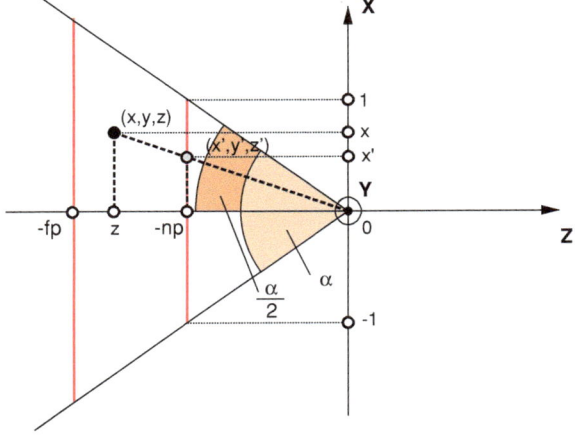

Let us assume that the projection matrix has the following form:

$$P = \begin{bmatrix} p_{11} & p_{12} & p_{13} & p_{14} \\ p_{21} & p_{22} & p_{23} & p_{24} \\ p_{31} & p_{32} & p_{33} & p_{34} \\ p_{41} & p_{42} & p_{43} & p_{44} \end{bmatrix}. \tag{4.30}$$

We want to project a point with the coordinates (x, y, z) onto a 2D plane and obtain a point with the coordinates (x', y', z'). As can be seen in Fig. 4.5, the projected x' and y' components can be computed using x (or appropriately y) and z:

$$\frac{\|z\|}{x} = \frac{\mathrm{np}}{x'} \tag{4.31}$$

$$x'' = \frac{x \cdot \mathrm{np}}{\|z\|} \tag{4.32}$$

$$x' = \frac{x \cdot \mathrm{np}}{\mathrm{ar} \cdot \|z\|} = \frac{x \cdot \mathrm{np}}{\mathrm{ar} \cdot (-1 \cdot z)} \tag{4.33}$$

$$\mathrm{tg}\left(\frac{\alpha}{2}\right) = \frac{1}{\mathrm{np}} \tag{4.34}$$

$$\mathrm{np} = \frac{1}{\mathrm{tg}\left(\frac{\alpha}{2}\right)} \tag{4.35}$$

$$x' = \frac{x}{\mathrm{ar} \cdot \mathrm{tg}\left(\frac{\alpha}{2}\right) \cdot (-1 \cdot z)} \tag{4.36}$$

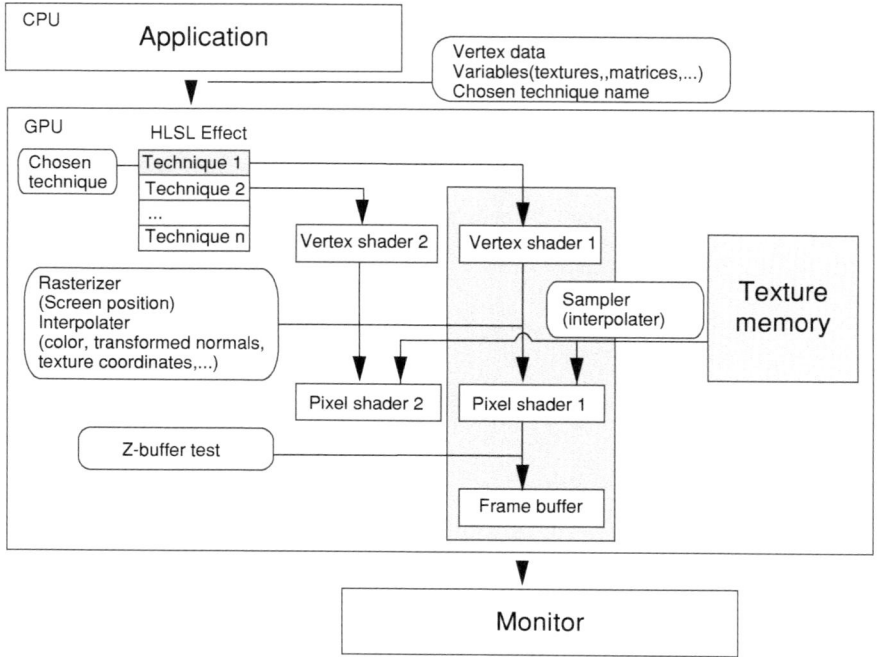

Fig. 4.6 XNA framework rendering pipeline

$$y' = \frac{y}{(-1 \cdot z) \cdot \text{tg}\left(\frac{\alpha}{2}\right)} .$$

Knowing (4.36) and (4.37), let us assume that:

$$p_{12} = p_{13} = p_{14} = p_{21} = p_{23} = p_{24} = p_{31} = p_{32} = p_{41} = p_{42} = p_{44} = 0.$$

$$p_{11} = \frac{1}{\text{ar} \cdot \text{tg}\left(\frac{\alpha}{2}\right)}, p_{22} = \frac{1}{\text{tg}\left(\frac{\alpha}{2}\right)}, p_{34} = -1. \tag{4.37}$$

z can be scaled to the range $[0, 1]$ by a linear equation (with the appropriate values of p_{33}, p_{43}) but we have to remember about the value of w_{h2} from (4.29) which is dependent from z (4.37) because $p_{34} = -1$. Knowing that, we get:

$$z' = \frac{z \cdot a + b}{-1 \cdot z} \tag{4.38}$$

$$\begin{cases} 1 = \frac{-\text{fp} \cdot a + b}{\text{fp}} \\ 0 = \frac{-\text{np} \cdot a + b}{\text{np}} \end{cases} \tag{4.39}$$

$$\begin{cases} 1 = -a + \frac{b}{fp} \\ 0 = -a + \frac{b}{np} \end{cases}$$

$$1 = \frac{b}{fp} - \frac{b}{np} = \frac{b \cdot np - b \cdot fp}{np \cdot fp} = \frac{b \cdot (np - fp)}{np \cdot fp} \tag{4.40}$$

$$b = \frac{np \cdot fp}{np - fp}$$

$$a = \frac{1}{np} \cdot \frac{np \cdot fp}{np - fp} = \frac{fp}{np - fp}$$

and finally:

$$z' = \frac{z \cdot \frac{fp}{np-fp} + \frac{np \cdot fp}{np-fp}}{-1 \cdot z}. \tag{4.41}$$

Finally, the projection matrix is as follows:

$$P = \begin{bmatrix} n_2 & 0 & 0 & 0 \\ 0 & n_1 & 0 & 0 \\ 0 & 0 & \frac{fp}{np-fp} & -1 \\ 0 & 0 & \frac{np \cdot fp}{np-fp} & 0 \end{bmatrix} \tag{4.42}$$

where:

$$n_1 = \frac{1}{tg\left(\frac{x}{2}\right)}$$

$$n_2 = \frac{n_1}{ar}.$$

4.2 Rendering Pipeline

In computer graphic terminology, the process of rendering a three-dimensional image to a two-dimensional image (raster) is called the rendering pipeline [9]. In contemporary graphic hardware, the three-dimensional data is represented as a set of vertices that are connected together to create basic primitives—triangles. Each vertex, beside its position in the three-dimensional space, might contain other information like ARGB color data (A is the opacity channel, the so-called alpha channel), normal values, or texture coordinates. During the rendering process, this additional data is linearly interpolated to the whole surface of the triangle. This makes it possible to draw a surface that is represented by a small number of vertices that can be highly magnified (a similar approach is utilized in two-dimensional vector graphics). The raster data used by the GPU is called texture and it is a one-, two-, or three-dimensional indexed array.

Nowadays, it is possible to create efficient programs that render huge datasets in real-time using high-level GPU languages (GLSL for open OpenGL, HLSL for DirectX, or CUDA for Nvidia GPU) but it is still crucial to know the exact GPU rendering pipeline for the chosen technology. Consequently, it is impossible to present the most interesting aspects of volume rendering algorithms independently of any particular technology. With this in mind, we will present some aspects of GPU-based programming, which are necessary to explain the most important details in the following paragraphs of this chapter. We will not go into details that are irrelevant or will not be explicitly mentioned later.

The technology that we use for the volumetric data visualization is the Microsoft XNA Framework, HLSL, and the C# language. The XNA rendering pipeline renders graphics by calling up the DirectX 9 rendering pipeline. The following Fig. 4.6 shows the subset of the DirectX 9 rendering pipeline used by the XNA Framework.

The application runs partially on the CPU and the GPU. The part on the CPU (the host) is responsible for loading data from the memory into the RAM and transporting data to the GPU (device) memory. The CPU program prepares vertex data: vertex memory buffers that provide storage for the untransformed model vertices; and the vertex declaration to describe the information (position, color, texture coordinates, normals, and so on) which is defined for each vertex. The host also controls the rendering pipeline behavior by setting the graphic device parameters (like, e.g., the alpha-blending mode) or inner HLSL script variables.

The source code GPU program resides inside the HLSL file (called the effect file). Each effect can have some global variables (like matrices, textures, floating point variables, etc.,). The particular code to be executed is organized with so-called techniques. The name of the technique to be executed is set by the host. Each technique consists of the Pixel Shader function and might include the Vertex Shader function. The Vertex Shader of an Effect transforms the vertices stored in the vertex buffer (commonly performs the world, view, and projective transforms). The output data from the Vertex Shader (transformed vertices) is then processed to compute the screen position of each pixel belonging to the processed triangle (rasterization). This process is preceded by, inter alia, clipping (removing triangles (or parts of triangles) that do not appear on the screen), back face culling (removes triangles that are not facing the camera—Fig. 4.7). The linear, bilinear, or trilinear interpolation is performed on additional vertex data like colors, transformed normals, textures, etc.

The Pixel Shader operates on raster data and does not have to be preceded by a Vertex Shader, but if it is, it has access to data from the previous rasterization and interpolation step. The Pixel Shader often computes artificial lighting of objects and covers surfaces with textures. A texture that resides in the device memory is

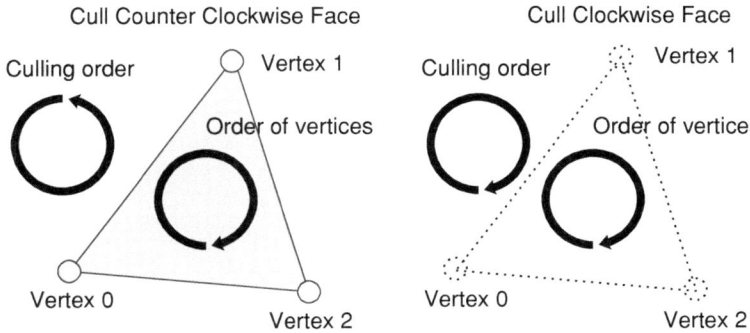

Fig. 4.7 Back face culling: vertices are ordered according to their indexes *(Vertex 0, Vertex 1, and Vertex 2)*. If they are ordered clockwise and the "cull counter-clockwise face" culling is enabled, the surface of the triangle is rendered. If, with the same order, the culling clockwise face is enabled, the triangle surface is not drawn

accessed by samplers which linearly interpolate the color value at given coordinates (the indexes of texture arrays are floating point values within the 0–1 range). The output data of the Pixel Shader is the color of a pixel which will appear in the frame buffer and ultimately on the screen.

4.3 GPU-Based Visualization Using the Direct Volume Rendering Technique

As described in the previous paragraph, the GPU-based visualization operates on vertices that are organized with triangles and a triangle is the basic (and the only three-dimensional) primitive that can be directly processed in HLSL. The task we want to accomplish is to visualize three-dimensional computed tomography data stored in two-dimensional slices. These slices might be stored in a three-dimensional array, as in Fig. 4.8, where the *X*- and *Y*- coordinates store information about the width and the height of the image and the *Z* coordinate determines the particular slice index. Each field in this array is called a voxel (a three-dimensional pixel) and it represents the averaged Hounsfield unit value of tissues contained inside the cuboid density.

In the practical medical visualization of tomography, it is often necessary to be able to instantly change the color and the opacity of some tissues in order to hide or show some anatomical structures that are of particular importance for the particular examination. For this reason, a visualization algorithms which would generate only the outer surfaces of body organs (for example by the marching cubes algorithm [10]) without storing data about these organs' interiors would not be sufficient.

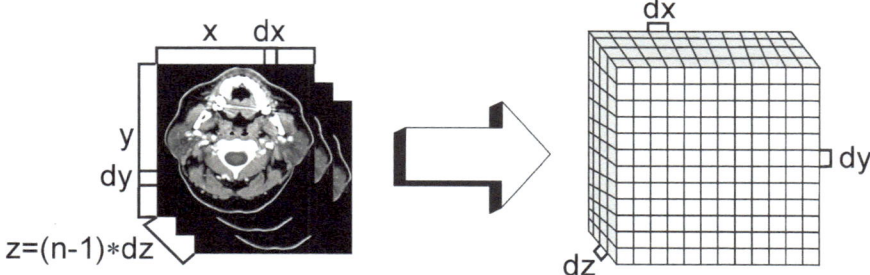

Fig. 4.8 A set of CT images storing volumetric data. Each voxel is dx × dy × dz in size. The data is stored in the GPU memory as a three-dimensional texture

Fig. 4.9 A three-dimensional cuboid primitive build of triangles. It consists of eight vertices that forming twelve triangles

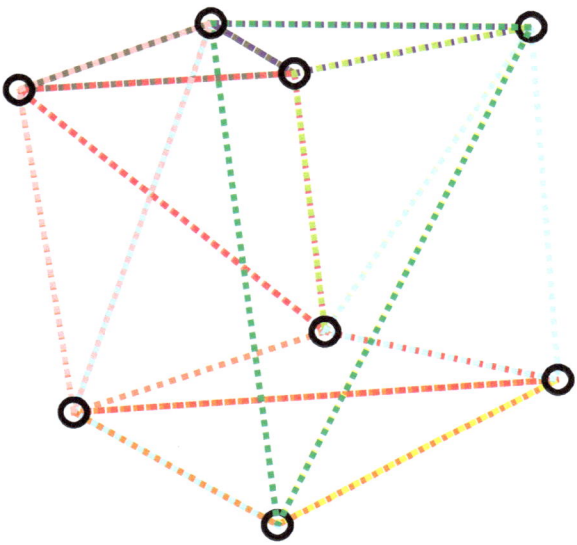

The most straightforward way to display this data is to represent each voxel by a cuboid primitive build of eight vertices and twelve triangles—Fig. 4.9. This approach, however, is not used in practice: in real data sets, it would require a huge number of primitives and the rendering speed would be too slow for any convenient interaction with the visualization. To obtain a high-speed visualization without losing the quality of the image it is necessary to organize the volumetric data in such a way that the GPU program could utilize hardware interpolation algorithms mentioned in the previous paragraph. The visualization algorithms which satisfy these conditions are called direct volume rendering methods because they display voxel data by evaluating an optical model describing how the volume emits, reflects, scatters, absorbs, and occludes light [11]. In contrast, indirect methods extract a surface description from volume data during the preprocessing step (we will not describe indirect algorithms in this book).

In essence, the role of the optical model is to describe how particles in the volume interact with light. For example, the most commonly used model [12–15] assumes that the volume consists of particles that simultaneously emit and absorb light (emission-absorption model).

The emission-absorption model is described elsewhere [11]. In computer graphics, emission is approximated by the color of a pixel (RGB) and the absorption by its opacity A. A discrete numerical solution is an iterative procedure that might be computed front to back or back to front.

Let us define:

$S = (r_S, g_S, b_S)$ the RGB color value in a particular place within the volume (the voxel color in a three-dimensional texture).

a_S the alpha value in a particular place within the volume (the voxel opacity in a three-dimensional texture).

$C = (r_C, g_C, b_C)$ the color value of a pixel in the final image

a_C the alpha value of a pixel in the final image.

Front to back blending:

$$
\left\{
\begin{array}{l}
C_1 = S_1 \\
a_{C1} = a_{S1} \\
\quad C_i = (1 - a_{Ci-1}) \cdot S_i \cdot a_{Si} + C_{i-1} \\
\quad a_{Ci} = (1 - a_{Ci-1}) \cdot a_{Si} + a_{Ci-1}
\end{array}
\right.
\tag{4.43}
$$

where $i = 2,\ldots, n$

1 is the index of the point at which the light ray enters the volume (in Fig. 4.10 any of f-points), n—is an index of the point in which the ray exits the volume (in Fig. 4.10 any of b-points).

Back to front blending:

$$
\left\{
\begin{array}{l}
C_1 = S_1 \\
a_{C1} = a_{S1} \\
\quad C_i = S_i \cdot a_{Si} + (1 - a_{Si}) \cdot C_{i-1} \\
\quad a_{Ci} = a_{Si} + (1 - a_{Si}) \cdot a_{Ci-1}
\end{array}
\right.
\tag{4.44}
$$

where $i = 2,\ldots,n$, 1 is an index of the point at which the ray exits the volume (in Fig. 4.10 any of b-points), n-is the index of the point at which the ray enters the volume (in Fig. 4.10 any of f-points). Points along the rays are sampled at a given interval (n has to be a finite number). In our case, this interval is constant during the rendering and depends of the size of visualized data.

Optical parameters of data to be displayed are computed by applying the so-called *transfer function*. The goal of the transfer function in visualization

Fig. 4.10 A diagram of the ray-casting algorithm. Data is contained inside a *cuboid*. Each ray begins at point O and the number of rays equals the dimension of the projection plane P. If the ray comes into the volumetric data at point fi, it leaves it at point bi. F stands for the front of the cuboid, b for its back. Values of pixel *colors* in P are computed using (4.43) or (4.44)

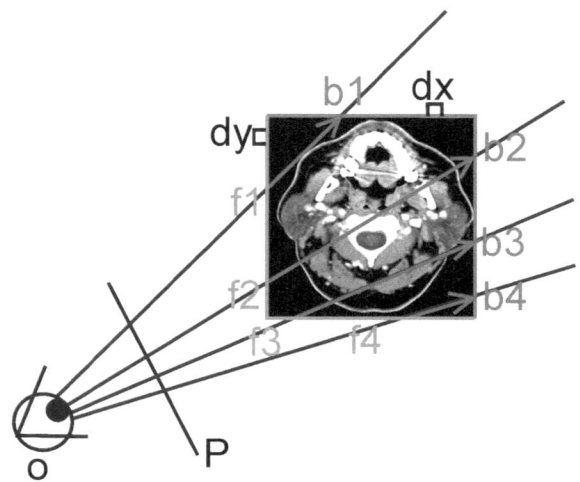

applications is to emphasize or *classify* features of interest in the data [15]. Transfer functions are usually implemented by *texture lookup tables*, though simple functions can also be computed in a Pixel Shader. A transfer function is used to mapping the Hounsfield Unit (HU) value of the volume to the RGBA palette (the Hounsfield scale value of a particular tissue to emission and absorption parameters). Plots of an example transfer function are presented in Fig. 4.11.

In order to enhance the shape and structure of rendered objects, artificial illumination has to be applied.

The most common local illumination model which calculates the light per pixel is the Phong lighting model [16]. The Phong model is made up of three parts: ambient, diffuse, and specular.

$$L = L_{ambient} + L_{diffuse} + L_{specular} \tag{4.45}$$

$$L_{ambient} = I_{ambient} \cdot K_{ambient} \tag{4.46}$$

where $I_{ambient}$ is the constant intensity of ambient light and $K_{ambient}$ is the coefficient of the ambient reflection of the surface. The ambient term is a constant which simulates indirect light on the parts of geometry where there is no direct light, or otherwise they would be completely black.

$$L_{diffuse} = \begin{cases} I_{diffuse} \cdot K_{diffuse} \cdot \cos(\alpha), & |\alpha| < 90° \\ 0 & \text{otherwise} \end{cases} \tag{4.47}$$

where $I_{diffuse}$ is the light source intensity, $K_{diffuse}$ is a material constant describing the color and α is the angle between the light source and the surface normal. The diffuse term calculates the reflection of light from a nonshiny surface, called a

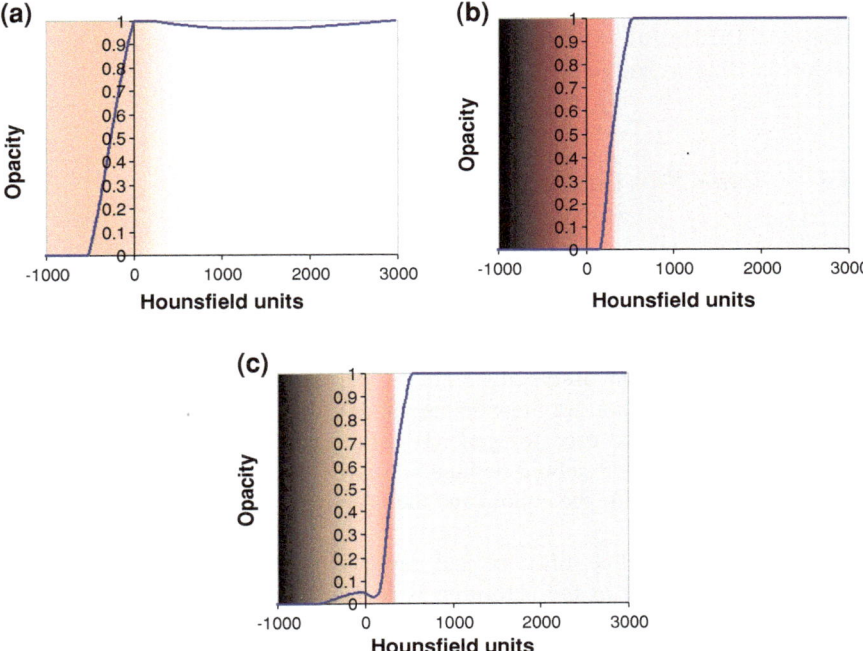

Fig. 4.11 Plots of an example transfer function (*blue line*). The *horizontal* axis is scaled in Hounsfield units, the *vertical* one shows the opacity of the tissue for a given HU. The *colors* in the background are RGB values of the tissue for the given HU, the visualization of the same volumetric data with transfer functions a, b and c is in Fig. 4.14

matte surface. The light is reflected at the same angle as it strikes the surface relative to the surface normal.

$$L_{\text{specular}} = \begin{cases} I_{\text{specular}} \cdot K_{\text{specular}} \cdot \cos^m(\beta), & |\beta| < 90° \\ 0 & \text{otherwise} \end{cases} \qquad (4.48)$$

where I_{specular} is the intensity of the incident light, K_{specular} is the specular reflection coefficient of the material, β is the angle between the reflection vector and the viewing vector and m controls the extension of the highlight. The specular term is added to simulate the shininess of surfaces, it creates highlights which give the viewer cues of light source positions and geometry details.

An essential part of the illumination model is the surface normal. In volume rendering, a surface normal is replaced by the gradient vector calculated at all points of interest. In our case we use L_{ambient} and L_{diffuse} components because they are sufficient for our task [13, 17]. The gradient operators we use are presented in Sect. 4.6.4.

The following paragraph presents the volume ray-casting algorithm and the texture-based algorithm. The example visualizations and numerical results are computed using a computed tomography angiography (CTA) image with the dimensions $(512 \times 512 \times 415)$ (415 axial slices, 512×512 pixels each). The viewport is 1024×768 in size.

4.3.1 Volume Ray-Casting

Each volume rendering algorithm based on physics evaluates the volume rendering integral even if viewing rays are not explicitly employed by the algorithm. An algorithm which directly simulates the travel of rays through the volume as presented in Fig. 4.10 is called volume ray-casting. Volume ray-casting simulates the travel of a ray through the observed volume, usually using the front–back approach (4.43). To begin rendering, we must define the so-called proxy geometry—a set of primitives which will be used for generating the volume. In the case of volume ray-casting, we will use a cuboid defined similarly to the one from Fig. 4.9. The volume data will be inside the cuboid and the visualization will be processed on its faces.

The rendering pipeline of a typical ray-casting algorithm is presented in Fig. 4.13. The first part of the algorithm is prepared on the CPU: if there is too much volume data to fit in the RAM in one part, it is divided into so-called bricks, with brick sorting arranging the bricks in the right order for rendering. This approach is optional and will be described at the end of this chapter. After setting the texture information and matrix data, the rest of the program is executed in parallel on the GPU. The listing of the HLSL implementation of that algorithm is in Sect. 4.6.2—Volume ray-casting rendering algorithm—HLSL code. In the Vertex Shader, the GPU applies transformations from Sect. 4.1 to vertex and texture coordinates. Then, in Pixel Shader, it computes the final pixel value according to (4.43) using the Ray Casting technique (see example). As mentioned above, to generate the two-dimensional image each pixel in the viewport must be filled with a color value, but it is not necessary to simulate all possible rays from point O to each pixel in the viewport. This is because the volume does not necessarily fill the observer's whole field of view. Consequently, we only need to find the pixels in the viewport which will be used as the entry and exit points of the ray running through the volume (f and b points from Fig. 4.10). In [18], the authors proposed a multi-pass approach in the first step of which they compute the coordinates of points f and b (Fig. 4.12). Both faces are computed using the same RenderFace technique (see example), but in one case, the clockwise back face culling is used, and in the other time the counterclockwise back face culling.

If the front and back faces are known, the ray direction dir can be computed easily. At each step of the following loop, the incoming HU value along the ray is replaced by RGBA parameters taken from the look-up table of the transfer function (two-dimensional texture Transfer). This scalar value mapping to physical quantities is often referred to as the classification [12]. A pixel is shaded according to Eq. (4.45). The gradient necessary for (4.47) is calculated using the central

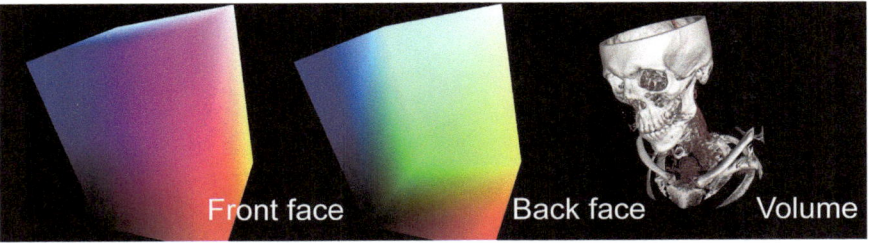

Fig. 4.12 In order to simplify the calculation of rays in the ray-casting algorithm, before applying (4.43), *the front and back faces* of the proxy geometry are rendered. The *front face* texture holds the coordinates of entry points of rays into the volume (*f*—points in Fig. 4.10) and the *back face* holds the coordinates of exit points of rays out of the volume (*f*—points in Fig. 4.10). These coordinates are in the space of the three-dimensional texture array, so the values are from the 0–1 interval. Each of the three coordinates is stored in a separate color component of the pixel. Results are stored in two-dimensional textures of the Front and the Back

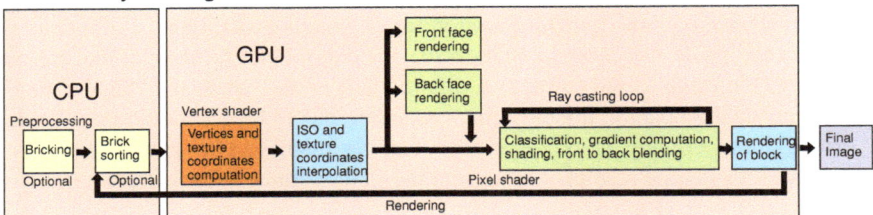

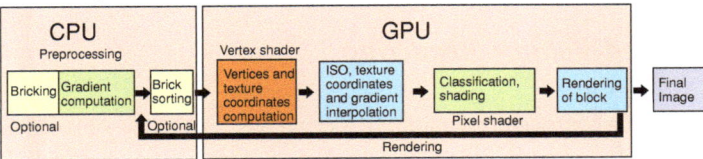

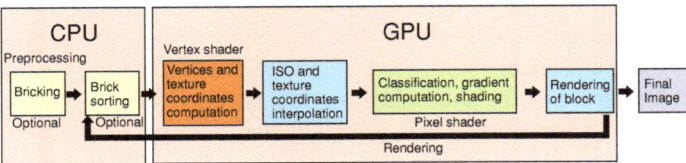

Fig. 4.13 The volume rendering pipeline of the volume ray-casting algorithm and the texture-based algorithm with view-aligned slices. The second algorithm is presented in two variants: with a precomputed gradient and with the dynamic computation of the gradient in the Pixel Shader

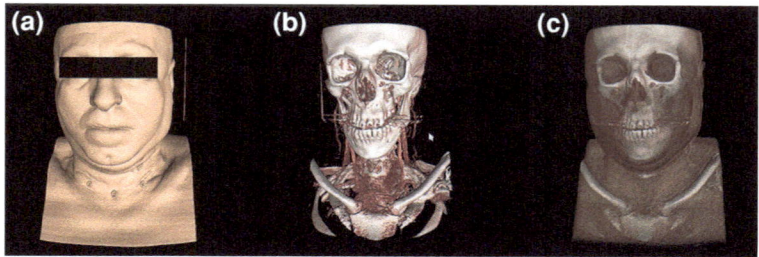

Fig. 4.14 The visualization of the same volumetric data with transfer functions from Fig. 4.11

difference schema. The loop ends if it reaches the maximal number of iterations (equal to the maximal number of sampled points along the ray at the given sample distance SampleDist), if the ray exits the volume or if the alpha parameter or the final alpha value gets high enough—in our case to 0.95. The last condition is called the early ray termination and is used to speed up the rendering. An additional approach that can be used to speed rendering up is the so-called empty space skipping. If we decide to apply it, we have to partition the volume into smaller cuboids and compute the transfer function for all voxels inside them. If the opacity of all voxels inside the cuboid equals zero, this cuboid can be skipped during the rendering. The main disadvantage of this method is that when the transfer functions changes the opacity, the checking procedure has to be computed once again.

Finally, the volume is rendered and can be displayed to system operator. Figure 4.14 shows the results of rendering the same volume using different transfer functions.

4.3.2 Texture-Based Volume Rendering

The second very popular approach to volume rendering also evaluates the volume rendering integral (this time (4.44)—back to front blending) but uses a completely different proxy geometry. The volume is rendered as a set of two-dimensional polygons which are close enough to each other to create the illusion of three-dimensionality. There are two variations of that algorithm: one with volume-aligned slices (polygons) and another with view-aligned slices. In the first one, the slices are in the fixed position of the data. Most commonly, there are three sets of polygons, first on the plane whose normal is perpendicular to versos of X- and Y-axis, the second whose normal is perpendicular to versos of Y and Z and the last whose normal is perpendicular to versos of X and Z. During the rendering, only one of this set is visible (the one for which the angle between the normal vector of the plane and the view direction vector is the smallest). This approach does not require using three-dimensional textures, but the rendering shows artifacts which are particularly visible when switching between sets of planes and when the angle between the normal and the view direction vector is close to the border value of the switching. Because of this drawback, the volume-aligned algorithm is not used anymore and has mostly been replaced with the view-aligned approach.

In the view-aligned approach, volumes are also represented by a proxy geometry consisting of two-dimensional polygons which are close to each other and contain pixels colors computed using (4.44), but the position of the slices is dynamically computed each time the position of the volume relative to the observer changes. The planes are generated as the intersection of a family of planes (4.49) and the edges of the cuboid representing the volume (the cuboid itself does not have to be visualized). What is interesting is the computation of the back to front equation, as it is not computed directly by the GPU program but is set in the blending attributes of the graphics hardware before the rendering procedure.

```
//C# code
GraphicsDevice.RenderState.SourceBlend = Blend.SourceAlpha;
GraphicsDevice.RenderState.DestinationBlend
    = Blend.InverseSourceAlpha;
```

That means that each new pixel S_i which we want to blend with background C_i is multiplied by the alpha of a new pixel a_{Si} and the background pixel is multiplied by $(1 - a_{Si})$. That corresponds exactly to formula (4.44).

The rendering pipeline for two versions of a view-aligned algorithm is presented in Fig. 4.13. The first one uses the precomputed gradient of volumetric data, the second one computes the gradient in a Pixel Shader. In the case of the precomputed version, the gradient information has to be stored inside the three-dimensional texture and transferred to the GPU (so this data occupies about four times more memory then the dynamically computed version) but it does not require computing the gradient in each pass of the Pixel Shader. Bricking, brick sorting, and the Vertex Shader perform operations similar to those in volume ray-casting.

The first step in both versions of the texture-based algorithm is to generate view-aligned slices. This operation is executed in the CPU. Let us assume that the observer is at point (0, 0, 0) of a Cartesian frame, he or she is looking in the direction of the Z-axis and does not change their position during the rendering procedure. After this assumption, each plane to which the vector linking the camera position with the beginning of the Cartesian frame is perpendicular is characterized by the equation:

$$z + d = 0 \qquad\qquad (4.49)$$

where z is a Z-axis coordinate and d is a real value.

Now it is easy to find vertices of a figure that arose from the plane intersecting the edges of the cuboid.

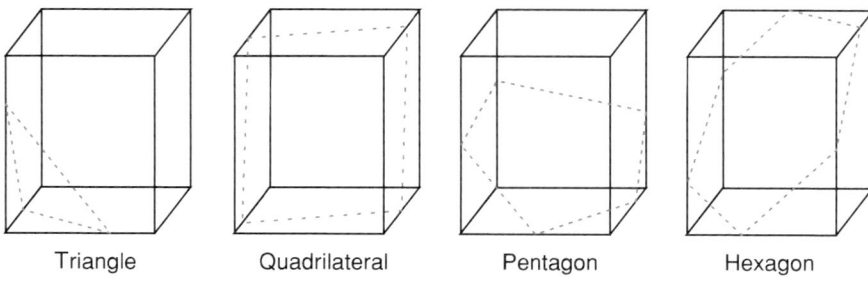

| Triangle | Quadrilateral | Pentagon | Hexagon |

Fig. 4.15 The possible shapes of polygons formed by the intersection of the plane and the cuboid edges

The algorithm proceeds as follows: for a given d and a given edge designated by points $V_1 = (x_1, y_1, z_1)$, $V_2 = (x_2, y_2, z_2)$, the edge has a common point with the plane if:

$$((z_1 < -d) \wedge (-d < z_2)) \vee ((z_2 < -d) \wedge (-d < z_1)) \tag{4.50}$$

If (4.50) is true, then the coordinates of the common point are as follows:

$$V_c = \begin{pmatrix} \dfrac{x_1 - x_2}{z_1 - z_2} \cdot (-d) + \left(x_1 - \dfrac{x_1 - x_2}{z_1 - z_2} \cdot z_1 \right), \\[2ex] \dfrac{y_1 - y_2}{z_1 - z_2} \cdot (-d) + \left(y_1 - \dfrac{y_1 - y_2}{z_1 - z_2} \cdot z_1 \right), \\[2ex] -d \end{pmatrix} \tag{4.51}$$

The possible shapes of polygons are shown in Fig. 4.15. It is very important to notice that all the possible polygons are convex.

The next step is to triangulate the obtained polygons. The triangulation is an operation of partitioning a figure into a set of disjunctive triangles (because triangles are the only three-dimensional primitive that can be rendered).

We have proposed a new triangulation algorithm whose implementation is presented in Sect. 4.6.1—Triangularization of volume slices—C# code. As the input data, we take the set of points defined by their coordinates which constitute vertices of polygons. We want to order them (for example in the clockwise sequence) to create a set of disjunctive triangles. The first operation of the algorithm is to sort the vertices according to their x coordinate value (Fig. 4.16 presents the schema of the algorithm with a right-handed coordinate system). Then we choose the left-most and the right-most vertices (if there are two of them we can choose either). Then we visit all vertices that are connected with the edges that are above and to the right of the left-most vertice (this is shown in the image of Fig. 4.16 as the arrow with index 1). When there are no more vertices satisfying this condition, we start from the right-most vertex and visit all vertices that are

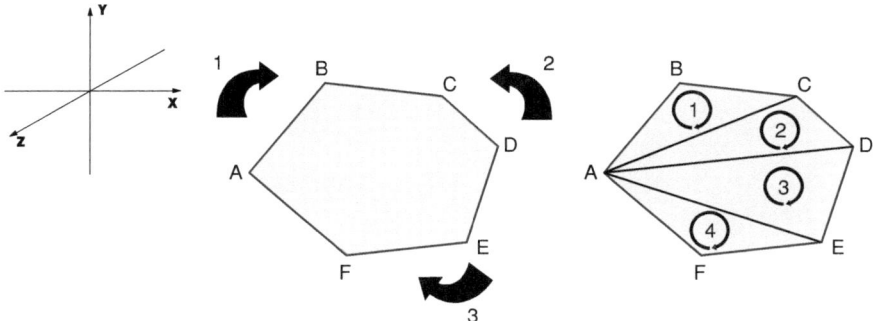

Fig. 4.16 The visualization of an example convex polygon triangulation algorithm (details in the text)

connected with right-most vertice by the edges that are above and to the left and were not visited before (arrow with the index 2). Then, we create a list of the visited vertices as follows: vertices from step 1 (A, B), vertices from step two in the reverse order (C, D) and all vertices that were left, ordered from right to left (E, F). Then we generate the triangles starting from the left-most vertex A by connecting it to the next two vertices which we have not yet used to create a triangle (A B C), (A C D), (A D E), (A E F). All of these triangles have vertices in the clockwise order.

In the texture-based algorithm, we generate a given number of polygons positioned in such a way that each of them is inside a cuboid holding the volumetric data. This means that if we increase the number of slices, the distance between them will shrink. An example result of a triangulation algorithm applied to a set of polygon slices is presented in Fig. 4.17.

After setting the texture information and matrix data, the rest of the program is executed in parallel on the GPU. The implementation of this algorithm is listed in Sect. 4.6.3—View-aligned slice rendering algorithm with gradient computation by the Pixel shader—HLSL code. We have used this particular HLSL to visualize data in many of our previous research projects [19–26]. The number of slices affects the quality of rendering results just as the sampling distance does volume ray-casting. Figure 4.18 shows the rendering results of an example volumetric dataset.

In the Pixel Shader, the HU value is classified using a transfer function stored in the Transfer look-up table. Then we add an acceleration technique that skips pixels with low alpha values (low alpha skipping) and which does not visually affect the quality of the image (Fig. 4.19). The algorithm then computes the gradient (we have shown a parallel implementation of the intermediate difference, the central difference and any 27-point gradient operator like the three-dimensional Sobel filter). After applying (4.47), the final color is produced. The same rendering is performed for each view-aligned slice starting from the last one (the farthest from the observer) to the first one (the closest to the observer). Both approaches—front

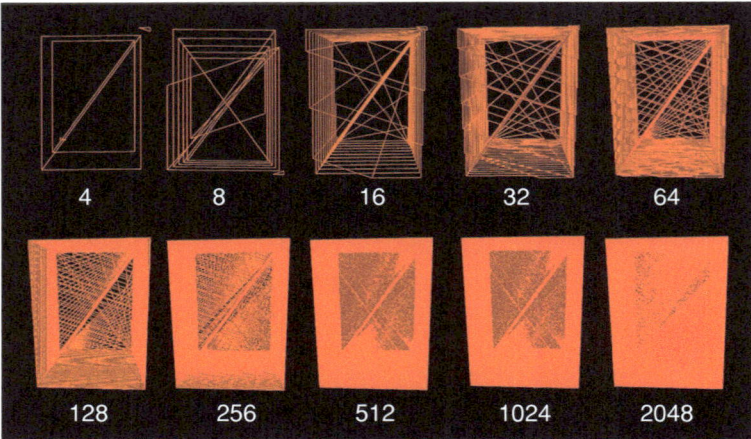

Fig. 4.17 Triangulating a set of polygons with a different number of primitives (4, 8, 16, 32, 64, 128, 256, 512, 1,024, and 2,048 slices)

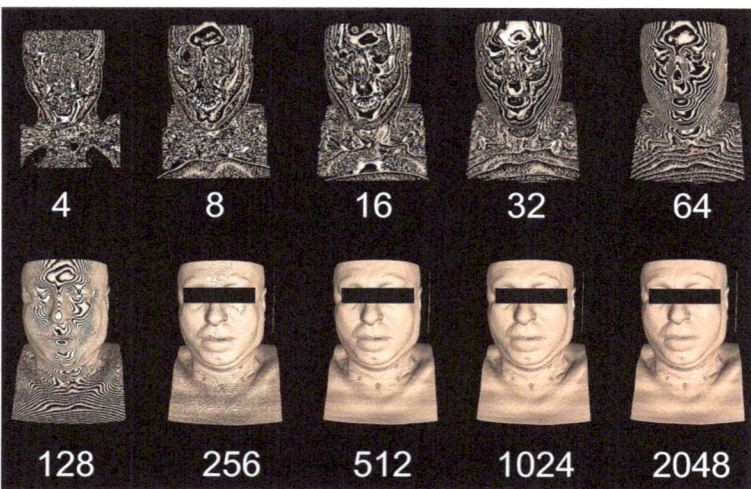

Fig. 4.18 The results of rendering a volume sized ($512 \times 512 \times 412$) with a different number of view-aligned slices. Face features become recognizable when the number of slices 256 or more. When the sampling exceeds the longest dimension of the data set (512) no rendering quality improvement can be observed

to back (with volume ray-casting) and back to front (with view-aligned slices) produce identical results when the same sampling distance (distance between slices) is set. For this reason, Fig. 4.14 can also be considered the results of a texture-based approach.

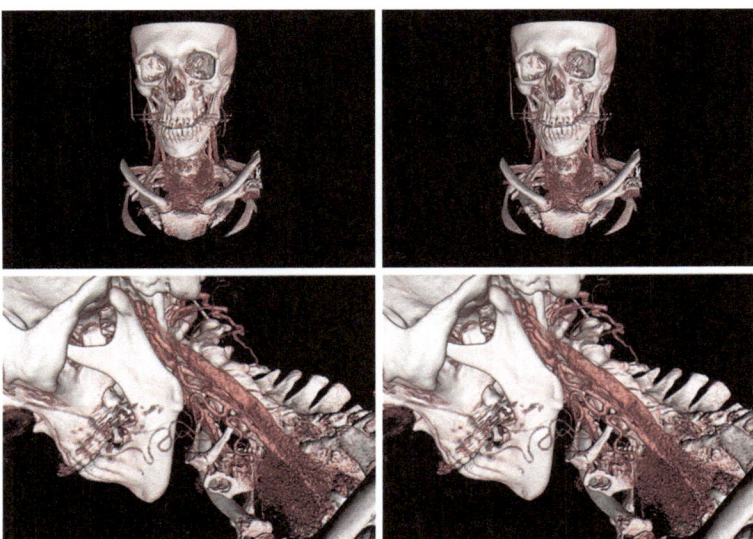

Fig. 4.19 Rendering CTA data with the same transfer function. The *bottom row* shows details. The right pair was processed using the low alpha skipping technique (the voxel with $a \leq 0.01$ was not visualized). The *left* pair illustrates the results of rendering without low alpha skipping. The visualizations do not show any noticeable differences

The next technique useful in data visualization consists in applying the so-called clipping plane, which limits the data set to be visualized. The most straightforward approach to creating the clipping effect is to limit the number of view-aligned slices rendered from the front that is observation, side (Fig. 4.20).

A factor which affects the realistic look ("reality") of the rendering is the gradient computation method that is selected. "Reality" is a factor that is quite hard to measure in an exact way. Figure 4.21 presents a visualization of a CTA image in which the lighting is computed using the gradient operators defined in Sect. 4.6.4. For our observation, the only visible differences are between the first images (the gradient computed with the intermediate difference method) and the rest of the set. The intermediate difference operator creates lighting artifacts that are easily visible compared to other methods. The illumination computed by the remaining operators is very similar.

Another problem that can appear during volume rendering is that the data size can exceed the GPU memory size. If so, the data has to be portioned into smaller blocks and each of these blocks should be loaded into the GPU texture memory from the RAM (or another storage location) and rendered separately. Parts of the volume should be drawn from the one whose middle point is the farthest from the position of the observer to the one whose middle point is the closest. The example polygon slices used for rendering large volumes are presented in Fig. 4.22.

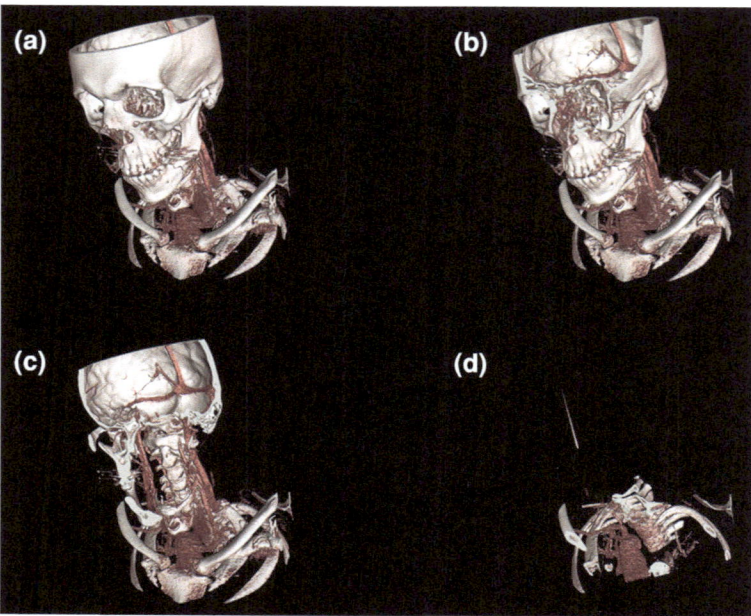

Fig. 4.20 The clipping plane effect achieved by limiting view-aligned slices from the front (observation) side

4.4 Superimposing 2D and 3D Data on Volumetric Images

Superimposition can be broadly defined as the process of combing multiple input images or some of their features into a single image, without causing a distortion, or a loss of information [27]. The aim of this process is to integrate both complementary and redundant information from multiple images to create a combined output image. Hence the new image generated should contain a more accurate description of the scene than any of the individual source images and be more suitable for human visual and machine perception.

In this book, we have covered two types of medical image modalities: two-dimensional computed tomography angiography (CTP) maps and three-dimensional CTA datasets. CTP maps do not require any specialized rendering technique to be properly displayed, but they could be more informative to a physician if they were presented in a three-dimensional environment. Thanks to this superimposition, the axial position of the slice can be more easily spotted and the interpretation of visualized brain structures is simplified. Figure 4.23 presents this kind of CTP on CTA superimposition.

The next problem we considered was how to visualize vascularization segmentation results. We wanted to present a three-dimensional rendering of the segmentation superimposed over the CTA volume. In our dataset it could not be

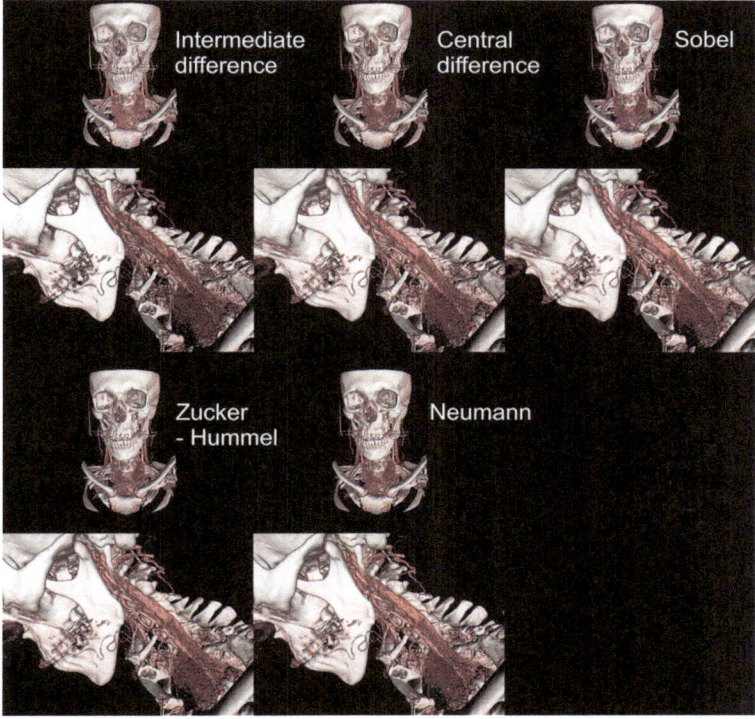

Fig. 4.21 Intermediate difference, central difference, Sobel, second row Zucker-Hummel, Neumann operators for computing gradients

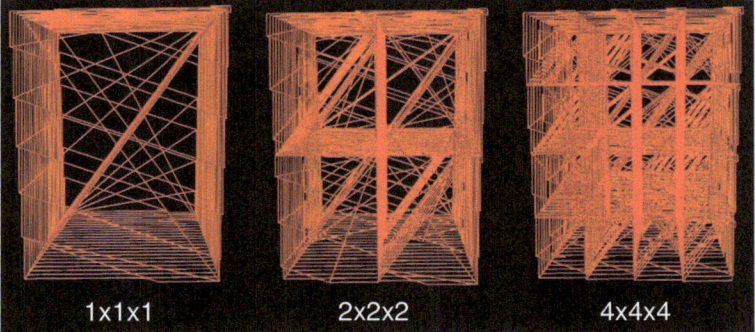

Fig. 4.22 The triangulation of a polygon set with different quantities of sub-volumes—blocks ($1 \times 1 \times 1$—one block of data; $2 \times 2 \times 2$—eight blocks, two for each dimension, $4 \times 4 \times 4$—64 blocks, four for each dimension). Each block consists of 32 view-aligned slices

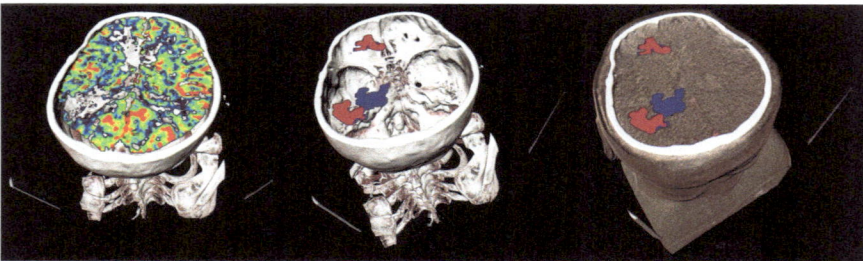

Fig. 4.23 A superimposition of a CTP image on a CTA image. The CTP image is rendered as the first top axial slice of a volumetric dataset. All image use the same CTA data, but the two on the *left* contain a transfer function from Fig. 4.11b and the third one from 4.11c. The first CTP image from the left is a cerebral blood flow (CBF) map, while the next two are prognostic maps generated for the CBF–CBV (cerebral blood volume) pair

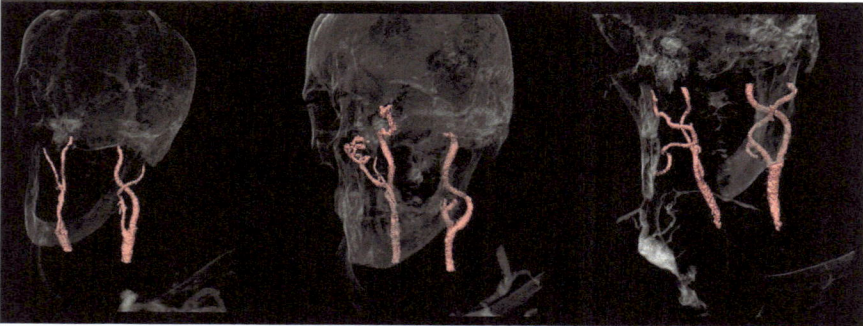

Fig. 4.24 The superimposition of vascularization segmentation results over CTA volumes. Both datasets are stored in a three-dimensional texture. The visualization now uses two transfer functions: the first for the CTA volume and the second for the segmentation volume. The transfer function for the CTA data is highly transparent while the transfer function for the segmentation is not transparent at all

done by just manipulating the transfer function to enhance blood vessels (if the right transfer function was sufficient to precisely enhance the vascularization, the segmentation might have been done by a simple thresholding). For this reason, we used a different approach: we put the segmentation results inside the same three-dimensional texture in which the HU values of the CTA are stored. This approach requires a lot of additional memory, but is very easy to write a single instruction multiple data–SIMD (HLSL) program that extends our visualization algorithm. The visualization now uses two transfer functions: the first for the CTA volume and the second for the segmentation volume. In the direct volume rendering procedure, RGBA values of voxels are computed in a single pixel shader procedure where the algorithm takes HU values from both three-dimensional textures. In Fig. 4.24, the transfer function for CTA data is highly transparent while the transfer function for the segmentation is not transparent at all. The condition in the

Table 4.1 A rendering speed comparison (FPS) between the volume ray-casting and texture-based approaches

	FPS with a given transfer function		
	A	B	C
Ray-casting with empty space skipping	30	12	17
Ray-casting without empty space skipping	14	11	11
Texture-based with precomputed gradient	8	8	8
Texture-based without alpha skipping	14	14	14
Texture-based with low alpha skipping	21	34	21

A, B, and C are transfer functions from Fig. 4.11. volume ray-casting

pixel shader examines if a particular voxel belongs to the segmented region. If it does, only the RGBA value of this voxel undergoes the color blending processing.

4.5 Rendering Speed Evaluation

The rest of this chapter will evaluate the speed of performing volume ray-casting and texture-based algorithms in the light of various parameters. As mentioned before, we will compare results using a CTA image sized $(512 \times 512 \times 415)$ with a 1024×768 viewport. Unless we stated that other parameters were used, numerical results are presented using the following: transfer function B from Fig. 4.11, the central difference gradient computation schema, low alpha skipping enabled, and a fixed position of the volume with respect to the observer. The assumed fixed position is important when comparing speeds of different approaches because the position of the volume might affects the rendering speed. The evaluation was carried out using two types of hardware configurations: a low-speed and a high-speed one. The results presented in Tables 4.1–4.8 are the averaged values from 30 s of rendering. As the standard deviation in each case was below 5 % of the average value, it is not shown in the Tables.

4.5.1 Evaluation on Low-Speed Hardware

The hardware was a consumer-quality PC with an Intel Core 2 Duo CPU 3.00 GHz processor, 3.25 GB RAM, and an Nvidia GeForce 9600 GT graphics card, running 32-bit Windows XP Professional. The computing power of this PC was comparable to current laptops.

The first experiment presented in Table 4.1 is a speed comparison between the volume ray-casting and the texture-based approach. We set the sampling distance to:

SampleDistance = 2*(dx, dy, dz)
and the number of slices for the texture algorithm to 256.

Table 4.2 A rendering speed comparison (FPS) of the texture-based algorithm with a precomputed gradient, without alpha skipping and with low alpha skipping as a function of the number of slices used in the visualization

Number of slices	Precomputed gradient			No alpha skipping			Low alpha skipping		
	A	B	C	A	B	C	A	B	C
4	728	728	728	1,107	1,106	1,107	1,498	2,020	1,501
8	280	280	280	458	458	459	667	985	670
16	130	130	130	219	219	219	328	493	329
32	64	64	64	108	108	108	163	248	164
64	32	32	32	54	54	54	81	126	82
128	16	16	16	27	27	27	41	63	41
256	8	8	8	14	14	14	21	34	21
512	4	4	4	7	7	7	11	19	11
1,024	2	2	2	4	4	4	6	9	6
2,048	1	1	1	2	2	2	3	4	3

A, B and C are transfer functions from Fig. 4.11

Empty space skipping can be seen to significantly affect the rendering speed if there are few half-transparent voxels (like in transfer function A). If the volume is highly transparent (case B) the speed gain is relatively small. A texture-based algorithm without alpha skipping is characterized by a constant rendering speed no matter which transfer function is used. The precomputed gradient method runs slower than the dynamic computation (caused by GPU hardware, not any algorithm) but this problem exceeds the scope of this book. If low alpha skipping is applied, this boosts the rendering speed of the texture-based method a lot. What is remarkable is that the ray-casting algorithm produces the best results if the data is not transparent (this is caused by the early ray termination condition in the rendering loop) while the texture-based algorithm is faster in highly transparent data (it can skip voxels that are too transparent to be visible in the final rendering).

Table 4.2 and Fig. 4.25 present the rendering speed of texture-based algorithms as a function of the number of slices used in the visualization. The horizontal axis is scaled logarithmically.

Once again, low alpha skipping greatly affects the rendering speed when it deals with a transfer function with many transparent and semi-transparent voxels (it is more than two times faster for transfer function B than in the approach without alpha skipping). The speed of the precomputed gradient and no alpha skipping approach is constant for different transfer functions if the number of slices stays the same. The gradient precomputation is the slowest approach because of the size of the volumetric data (the problem with gradient precomputation was mentioned before).

Table 4.3 and Fig. 4.26 (left) show a comparison of the rendering speed of a texture-based algorithm visualizing data partitioned into specific numbers of blocks. The horizontal axis is scaled logarithmically.

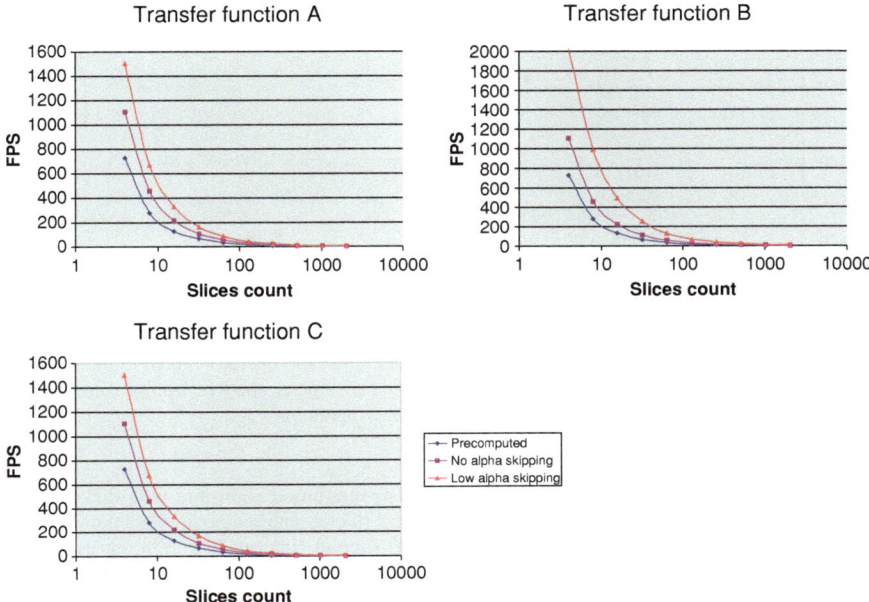

Fig. 4.25 A rendering speed comparison (FPS) of the texture-based algorithm with a precomputed gradient without alpha skipping and with low alpha skipping as a function of the number of slices used in the visualization

Table 4.3 A rendering speed comparison (FPS) of a texture-based algorithm visualizing data paritioned into specific numbers of blocks as a function of the number of view-aligned slices

Number of slices	$1 \times 1 \times 1$	$2 \times 2 \times 2$	$4 \times 4 \times 4$	$8 \times 8 \times 8$
4	2,020	1,100	168	22
8	985	520	103	13
16	493	252	57	8
32	248	124	31	4
64	126	62	16	2
128	63	31	9	1
256	34	16	5	0 (< 1)
512	19	8	3	0 (< 1)
1,024	9	4	2	0 (< 1)
2,048	4	3	1	0 (< 1)

The rendering speed decreases non-linearly along with the growing number of blocks. It should be remembered that when $4 \times 4 \times 4$ partitioning is used, we need four times fewer slices in each block to show the data with the same quality as in $1 \times 1 \times 1$ and two times fewer than in $2 \times 2 \times 2$. This is clearly visible in Fig. 4.22. However, if we want to keep the same rendering quality, loading more blocks from the RAM to the GPU texture memory is slower than rendering the

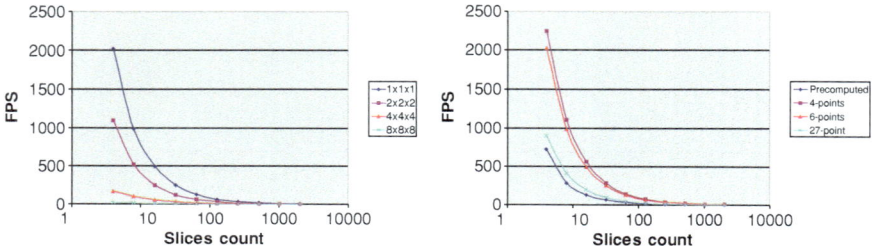

Fig. 4.26 *Left* rendering speed comparison (FPS) of a texture-based algorithm with a precomputed gradient without alpha skipping and with low alpha skipping as a function of the number of slices used in the visualization. *Right* rendering speed comparision (FPS) of a texture-based algorithm with different gradient computation methods and operators: precomputed (larger data set, no operations in pixel shader), and computed in a pixel shader: 4-point (intermediate difference), 6-point (central difference), 27-point (Sobel operator)

Table 4.4 Rendering speed comparison (FPS) of a texture-based algorithm with different gradient computation methods and operators: precomputed (larger data set, no gradient computing in the pixel shader), and computed in the pixel shader: 4-point (intermediate difference), 6-point (central difference), 27-point (Sobel operator)

Number of slices	Precomputed	4-point	6-point	27-point
4	728	2,245	2,020	903
8	280	1,109	985	407
16	130	562	493	192
32	64	285	248	95
64	32	144	126	47
128	16	72	63	23
256	8	36	34	12
512	4	19	19	7
1,024	2	9	9	3
2,048	1	5	4	2

entire data at once (for example the FPS of $1 \times 1 \times 1$ with 1,024 slices > FPS of $2 \times 2 \times 2$ with 512 > FPS of $8 \times 8 \times 8$ with 256).

Table 4.4 and Fig. 4.26 (right) show the rendering speed comparison of a texture-based algorithm with different approaches to gradient computation (as presented in Fig. 4.21).

It is noticeable that the more points we need for computing the gradient, the slower the algorithm becomes (the problem with gradient precomputation has been mentioned before). The difference between a 4-point and a 6-point operator decreases as the number of slices, reaches a value sufficient for reliably visualizing the CTA (256 and more).

Table 4.5 Rendering speed comparison (FPS) of the volume ray-casting and texture-based approaches

	FPS with a given transfer function		
	A	B	C
Ray-casting with empty space skipping	276	105	138
Ray-casting without empty space skipping	129	79	92
Texture-based with precomputed gradient	49	49	49
Texture-based without alpha skipping	97	97	97
Texture-based with low alpha skipping	114	222	112

A, B and C are transfer functions from Fig. 4.11

4.5.2 Evaluation on High-Speed Hardware

The hardware was a consumer-quality PC with an Intel Core i7-4470 CPU 3.40 GHz processor, 8 GB RAM, and an Nvidia GeForce GTX 770 graphics card, running 64-bit Windows 7 Home premium. This PC is of an up-to-date hardware configuration (purchased in mid-2013).

We used exactly the same benchmarks as in the previous section. The results obtained confirmed the observations we made for low-speed hardware. Consequently, the discussion of results from Sect. 4.5.1 applies to this section as well and we have decided not to repeat it.

The first experiment presented in Table 4.5 is a speed comparison between the volume ray-casting and the texture-based approach. We set the sampling distance to:

SampleDistance = 2*(dx, yx, dz)
and the number of slices for the texture algorithm to 256.

Table 4.6 and Fig. 4.27 present the rendering speeds of texture-based algorithms as a function of the number of slices used in the visualization. The horizontal axis is scaled logarithmically.

Table 4.7 and Fig. 4.28 (left) show a comparison of the rendering speed of a texture-based algorithm that visualizes data paritioned into given numbers of blocks. The horizontal axis is logarithmic.

Table 4.8 and Fig. 4.28 (right) present a comparison of the rendering of a texture-based algorithm using different approaches to gradient computation (as presented in Fig. 4.21).

Table 4.6 A rendering speed comparison (FPS) of a texture-based algorithm with a precomputed gradient without alpha skipping and with low alpha skipping as a function of the number of slices used in the visualization

Number of slices	Precomputed gradient			No alpha skipping			Low alpha skipping		
	A	B	C	A	B	C	A	B	C
4	2,445	2,445	2,445	5,989	5,989	5,989	6,320	6,268	6,310
8	1,550	1,550	1,550	4,333	4,333	4,333	4,589	5,511	5,266
16	758	758	758	1,996	1,996	1,996	2,143	3,671	2,588
32	378	378	378	902	902	902	873	1,908	1,127
64	192	192	192	420	420	420	424	974	474
128	98	98	98	197	197	197	207	488	226
256	49	49	49	97	97	97	105	230	113
512	25	25	25	50	50	50	54	112	60
1,024	13	13	13	27	27	27	28	57	31
2,048	6	6	6	13	13	13	14	29	15

A, B and C are transfer functions from Fig. 4.11

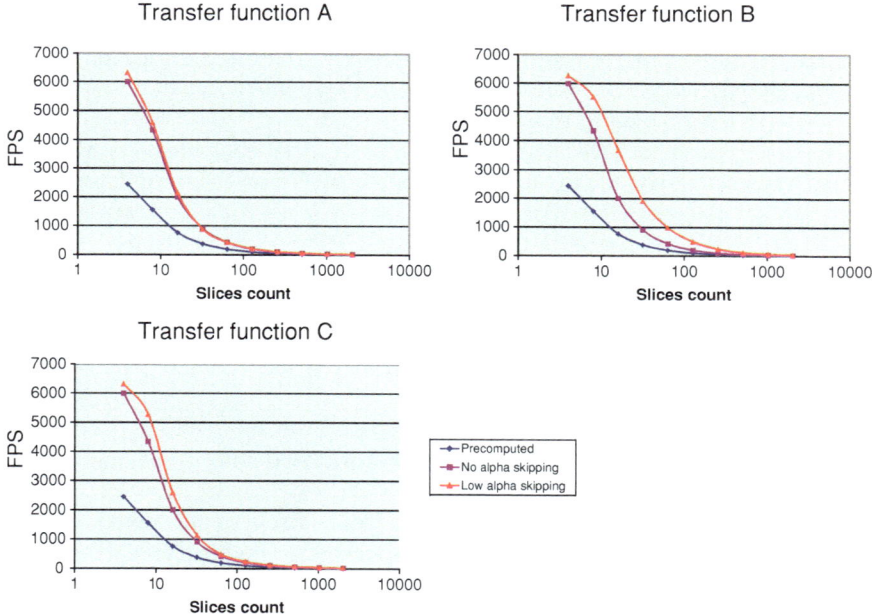

Fig. 4.27 A rendering speed comparision (FPS) of a texture-based algorithm with a precomputed gradient without alpha skipping and with low alpha skipping as a function of the number of slices used in the visualization

Table 4.7 A rendering speed comparison (FPS) of a texture-based algorithm visualizing data paritioned into given numbers of blocks as a function of the number of view-aligned slices

Number of slices	$1 \times 1 \times 1$	$2 \times 2 \times 2$	$4 \times 4 \times 4$	$8 \times 8 \times 8$
4	6,268	2,132	352	48
8	5,511	1,471	217	30
16	3,671	904	123	17
32	1,908	509	66	9
64	974	276	34	5
128	488	144	18	3
256	230	73	9	2
512	112	37	5	1
1,024	57	19	3	0 (<1)
2,048	29	10	2	0 (<1)

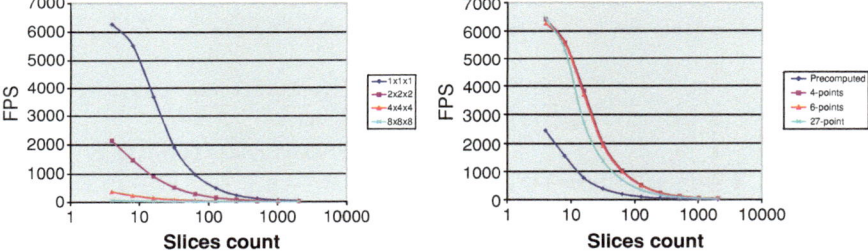

Fig. 4.28 On the *left* a rendering speed comparison (FPS) of a texture-based algorithm with a precomputed gradient without alpha skipping and with low alpha skipping as a function of the number of slices used in the visualization. On the *right* a rendering speed comparison (FPS) of a texture-based algorithm with different gradient computation methods and operators: precomputed (larger data set, no operations in the pixel shader), and computed in the pixel shader: 4-point (intermediate difference), 6-point (central difference), 27-point (Sobel operator)

Table 4.8 A rendering speed comparison (FPS) of a texture-based algorithm with different gradient computation methods and operators: precomputed (larger data set, no gradient computing in the pixel shader), and computed in the pixel shader: 4-point (intermediate difference), 6-point (central difference), 27-point (Sobel operator)

Number of slices	Precomputed	4-point	6-point	27-point
4	2,445	6,412	6,268	6,452
8	1,550	5,575	5,511	5,285
16	758	3,810	3,671	2,695
32	378	1,997	1,908	1,362
64	192	1,020	974	686
128	98	511	488	338
256	49	241	230	166
512	25	117	112	83
1,024	13	58	57	42
2,048	6	29	29	21

4.6 Implementations

4.6.1 Triangularization of Volume Slices: C# Code

```
public static VertexPositionTexture[]Triangularization(
      ArrayList pointCollection)
{
      ArrayList sortedArrayList = SortPoints(pointCollection);
        int triangleCount = sortedArrayList.Count - 2;
        VertexPositionTexture[] vpt =
              new VertexPositionTexture[3 * triangleCount];

      //Connect vertices and create traignels
        for (int a = 0; a < triangleCount; a++)
        {
                      vpt[3 * a].Position = (Vector3)sortedArrayList[0];
                      vpt[(3 * a) + 1].Position
                          = (Vector3)sortedArrayList[a + 1];
                      vpt[(3 * a) + 2].Position
                          = (Vector3)sortedArrayList[a + 2];
        }
        return vpt;
}

//Compare with Figure 5.16
private static ArrayList SortPoints(ArrayList pointCollection)
{
      ArrayList sortedArrayList = new ArrayList();
        ArrayList sortedArrayListHelp = new ArrayList();
        //sort points from left to right along X axis
        pointCollection.Sort(new IComparerX());
        Vector3 mostLeftest = (Vector3)pointCollection[0];
        Vector3 mostRightest
              = (Vector3)pointCollection[pointCollection.Count - 1];

        Vector3 current = mostLeftest;
        //from left to right and up
        Vector3 mostRightestAndUp;
```

```
for (int a = 0; a < pointCollection.Count; a++)
{
        if (current.Y <= ((Vector3)pointCollection[a]).Y)
        {
                sortedArrayList.Add(pointCollection[a]);
                current = (Vector3)pointCollection[a];
                pointCollection.RemoveAt(a);
                a--;
        }
}
mostRightestAndUp = current;
current = mostRightest;
//from right to left and up
for (int a = pointCollection.Count - 1; a >= 0; a--)
{
                if (current.Y <= ((Vector3)pointCollection[a]).Y
        && mostRightestAndUp.X <= ((Vector3)pointCollection[a]).X)
        {
                sortedArrayListHelp.Add(pointCollection[a]);
                current = (Vector3)pointCollection[a];
                pointCollection.RemoveAt(a);
          }
}
for (int a = sortedArrayListHelp.Count - 1; a >= 0; a--)
{
                sortedArrayList.Add(sortedArrayListHelp[a]);
 }
//add rest of the elements from right to left
while (pointCollection.Count > 0)
        {
        sortedArrayList.Add(pointCollection[pointCollection.Count
                - 1]);
        pointCollection.RemoveAt(pointCollection.Count - 1);
}
return sortedArrayList;
}


private class IComparerX : IComparer
    {
        int IComparer.Compare(object a, object b)
                {
            Vector3 c1 = (Vector3)a;
            Vector3 c2 = (Vector3)b;
            if (c1.X > c2.X) return 1;
            if (c1.X < c2.X) return -1;
            else return 0;
                }
    }
```

4.6.2 *Volume Ray-Casting Rendering Algorithm: HLSL Code*

```
//---------------------------
//Variables
//---------------------------

//Transform matrix
float4x4 WorldViewProj;
//Distance between slices on ray
float3 SampleDist;
//Maximal number cf iterations
int Iterations;
//Scaling factor of the rendered data
float4 ScaleFactor;

//Direction of ligt
float3 LightDirection = float3(0, 1, 1);
//Sampling along dimensions
float dX;
float dY;
float dZ;


//---------------------------
//Textures and samplers
//---------------------------

//Front and back face
texture2D Front;
texture2D Back;
//Data
texture3D Volume;
//Transfer function
texture2D Transfer;


sampler2D FrontS = sampler_state
{
     Texture = <Front>;
     MinFilter = POINT;
```

```
        MagFilter = POINT;
        MipFilter = LINEAR;

        AddressU = Border;              // border sampling in U
        AddressV = Border;              // border sampling in V
        BorderColor = float4(0,0,0,0);  // outside of border should be black
};

sampler2D BackS = sampler_state
{
        Texture = <Back>;
        MinFilter = POINT;
        MagFilter = POINT;
        MipFilter = LINEAR;

        AddressU = Border;              // border sampling in U
      AddressV = Border;                // border sampling in V
      BorderColor = float4(0,0,0,0);    // outside of border should be black
};

sampler3D VolumeS = sampler_state
{
        Texture = <Volume>;
        MinFilter = LINEAR;
        MagFilter = LINEAR;
        MipFilter = LINEAR;

        AddressU = Border;              // border sampling in U
        AddressV = Border;              // border sampling in V
        AddressW = Border;
        BorderColor = float4(0,0,0,0);  // outside of border should be black
};

sampler1D TransferS = sampler_state
{
        Texture = <Transfer>;
        MinFilter = LINEAR;
        MagFilter = LINEAR;
        MipFilter = LINEAR;

        AddressU  = CLAMP;
        AddressV  = CLAMP;
};

struct VertexShaderInput
```

```
      {
            float4 Position : POSITION0;
            float2 texC                 : TEXCOORD0;
      };


      struct VertexShaderOutput
      {
            float4 Position           : POSITION0;
            float3 texC               : TEXCOORD0;
            float4 pos                : TEXCOORD1;
      };


      //----------------------------
      //Helper functions
      //----------------------------


      //Helper function for gradient
      float  compGradFragment(float  cordX1,  float  cordX2,  float  cordY1,  float
cordY2, float cordZ1, float cordZ2)
      {
            cordX1 = saturate(cordX1);
            cordX2 = saturate(cordX2);
            cordY1 = saturate(cordY1);
            cordY2 = saturate(cordY2);
            cordZ1 = saturate(cordZ1);
            cordZ2 = saturate(cordZ2);


            return  (tex3Dlod(VolumeS,  float4(cordX2,  cordY2,  cordZ2,  0)).x  -
tex3Dlod(VolumeS, float4(cordX1, cordY1, cordZ1, 0)).x);
      }


      //----------------------------
      //Computes gradient with central difference schema
      //----------------------------
      float3 compGradCD(float cordX, float cordY, float cordZ)
      {
            float3 grad = float3(0, 0, 0);
            grad.x = compGradFragment(cordX - dX, cordX + dX,
                        cordY, cordY, cordZ, cordZ);
            grad.y = compGradFragment(cordX, cordX,
                        cordY - dY, cordY + dY, cordZ, cordZ);
            grad.z = compGradFragment(cordX, cordX,
                        cordY, cordY, cordZ - dZ, cordZ + dZ);
            return grad;
      }
```

```
//----------------------------
//Main vertex shader
//----------------------------
VertexShaderOutput RayCastingVS(VertexShaderInput input)
{
     VertexShaderOutput output;
     float4 pHelp = input.Position;
     pHelp.x = pHelp.x - .50f;
     pHelp.y = pHelp.y - .50f;
     pHelp.z = pHelp.z - .50f;

     output.Position = mul(pHelp * ScaleFactor, WorldViewProj);

     output.texC = input.Position.xyz;
     output.pos = output.Position;
     return output;
}


//----------------------------
//Renders front and back face (see Figure 5.12)
//----------------------------
float4 FacePS(VertexShaderOutput input) : COLOR0
{
    return float4(input.texC, 1.0f);
}


//----------------------------
//Main ray casting pixel shader
//----------------------------
float4 RayCastingPS(VertexShaderOutput input) : COLOR0
{
     //Calculates projective texture coordinates
     //used to project the front and back position textures onto the cube
     float2 texC = input.pos.xy /= input.pos.w;
     texC.x =  0.5f*texC.x + 0.5f;
     texC.y = -0.5f*texC.y + 0.5f;
     float3 front = tex2D(FrontS, texC).xyz;
     float3 back = tex2D(BackS, texC).xyz;
     float3 dir = normalize(back - front);
     float4 pos = float4(input.texC, 0);
     float4 dst = float4(0, 0, 0, 0);
     float4 src = 0;

     float4 value = 0;
```

```
        float3 L = LightDirection;
        L = normalize( L );

        //Computes sampling distance along the ray
        float3 Step = dir * SampleDist;
        for(int i = 0; i < Iterations; i++)
        {
                pos.w = 0;
                //Get HU value of voxel on the ray
                value = tex3Dlod(VolumeS, pos);
                //Get the rgba value of voxel from transfer function
                src = tex1Dlod(TransferS, value.x);

                float3 grad = compGradCD(pos.x, pos.y, pos.z);
                if (any(grad))
                        grad = normalize(grad);
                else
                        grad = 0;
                //Computes diffuse component (5.47)
                float diffuse = dot(grad, L);
                //Computes Phong model (5.45) without specular component
                src.rgb = diffuse * src.rgb + (.25f * src.rgb);
                //Front to back blending (5.43)
                src.rgb *= src.a;
                dst = (1.0f - dst.a)*src + dst;
                //Early ray termination
                if(dst.a >= .95f)
                        i = Iterations;
                else
                {
                        //Move along the ray
                        pos.xyz += Step;
                        //Break if the position is greater than <1, 1, 1>
                        if(pos.x > 1.0f || pos.y > 1.0f || pos.z > 1.0f)
                                i = Iterations;
                }
        }
        return dst;
}

//--------------------------
//Renders front and back face (see Figure 5.12)
//--------------------------
technique RenderFace
```

```
{
    pass Pass1
    {
        VertexShader = compile vs_2_0 RayCastingVS();
        PixelShader = compile ps_2_0 FacePS();
    }
}

//---------------------------
//Main technique
//---------------------------

technique RayCasting
{
    pass Pass1
    {
        VertexShader = compile vs_3_0 RayCastingVS();
        PixelShader = compile ps_3_0 RayCastingPS();
    }
}
```

4.6.3 View-Aligned Slice Rendering Algorithm with Gradient Computation in the Pixel Shader: HLSL Code

```
//---------------------------
//Variables
//---------------------------
float4x4 World;
float4x4 View;
float4x4 Projection;
//Data
texture3D Volume;
//Direction of light
float3 LightDirection;

//Coordinates of cube egdes
float MaxZ;
float MinZ;
float MaxX;
float MinX;
float MaxY;
float MinY;
```

```
//Sampling along dimensions
float dX;
float dY;
float dZ;

//2 * dx, 2 * dy, 2 * dz
float dX2;
float dY2;
float dZ2;
//Matrix for 27-points gradient operators
float convolutionMatrix [3 * 3 * 3 * 3];

//---------------------------
//Textures and samplers
//---------------------------

Texture Transfer;
sampler TransferS = sampler_state {
texture = <Transfer>;
magfilter = LINEAR;
minfilter = LINEAR;
mipfilter=LINEAR;
AddressU = mirror;
AddressV = mirror;
};


sampler3D VolumeS = sampler_state
{
     Texture = <Volume>;
     MinFilter = LINEAR;
     MagFilter = LINEAR;
     MipFilter = LINEAR;

     AddressU = Mirror;               // border sampling in U
     AddressV = Mirror;               // border sampling in V
     AddressW = Mirror;
     BorderColor = float4(0,0,0,0);   // outside of border should be black
};


struct VertexShaderInput
{
     float4 Position : POSITION0;
```

```
      float2 texC                : TEXCOORD0;
};

struct VertexShaderOutput
{
      float4 Position : POSITION0;
      float3 texC      : TEXCOORD0;

};

//---------------------------
//Helper functions
//---------------------------

float compGradFragment(float cordX1, float cordX2,
      float cordY1, float cordY2, float cordZ1, float cordZ2)
{
      cordX1 = saturate(cordX1);
      cordX2 = saturate(cordX2);
      cordY1 = saturate(cordY1);
      cordY2 = saturate(cordY2);
      cordZ1 = saturate(cordZ1);
      cordZ2 = saturate(cordZ2);

    return (tex3Dlod(VolumeS, float4(cordX2, cordY2, cordZ2, 0)).x
      - tex3Dlod(VolumeS, float4(cordX1, cordY1, cordZ1, 0)).x);
}

//Computes gradient with central difference schema
float3 compGradCD(float cordX, float cordY, float cordZ)
{
      float3 grad = float3(0, 0, 0);
      grad.x = compGradFragment(cordX - dX, cordX + dX,
              cordY, cordY, cordZ, cordZ);
      grad.y = compGradFragment(cordX, cordX,
              cordY - dY, cordY + dY, cordZ, cordZ);
      grad.z = compGradFragment(cordX, cordX,
              cordY, cordY, cordZ - dZ, cordZ + dZ);
      return grad;
}

//Computes gradient with intermediate difference schema
float3 compGradID(float cordX, float cordY, float cordZ)
{
      float3 grad = float3(0, 0, 0);
```

```
        float cV = tex3Dlod(VolumeS, float4(cordX, cordY, cordZ, 0)).x;
        float xV = tex3Dlod(VolumeS, float4(cordX - dX, cordY, cordZ, 0)).x;
        float yV = tex3Dlod(VolumeS, flcat4(cordX, cordY - dY, cordZ, 0)).x;
        float zV = tex3Dlod(VolumeS, float4(cordX, cordY, cordZ - dZ, 0)).x;

        grad.x = cV - xV;
        grad.y = cV - yV;
        grad.z = cV - zV;
        return grad;
}


//Coputes gradient using convolution with 27-points gradient kernel
float3 compGradConvolution(float cordX, float cordY, float cordZ)
{
        float3 grad = float3(0, 0, 0):
        int a, b, c;

        for (a = -1; a <= 1; a++)
             for (b = -1; b <= 1; b++)
                  for (c = -1; c <= 1; c++)
              {
                    int help = ((a + 1) * 9) + ((b + 1) * 3)
                           + (c + 1);
                    grad.x = grad.x
                           + tex3Dlod(VolumeS, float4(cordX + (a * dX),
                           ccrdY  + (b * dY), cordZ + (c * dZ), 0)).x
                                    * convolutionMatrix[help];
                    grad.y = çrad.y
                           + tex3Dlod(VolumeS, float4(cordX + (a * dX),
                            cordY  + (b * dY), cordZ + (c * dZ), 0)).x
                                    * convolutionMatrix[27 + help];
                    grad.z = grad.z
                    + tex3Dlcd(VolumeS, float4(cordX + (a * dX),
                    cordY  + (b * dY), cordZ + (c * dZ), 0)).x
                                    * convolutionMatrix[54 + help];
              }
        return grad;
}


//---------------------------
//Main vertex shader
//---------------------------


VertexShaderOutput TechniqueAlignedVS(VertexShaderInput input)
{
```

```
        float4 inputHelp = input.Position;

        VertexShaderOutput output;
        float4 worldPosition = mul(inputHelp, World);
        float4 viewPosition = mul(worldPosition, View);
        output.Position = mul(viewPosition, Projection);

        float A = (dX2 -1)/(MinX - MaxX);
        float B = dX -(A *MinX);
        float x = A * input.Position.x + B;

        A = (dY2 -1)/(MinY - MaxY);
        B = dY -(A *MinY);
        float y = A * input.Position.y + B;


        A = (dZ2 -1)/(MinZ - MaxZ);
        B = dZ -(A *MinZ);
        float z = A * input.Position.z + B;

        //coordinates of texture
        output.texC = float3(saturate(x) , saturate(y) , saturate(z));
        return output;
}


//---------------------------
//Main pixel shader
//---------------------------
float4 TechniqueAlignedPS(VertexShaderOutput PSIn) : COLOR0
{
        //HU value of voxel
        float4 pos = float4(PSIn.texC, 0);
        float4 value = tex3Dlod(VolumeS, pos);
        float2 coord = float2(value.x,0.0f);
        float4 src = 0;
        //Get the rgba value of voxel from transfer function
        src = tex2D(TransferS, coord);
        //low-alpha skipping
        if (src.a > 0.01f)
        {
                float3 L = LightDirection;
                L = normalize( L );
                float3 grad = float3(0, 0, 0);
                grad = compGradCD(PSIn.texC.x, PSIn.texC.y, PSIn.texC.z);
                //or
```

```
                //grad = compGradID(PSIn.texC.x, PSIn.texC.y, PSIn.texC.z);
                //or
                //grad = compGradConvolution(PSIn.texC.x, PSIn.texC.y,
                //         PSIn.texC.z);
                if (any(grad))
                {
                        grad = normalize(grad);
                }
                else
                        grad = 0;
                //Computes diffuse component (5.47)
                float diffuse = dot(grad, L);
                //Computes Phong model (5.45) without specular component
                src.rgb = (diffuse * src.rgb) + (.25f * src.rgb);
        }
        return src;
}


//--------------------------
//Pixel shader without light component
//It is used for rendering slice that is the closest to observer
//--------------------------

float4 TechniqueAlignedPS_NoLight(VertexShaderOutput PSIn) : COLOR0
{
float4 pos = float4(PSIn.texC, 0);
float4 value = tex3Dlod(VolumeS, pos);
//index the transfer function with the HU-value (value.a)
//and get the rgba value for the voxel
float2 coord = float2(value.x,0.0f);
float4 src = 0;
src = tex2D(TransferS, coord);
        return src;
}


//--------------------------
//Main technique
//--------------------------

technique TechniqueAligned
{
        pass Pass0
        {
                VertexShader = compile vs_3_0 TechniqueAlignedVS();
                PixelShader  = compile ps_3_0 TechniqueAlignedPS();
```

```
            }
    }


//---------------------------
//Technique that is used for rendering slice
//that is the closest to observer
//---------------------------

technique TechniqueAlignedNoLight
{
        pass Pass0
        {
                VertexShader = compile vs_3_0 TechniqueAlignedVS();
                PixelShader  = compile ps_3_0 TechniqueAlignedPS_NoLight();
        }
}
```

4.6.4 Three-Dimensional Discrete Gradient Operators

The surface normal forms an essential part of the illumination model. In direct volume rendering, a surface normal is often replaced by a gradient vector calculated at all points of interest:

$$\nabla f(x, y, z) = \left(\frac{df}{dx}, \frac{df}{dy}, \frac{df}{dz} \right). \tag{4.52}$$

There are several methods for numerical gradient calculation. The following are the most common:

- Intermediate difference operator:

$$\nabla f(x_i, y_j, z_k) = \begin{pmatrix} f(x_i + 1, y_j, z_k) - f(x_i, y_j, z_k), \\ f(x_i, y_j + 1, z_k) - f(x_i, y_j, z_k), \\ f(x_i, y_j, z_k + 1) - f(x_i, y_j, z_k) \end{pmatrix} \tag{4.53}$$

- Central difference operator:

$$\nabla f(x_i, y_j, z_k) = \frac{1}{2} \begin{pmatrix} f(x_i + 1, y_j, z_k) - f(x_i - 1, y_j, z_k), \\ f(x_i, y_j + 1, z_k) - f(x_i, y_j - 1, z_k), \\ f(x_i, y_j, z_k + 1) - f(x_i, y_j, z_k - 1) \end{pmatrix} \tag{4.54}$$

- Three-dimensional kernel of Neumann gradient operator [28]:

$$
\nabla_x := \frac{1}{52}\left(
\begin{pmatrix} -2 & 0 & 2 \\ -3 & 0 & 3 \\ -2 & 0 & 2 \end{pmatrix}
\begin{pmatrix} -3 & 0 & 3 \\ -6 & 0 & 6 \\ -3 & 0 & 3 \end{pmatrix}
\begin{pmatrix} -2 & 0 & 2 \\ -3 & 0 & 3 \\ -2 & 0 & 2 \end{pmatrix}
\right)
$$

$$
\nabla_y := \frac{1}{52}\left(
\begin{pmatrix} 2 & 3 & 2 \\ 0 & 0 & 0 \\ -2 & -3 & -2 \end{pmatrix}
\begin{pmatrix} 3 & 6 & 3 \\ 0 & 0 & 0 \\ -3 & -6 & -3 \end{pmatrix}
\begin{pmatrix} 2 & 3 & 2 \\ 0 & 0 & 0 \\ -2 & -3 & -2 \end{pmatrix}
\right)
$$

$$
\nabla_z := \frac{1}{52}\left(
\begin{pmatrix} -2 & -3 & -2 \\ -3 & -6 & -3 \\ -2 & -3 & -2 \end{pmatrix}
\begin{pmatrix} 0 & 0 & 0 \\ 0 & 0 & 0 \\ 0 & 0 & 0 \end{pmatrix}
\begin{pmatrix} 2 & 3 & 2 \\ 3 & 6 & 3 \\ 2 & 3 & 2 \end{pmatrix}
\right)
$$

$$(4.55)$$

- Three-dimensional kernel of Zucker-Hummel operator [29]:

$$
\nabla_x := \left(
\begin{pmatrix} -\frac{\sqrt{3}}{3} & 0 & \frac{\sqrt{3}}{3} \\ -\frac{\sqrt{2}}{2} & 0 & \frac{\sqrt{2}}{2} \\ -\frac{\sqrt{3}}{3} & 0 & \frac{\sqrt{3}}{3} \end{pmatrix}
\begin{pmatrix} -\frac{\sqrt{2}}{2} & 0 & \frac{\sqrt{2}}{2} \\ -1 & 0 & 1 \\ -\frac{\sqrt{2}}{2} & 0 & \frac{\sqrt{2}}{2} \end{pmatrix}
\begin{pmatrix} -\frac{\sqrt{3}}{3} & 0 & \frac{\sqrt{3}}{3} \\ -\frac{\sqrt{2}}{2} & 0 & \frac{\sqrt{2}}{2} \\ -\frac{\sqrt{3}}{3} & 0 & \frac{\sqrt{3}}{3} \end{pmatrix}
\right)
$$

$$
\nabla_y := \left(
\begin{pmatrix} \frac{\sqrt{3}}{3} & \frac{\sqrt{2}}{2} & \frac{\sqrt{3}}{3} \\ 0 & 0 & 0 \\ -\frac{\sqrt{3}}{3} & -\frac{\sqrt{2}}{2} & -\frac{\sqrt{3}}{3} \end{pmatrix}
\begin{pmatrix} \frac{\sqrt{2}}{2} & 1 & \frac{\sqrt{2}}{2} \\ 0 & 0 & 0 \\ -\frac{\sqrt{2}}{2} & -1 & -\frac{\sqrt{2}}{2} \end{pmatrix}
\begin{pmatrix} \frac{\sqrt{3}}{3} & \frac{\sqrt{2}}{2} & \frac{\sqrt{3}}{3} \\ 0 & 0 & 0 \\ -\frac{\sqrt{3}}{3} & -\frac{\sqrt{2}}{2} & -\frac{\sqrt{3}}{3} \end{pmatrix}
\right)
$$

$$
\nabla_z := \left(
\begin{pmatrix} -\frac{\sqrt{3}}{3} & -\frac{\sqrt{2}}{2} & -\frac{\sqrt{3}}{3} \\ -\frac{\sqrt{2}}{2} & -1 & -\frac{\sqrt{2}}{2} \\ -\frac{\sqrt{3}}{3} & -\frac{\sqrt{2}}{2} & -\frac{\sqrt{3}}{3} \end{pmatrix}
\begin{pmatrix} 0 & 0 & 0 \\ 0 & 0 & 0 \\ 0 & 0 & 0 \end{pmatrix}
\begin{pmatrix} \frac{\sqrt{3}}{3} & \frac{\sqrt{2}}{2} & \frac{\sqrt{3}}{3} \\ \frac{\sqrt{2}}{2} & 1 & \frac{\sqrt{2}}{2} \\ \frac{\sqrt{3}}{3} & \frac{\sqrt{2}}{2} & \frac{\sqrt{3}}{3} \end{pmatrix}
\right)
$$

$$(4.56)$$

- Three-dimensional kernel of Sobel operator [30]:

$$
\nabla_x := \left(
\begin{pmatrix} -1 & 0 & 1 \\ -3 & 0 & 3 \\ -1 & 0 & 1 \end{pmatrix}
\begin{pmatrix} -3 & 0 & 3 \\ -6 & 0 & 6 \\ -3 & 0 & 3 \end{pmatrix}
\begin{pmatrix} -1 & 0 & 1 \\ -3 & 0 & 3 \\ -1 & 0 & 1 \end{pmatrix}
\right)
$$

$$
\nabla_y := \left(
\begin{pmatrix} 1 & 3 & 1 \\ 0 & 0 & 0 \\ -1 & -3 & -1 \end{pmatrix}
\begin{pmatrix} 3 & 6 & 3 \\ 0 & 0 & 0 \\ -3 & -6 & -3 \end{pmatrix}
\begin{pmatrix} 1 & 3 & 1 \\ 0 & 0 & 0 \\ -1 & -3 & -1 \end{pmatrix}
\right)
$$

$$
\nabla_z := \left(
\begin{pmatrix} -1 & -3 & -1 \\ -3 & -6 & -3 \\ -1 & -3 & -1 \end{pmatrix}
\begin{pmatrix} 0 & 0 & 0 \\ 0 & 0 & 0 \\ 0 & 0 & 0 \end{pmatrix}
\begin{pmatrix} 1 & 3 & 1 \\ 3 & 6 & 3 \\ 1 & 3 & 1 \end{pmatrix}
\right)
$$

$$(4.57)$$

References

1. Nitschke B (2007) Professional XNA Game Programming: For Xbox 360 and Windows. Wiley Publishing, Inc. 10475 Crosspoint Boulevard Indianapolis, IN 46256, ISBN: 978-0-470-12677-6
2. Grootjans R (2009) XNA 3.0 Game Programming Recipes: A Problem-Solution Approach. ISBN-10: 143021855X
3. Jaegers K (2010) XNA 4.0 Game Development by Example: Beginner's Guide, Packt Publishing, ISBN-10: 1849690669
4. Reed A (2010) Learning XNA 4.0. O'Reilly Media. 1005 Gravenstein Highway North, Sebastopol, CA 95472
5. Carter C (2009) Microsoft® XNA™ game studio 3.0, 1st edn. Sams Publishing. 800 East 96th Street, Indianapolis, Indiana 46240 USA
6. Official website of MonoGame technology. http://www.monogame.net
7. Official documentation of MonoGame technology https://github.com/mono/MonoGame/wiki
8. Hefferon J (2009) Linear algebra. Virginia Commonwealth University Mathematics. http://joshua.smcvt.edu/linearalgebra/
9. The XNA Rendering Pipeline. http://msdn.microsoft.com/en-us/library/dd0417%28v=xnagamestudio.31%2.aspx
10. Lorensen WE, Cline HE (1987) Marching cubes: a high resolution 3D surface construction algorithm. Comput Graph 21(4):163–169
11. Nelson M (1995) Optical models for direct volume rendering. J IEEE Trans Visual Comput Graph 1(2):99–108
12. Engel K, Hadwiger M, Kniss J, Rezk-Salama C, Weiskopf D (2006) Real-time volume graphics 1st edn. A K Peters, ISBN: 1-56881-266-3
13. Hachaj T, Ogiela MR (2012) Visualization of perfusion abnormalities in augmented reality with GPU-based volume rendering algorithm. Comput Graph 36(3):163–169
14. http://graphicsrunner.blogspot.com/. Online tutorial about volume ray casting with code examples
15. Randima F (2004) GPU gems part 6—part VI: beyond triangles. Addison Wesley Pub Co Inc., ISBN-10: 0321228324
16. Phong BT (1975) Illumination for computer generated pictures. Commun ACM 18(6):311–317
17. Hachaj T, Ogiela MR (2011) Augmented reality approaches in intelligent health technologies and brain lesion detection. Availability, reliability and security for business, enterprise and health information systems. Lect Notes Comput Sci 6908:135–148
18. Krüger J, Westermann R (2003) Acceleration techniques for GPU-based volume rendering. In: Proceedings of IEEE visualization. pp 287–292
19. Hachaj T, Ogiela MR (2012) Segmentation and visualization of tubular structures in computed tomography angiography. Lect Notes Artif Intell 7198:495–503
20. Hachaj T, Ogiela MR (2012) Evaluation of carotid artery segmentation with centerline detection and active contours without edges algorithm. Lect Notes Comput Sci 7465:469–479
21. Ogiela MR, Hachaj T (2012) The automatic two-step vessel Lumen segmentation algorithm for carotid bifurcation analysis during perfusion examination. In: Watada J, Watanabe T, PhillipsWren G (eds) Intelligent decision technologies (IDT'2012), vol 2. Smart innovation systems and technologies, vol 16, pp 485–493
22. Ogiela MR, Hachaj T (2013) Automatic segmentation of the carotid artery bifurcation region with a region-growing approach. J Electron Imaging 22(3):033029. doi:10.1117/1.JEI.3.033029
23. Hachaj T, Ogiela MR (2012) Framework for cognitive analysis of dynamic perfusion computed tomography with visualization of large volumetric data. J Electron Imaging 21(4):043017. doi:10.1117/1.JEI.21.4.043017

24. Hachaj T (2014) Real time exploration and management of large medical volumetric datasets on small mobile devices—evaluation of remote volume rendering approach. Int J Inform Manage 34:336–343. doi:10.1016/j.ijinfomgt.2013.11.005
25. Hachaj T, Ogiela MR (2010) Augmented reality interface for visualization of volumetric medical data. Adv Intell Soft Comput 84:271–277 (Springer, Berlin, Heidelberg)
26. Hachaj T (2012) Pattern classification methods for analysis and visualization of brain perfusion CT maps. Comput Intell Parad Adv Pattern Classif 386:145–170
27. Yang Y, Park DS, Huang S, Rao N (2010) Medical image fusion via an effective wavelet-based approach. EURASIP J Adv Signal Process 2010:44
28. Neumann L, Csébfalvi B, König A, Gröller E (2000) Gradient estimation in volume data using 4D linear regression. Comput Graph Forum 19(3):351–358
29. Ballard DH, Brown CM (1982) Computer vision. Prentice Hall, INC. Englewood Cliffs, New Jersey 07632
30. Sobel I (1996) An isotropic $3 \times 3 \times 3$ volume gradient operator. Hewlett-Packard's Voxelator V-3 CD-ROM

Chapter 5
Natural User Interfaces for Exploring and Modeling Medical Images and Defining Gesture Description Technology

A Natural User Interface (NUI) is a type of human–machine interaction based on the automatic analysis of the user's natural behavior. These human actions are interpreted by the machine as commands that control system operations. Natural behavior is a group of activities performed by humans in everyday life to interact with their animated and unanimated environment. The main purpose of using the NUI is to simplify the access to the computer. NUI is to support intuitive inter-action methods that are very easy to teach. Users who have never been exposed to a particular application before should, with help of the NUI, handle it much faster than if they were to use a traditional graphic user interface (GUI) with a mouse or keyboard.

The most popular "natural behavior" uses in computer methods include eye tracking [1], facial expression identification [2], full body pose recognition [3], human pose tracking [4], detecting and recognizing hand postures [5], gesture-based interaction by multitouch interfaces [6], emotion analysis [7], natural interfaces using augmented reality (AR) [8], head tracking [9], voice interface [10].

If we look at the NIU from the perspective of a computer, it has to take over the role of a human interlocutor or simulate the reactions of an unanimated object (for example digital documents might be browsed like a paper book on a touchscreen). Hence the computer has to, more or less, imitate the process of world perception that is carried out by humans. Human beings gather data from their environment using their five senses: touch, sight, hearing, taste, and smell. A computer can be equipped with sensors that can acquire these types of signals, but obviously not all of them are useful for the NUI. Figure 5.1 presents three basic types of natural user interfaces. The division is based on the human sense to which a particular group of methods corresponds. For quite obvious reasons taste and smell are unsuitable for everyday human–computer interaction. On the other hand touch (touch user interface—TUI), sight (vision user interface—VUI) and hearing (audio user interface—AUI) can be handled quite well.

Table 5.1 shows the relationship between the three above NUI, and also key facts that must be taken into consideration when tailoring data analysis and rec-ognition methods before deploying these interfaces in a computer system. Audio

M. R. Ogiela and T. Hachaj, *Natural User Interfaces in Medical Image Analysis,*   205
Advances in Computer Vision and Pattern Recognition,
DOI: 10.1007/978-3-319-07800-7_5,
© Springer International Publishing Switzerland 2015

(a)   **(b)**

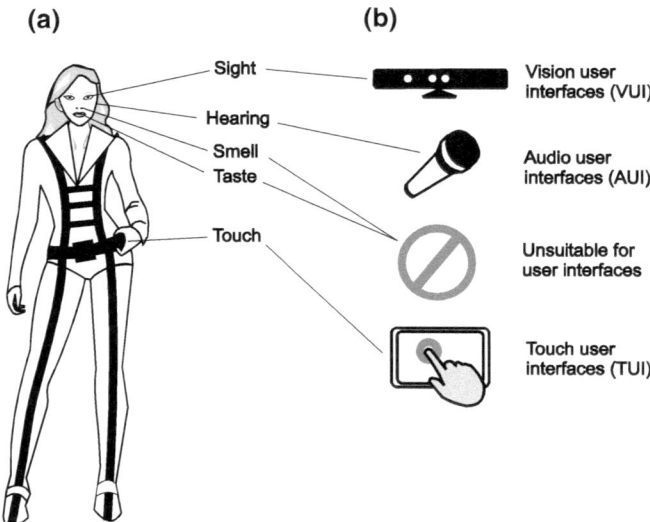

Fig. 5.1 Three basic types of natural user interfaces. The division is based on the human sense to which a particular group of methods corresponds. **a** The five senses, **b** natural user interfaces (*NUI*)

user interfaces are only mentioned to make the NUI division complete but their methods will not be discussed in this book. Should the reader be interested in AUI, they should start by reviewing the state of the art publications in this field, for example [11–15].

If readers are not convinced of the usefulness of the NUI approach, let us remind them of the evolution of computer interfaces over the last approximately 30 years. At the beginning of this period, computers were managed mostly via text-based interfaces in which all information was read from the screen and commands were input via a keyboard (for example in DOS). To operate the system efficiently, the user had to know many commands by heart, know additional command line options etc. Later more and more OSs introduced GUIs with icons and unified graphical appearance (predefined components and layouts) which often reduced the time that had to pass between the first contact with the software and using it for work. Voice command interactions have now been present for many years in cell phones, for example to speed up the dialing. Of course, many applications still allow shortcuts, keyboard commands and scripts as the most precise (but often the hardest to learn) type of interaction. Most prototypes of NUI systems presented in Table 5.1 were proposed many years ago, but due to the cost of the technology, they could not have been commercialized on a large scale. Nowadays, relatively cheap mobile devices equipped with multimedia hardware like microphones and cameras are the popular targets of customer interest. With this in mind we can conclude that potential users are interested in functionalities that are provided to them in this hardware, including NUI services. This interest

Table 5.1 The distinction between natural user interface approaches

	TUI	VUI	AUI
Signal dimensionality (per channel)	Mostly two-dimensional; sometimes three-or more dimensional when pressure or velocity measurements are available	Mostly two or three-dimensional	Mostly one-dimensional
Basis of interaction	Gesture recognition, touch-based screen cursor control	Hand, head, full body, finger and eye tracking, marker tracking, facial expression recognition, gesture recognition, rarely remote screen cursor controlling	Speech synthesis, speech recognition
Most popular registration devices	Touch pad, touch screen	RGB cameras, IR cameras (microsoft Kinect, leap motion controller), wireless three-dimensional manipulators (Nintendo Wii remote, Sony move controller)	Various audio registration devices (microphones)
Advantages	Very intuitive	Does not require touch-contact with registration device	Does not require touch-contact with registration device
Limitations	Requires touch-contact with the registration device, may be quite inaccurate when based only on finger touch, for precise manipulation a touch pen is required	Might require special lighting or environmental conditions to work properly, the accuracy decreases dramatically as distance grows, making precise screen cursor manipulation almost impossible	Might require special environmental conditions to work properly, voice commands and responses might be annoying for other people, one user might disrupt work of other AUI users, with distance the accuracy decreases, precise screen cursor manipulation is impossible

The section on "most popular devices" takes into account technologies that do not require specially designed environments to function (like motion capture) and are more or less "mobile" gives noticeable feedback to the industry and to scientific research on new applications for these multimedia sensors. It must be emphasized that the aim of a NUI is not to replace traditional interfaces like the keyboard or the mouse (because at present, the NUI lack the precision required to totally replace traditional input devices) but to simplify operating a computer or to be used in situations in which access to a mouse or a keyboard is difficult or impossible.

This chapter will present several applications of TUI and VUI in medical imaging systems. We will also mention important aspects and techniques of overcoming hardware limitations that make pattern recognition methods applicable to NUI using off-the-shelf sensors.

5.1   Touch User Interfaces

Nowadays, TUIs are mostly based on multitouch sensing surfaces. Touch user interfaces are among the most popular natural user interfaces used in almost all contemporary mobile devices like tablets, smartphones, cellphones, and many others. This is mainly because this interface is the most intuitive type of a NUI. In a TUI—based application, the behavior of the GUI imitates the reaction of a real world object to being touched by the user. Very often, the OS desktop simulates a real-life desktop that has different objects placed around it. We can, for example, drag these objects around the virtual desktop, activate them by clicking them or, for instance, browse multimedia galleries with a "swiping" finger move. This interface may not be accurate when operated with fingers, but the interaction does not require high-precision. TUI users do not need good coordination of movements (which is required when using, e.g., a mouse). Because a TUI is combined with an icon-based GUI, literacy is often not required. What is still in greater contrast to an AUI (which might erroneously be considered as easy to communicate with) it does not require the user to be able to speak fluently and comprehend words. We can clearly observe the potential of TUI while watching small children very quickly learn basic TUI functions necessary to operate mobile devices (see Fig. 5.2), sometimes even before they can clearly say their thoughts out loud.

5.1.1   Remote Volume Rendering on Mobile Devices

As personal healthcare is among the most important aspects of everyone's life, computer methods that have been proven to have technical and scientific potential are quickly developed and utilized in medicine [16]. The NUI is no exception. For example, more and more physicians want to have access to radiological images and reports on their PDAs (personal digital assistants) or smartphones. That is because a PDA gives them quick access to patients' health records without having to access data from larger and less mobile high-performance workstations. What is

Fig. 5.2 Two and a half year old child explores a multimedia gallery via a TUI

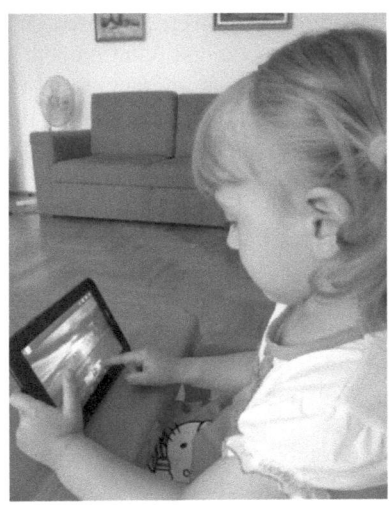

most important, and has been shown in [17], volumetric data interpretation of selected illnesses on PDSs might be as accurate as the interpretation of that data displayed on the PACS (picture archiving and communication) terminals. It can be concluded that mobile devices have the potential to expand radiologists' availability for consultation and expedite emergency patient management.

Most PDAs have TUIs in order to minimize their size and increase their portability. However, the small sizes of PDAs coupled with the need of low-power consumption today represent the main drivers limiting the computational power of these mobile devices. This limitation becomes a serious problem when dealing with image data, and particularly with volumetric images like CT (computed tomography). Many state of the art mobile devices (even cell phones) have programmable GPUs, but they do not support crucial hardware functionalities (like sufficient GPU RAM size, volumetric texturing, etc.,—for more details see Chap. 4 and [18]) which would enable the real-time visualization of medical data. For this reason, instead of transferring the whole image dataset to the client computer (the viewing station), the PDA frequently only acts as an interface to the remote server performing all the rendering procedures [19]. The user enters commands for the server through their personal interface displayed on their PDA. Only the final image, the product of image processing on the server, is transferred to the client and displayed on its screen.

Remote visualization is not a new idea. Before GPUs became capable of efficient SIMD (single instruction multiple data) processing, visualizations had to be done on a CPU in a MIMD (multiple instruction multiple data) architecture at supercomputer centers [20–23]. More recently, when single workstations with off-the-shelf GPU could deal with volume rendering of patient's data, the aim of research was not how to render the data but how to make the visualization accessible on various low-power devices. Many commercial solutions and scientific papers were proposed on this subject. For example, [24] adopts a remote rendering mode and point models and then proposes a transmission and rendering approach that can interact in real-time. At first, improved simple algorithms based on moving least squares and the display resolution of mobile devices is proposed. Then, a hierarchy selection of point models and a QoS transmission control strategy are given based on the interest area of the operator, the interest degree of the object in the virtual environment and the rendering error. Paper [25] presents a novel approach based on a controller that can automatically adjust 3D data streaming parameters using feedback measures from the client device. Experimental results prove the effectiveness of this solution in coping with bandwidth changes, thus providing high-Quality of Service (QoS) in remote visualizations. Cloud computing technology is a solution that can process a very large amount of information without adding to each client user's processing cost. In paper [26], authors propose an interactive rendering system for large 3D mesh models stored on a remote environment through a network of relatively small capacity machines, based on the cloud computing concept. Proposed system uses both model- and image-based rendering methods for efficient load balancing between a server and clients. On the server, the 3D models are rendered by the model-based method using a hierarchical data structure with Level of Detail (LOD). On the client, an arbitrary view is constructed using a novel image-based method, referred to as the Grid-Lumigraph, which blends colors from sampling images received from the server. Consequently, application services rendering remote medical images and electronic health records (EHR) have become a hot topic and stimulated increased interest in studying this subject in recent years. In paper [27], authors propose an EHR sharing and integration system in healthcare clouds and analyze the arising security and privacy issues in the access to and management of EHRs. In [28] authors present an interactive virtual colon navigation system on a PDA that is a client-server system over a wireless network. To improve the quality of the rendering results on the PDA, the overall rendering speed, and the user interactivity, the authors proposed three novel methods and adapt a GPU-based direct volume rendering technique. The image is rendered on a server with a direct volume rendering ray casting algorithm and are send to the client (PDA) on request from the device. The client sends a request for a series of consecutive frames. In the proposed method, the previous touch pen position and the current one are sent to the server from the client as the start position and the end position, respectively. Then the server computes several evenly spaced positions between the two positions, generating rendering frames for these positions and the end position, and transferring them to the client. The number of those positions was determined experimentally. In order to transfer data, first the server generates a rendering result as a 2D image and its vector data, which can be drawn rapidly on the client, such as lines and points. The rendered 2D image is then compressed by an image compression method, such as JPEG. Second, it sends the compressed 2D image and the vector data separately to the client. Finally, the client decompresses the compressed 2D image, displays it and draws the vector data on top of the image. Authors in [29] aim to develop a system that enables users in different regions to share a working environment for collaborative visualization with the potential for exploring huge medical datasets. The system consists of three major components: a mobile client (PDA), a gateway, and a parallel rendering server. The mobile client serves as a front end and enables users to choose the visualization and control parameters interactively and cooperatively. The gateway handles requests and responses between mobile clients and the rendering server for efficient communication. Through the gateway, it is possible to share working environments between users, allowing them to work together in a computer-supported cooperative work (CSCW) mode. Finally, the parallel rendering server is responsible for performing heavy visualization tasks. Paper [30] proposes an optimized image compositing scheme with a linear pipeline and adaptive transport to support efficient image delivery to a remote client. The proposed scheme arranges an arbitrary number of parallel processors within a cluster in a linear order and divides the image into a carefully selected number of segments, which flow through the linear in-cluster pipeline and wide-area networks to the remote client consecutively.

In the next section we will present an architecture description and an evaluation of the performance of a system that can be used for the real-time exploration and management of large medical volumetric datasets with low-power mobile devices like tablets or even cell phones.

5.1.2 *Exploration of Volumetric Datasets on Mobile Devices with TUI*

In our paper [31], we have proposed a prototype system enabling the real-time exploration of large medical volumetric datasets on small mobile devices using the remote volume rendering approach. In this paragraph we will briefly summarize its architecture and evaluation results.

The proposed system consists of two types of applications: client-side applications (rendering client) and one server-side application (rendering server). The client displays rendered volumes in two resolutions: low during interaction and full after interaction ends. In addition, the number of requests from the client has to be limited because the input interface would generate too many requests and the in-response outgoing data from the server could cause network latency.

The role of client applications is to supply physicians with a TUI for exploring volumetric medical data (Fig. 5.3). The role of the server is to receive orders from clients for remotely rendering 3D images and sending them back 2D results. The schema of the discussed system is shown in Fig. 5.4. In our proposal, the rendering client is an Android multithread application using OpenGL libraries for 2D data visualization. Android OS (our implementation requires at least the API level 10) is supported by multiple cellphones, smartphones, tablets, etc. which can be used as PDAs. The First thread is the GUI thread processing the event caused by the touch screen. If the user wants to change the orientation of the observed volume (for example rotate it), a new linear transfer matrix is computed. Matrix coefficients are

Fig. 5.3 TUI gestures used for exploring a volumetric image. At first glance, these are typical touch-screen gestures like dragging for X, Y axis translations, pinching and spreading for Z axis translations, dragging with "tap and hold" a virtual button for X, Y axis rotations

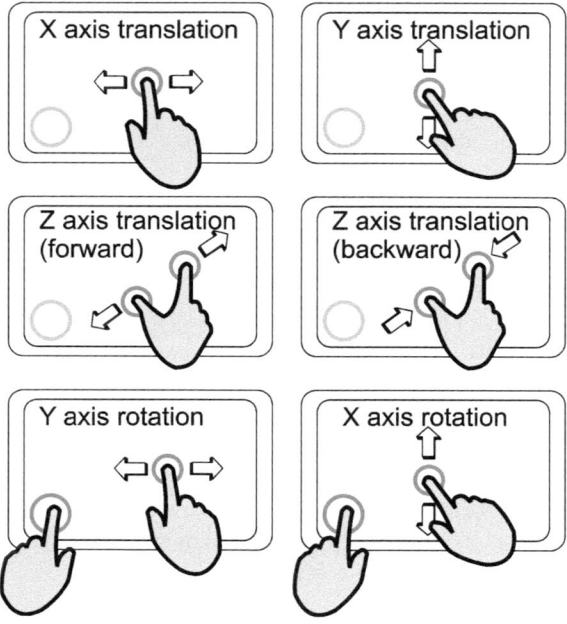

sent to the Rendering server with a request to create 2D projections of 3D data of a limited resolution. If the rendering request is send, the code in the thread sets the value of SIR (send render response) to 1. To limit the number of rendering requests, the following condition was used:

The request is send to the server only if

$$\sqrt{\left(\frac{\Delta x}{\text{screen width}}\right)^2 + \left(\frac{\Delta y}{\text{screen height}}\right)^2} > T \tag{5.1}$$

Where Δx, Δy is the relative distance (in pixels) along the vertical and horizontal axis, respectively, that the user's finger "traveled" in the drag mode over the touchscreen. The screen width and height represent the resolution of the screen. Δx, Δy values cumulate during the interaction and are set to 0 each time the request is sent to server.

The rotation and translation coefficients of the linear matrix are computed proportionally to Δx, Δy and are inversely proportional to the distance from the volume to the observer. The closer the user is to the observed volume, the more precise the interactions become. Our application's TUI facilitates X, Y, and Z axis translations and rotations around axes X and Y (see Fig. 5.3).

The second thread is Socket thread number 1. Its function is to initiate the connection with the rendering server, and every time new data arrives from the server, to create a new texture that can be visualized on the screen using the OpenGL library. The Socket thread 2 is used to send a request to the server to

Rendering client

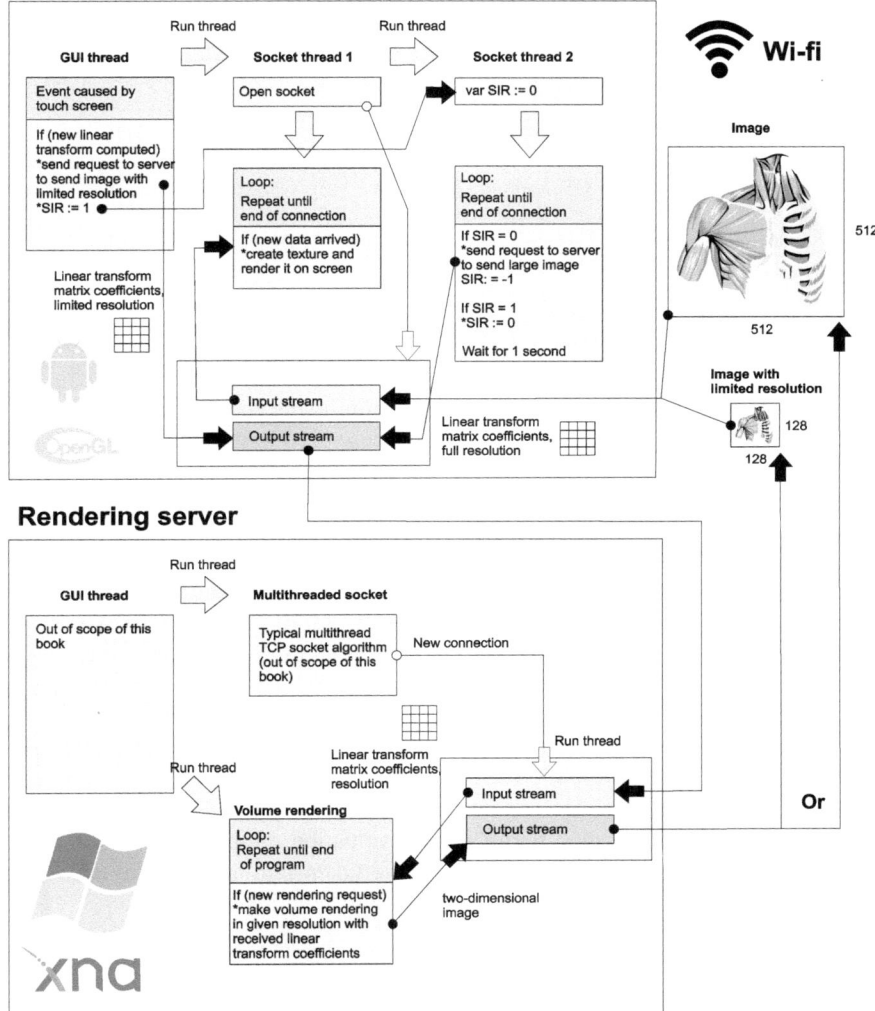

Fig. 5.4 The schema of a system enabling a real-time exploration of large medical volumetric datasets on small mobile devices using the remote volume rendering approach. Described in the text

create 2D projections of 3D data at the full resolution. The code in this thread operates in a loop. The request is sent if the SIR value equals 0 and then the server changes the SIR value to -1. If the SIR value equals 1, the server changes it to 0. Each iteration of the loop ends with an instruction that pauses the thread for 1 s. For this reason, the request for the full resolution image is sent no earlier than one second after the user stops interacting with the TUI.

Table 5.2 Hardware and OS parameters of devices used for evaluating the proposed remote rendering system

Server	Cell phone	Tablet
PC class computer	Model: Samsung Galaxy Y GT-S5360	Model: Samsung GALAXY Tab 2 7.0
OS 32-bit Windows 7 OS RAM 3.25 GB	Released 2011, October	Released 2012, April
CPU Intel Core 2 Duo CPU 3.00 GHz	OS Android OS, v2.3.6 (Gingerbread)	OS Android 4.1.1 (Jelly Bean)
GPU Nvidia GeForce	Display: 240 × 320 pixels, 3.0 inches	Display: 600 × 1024 pixels, 7.0 inches
GTX 770	RAM 512 MB	RAM 1 GB
	CPU 830 MHz	CPU 1.0 GHz dual-core

The rendering server is a Windows application using the XNA framework to perform the volume rendering with algorithms described in the Chap. 4. It consists of a GUI thread (which is irrelevant in this description), a multithreaded server socket, multiple run threads and a rendering thread. The multithreaded TCP/IP server is used for the communication between clients and the server. It starts a new run thread every time a new client connects to server. Run thread operates the incoming transmission from the client, containing the linear transform matrix and information about the requested output image resolution (low or full). Then, the run thread performs rendering with the volume rendering thread and sends back the requested visualization to the client. The communication in our solution is based on Wi-Fi LAN.

We have evaluated the performance of our system on a PC class computer as a rendering server and two mobile devices: a cell phone and tablet. The hardware and OS parameters of these devices are presented in Table 5.2. Figure 5.5 contains pictures taken during a system performance evaluation on these devices.

To test the algorithm performance, we have taken into account the following parameters:

- Drawing—the speed of drawing a texture on a screen measured in fps (frames per second).
- Loading—the loading time of a texture into the GPU RAM from the RAM measured in $s \cdot 10^{-2}$.
- Response—the time that passes between touching a client screen (changing linear transform coefficients), sending a rendering request from the device to the server and receiving an image with the updated position according to new transform from the server. Time measured in $s \cdot 10^{-2}$.
- Overall time—the sum of the Loading and Response times measured in fps.

Tables 5.3 and 5.4 present results of a system evaluation performed on a cellphone and a tablet. The presented values are averaged over 30 s of the inter-action. Because in each case the standard deviation was below 5 % of the average value we did not show it in tables.

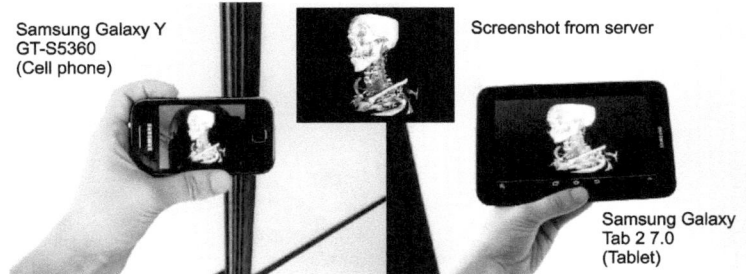

Samsung Galaxy Y
GT-S5360
(Cell phone)

Screenshot from server

Samsung Galaxy
Tab 2 7.0
(Tablet)

Fig. 5.5 A picture taken during the evaluation of system performance on devices presented in Table 5.2. The displayed data is 3D CTA (CTA). *From left to right* remote visualization on a cellphone screen, a screenshot from the rendering server and remote visualization on a tablet screen

Table 5.3 The results of a system evaluation performed on a cell phone

Phone

Texture size (pixels)	Drawing (fps)	Loading to memory $(s \cdot 10^{-2})$	Response $(s \cdot 10^{-2})$	Overall time (fps)
64^2	60.0	1.7	1.8	28.6
128^2	60.0	2.1	4.8	14.5
256^2	60.0	5.9	16.7	4.4
512^2	60.0	16.7	50.0	1.5
1024^2	60.0	47.0	142.2	0.5

Table 5.4 The results of a system evaluation performed on a tablet

Tablet

Texture size (pixels)	Drawing (fps)	Loading to memory $(s \cdot 10^{-2})$	Response $(s \cdot 10^{-2})$	Overall time (fps)
64^2	60.0	1.7	1.8	28.6
128^2	60.0	1.7	4.3	16.7
256^2	60.0	3.1	16.0	5.2
512^2	60.0	11.1	46.8	1.7
1024^2	60.0	19.4	130.7	0.7

The drawing speed for the cell phone and the tablet is 60 fps irrespective of the texture size. 60 fps is the maximum speed to which the OpenGL rendering refreshing frequency is adjusted to prevent performance fluctuations. Both the loading and response speeds depend on the texture size. The response speed increases faster than the loading speed because data processing requires results to be transferred over the LAN which is the bottleneck of the solution. The differences in the overall processing time between the cell phone and the tablet are not much (see Fig. 5.6): for the texture resolution of 64×64 pixels they are identical

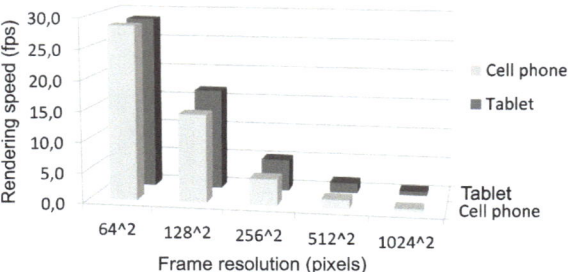

Fig. 5.6 The differences in overall processing time (*remote rendering speed in fps*) between a cell phone and a tablet

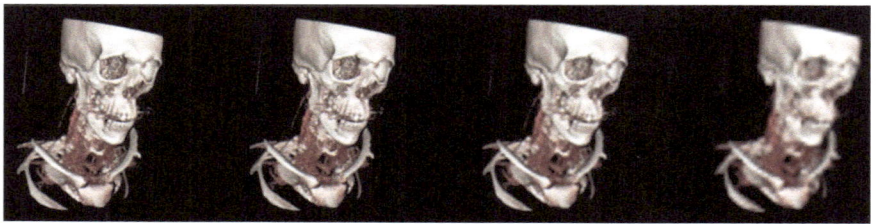

Fig. 5.7 The direct volume rendering of a CTA with size $512 \times 512 \times 415$ used to evaluate the system. The presented images have different baseline resolutions rescaled to 512×512, namely, from left to right 512×512, 256×256, 128×128 and 64×64

but they begin to differ as the resolution increases. For the texture size of 1024×1024 pixels, the solution operates 40 % faster on the tablet.

Because the response time is less dependent on device hardware parameters than on the size of data to be transferred over the web, it is crucial for the system performance to use a low-resolution image during the TUI interaction and a full resolution image after the interaction is completed. In order to obtain an overall time at the level of 30 fps which seems to be reasonable for this type of a solution, the limited image frame resolution has to be at the level of 64×64. Obviously, this image is then rescaled by hardware interpolation to fit the screen of the TUI device. As Fig. 5.7 shows, an image sized 64×64 rescaled by hardware interpolation to 512×512 does not lack much in its overall quality, but it does lack some details. The 512×512 full resolution is sufficient for the considered Computed Tomography Angiography (CTA) dataset because its largest dimension equals 512.

5.2 Vision User Interface

Vision user interfaces use a different image processing and analysis method to generate features. These features (like, e.g., the coordinates of hands) can then be used directly as the input for the system to remotely steer the graphical interface.

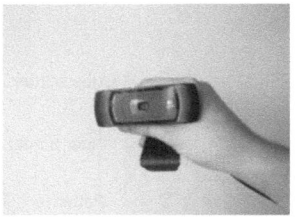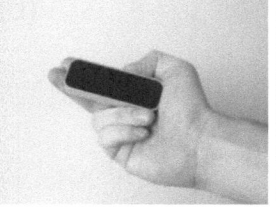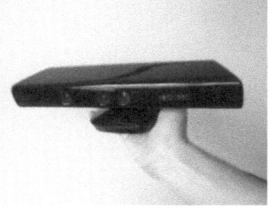

Fig. 5.8 Examples of multimedia USB devices that can be used to create vision user interfaces: Logitech Webcam C920 HD PRO, Leap Motion and Microsoft Kinect

These features may also be utilized by various pattern classification methods in order to identify the user's activities, e.g., gestures (hand waving, nodding) or even complex movement sequences (like karate techniques). Various RGB and infrared (IR) cameras most often serve as image acquisition devices for VUI systems. Contemporary off-the-shelf multimedia hardware supports systems with video data streams of a 30 fps frequency which were shown to be sufficient for analyzing a moderate speed of user interaction. No need to touch any remote controller, the intuitiveness of gestures and a "taste of novelty" seem to be the most impotent factors making the VUI so interesting to consumers. Figure 5.8 presents popular vision-based multimedia devices we have used in our research and commercial projects. These are a USB-connectable RGB web camera, an IR based Leap Motion sensor and a NUI controller—Microsoft Kinect.

For many years, low-cost RGB cameras have been built-in components of portable devices like laptops or smartphones. It is also highly probable that miniaturized IR sensors like those present in Fig. 5.8 will soon become the standard equipment of mobile computers.

5.2.1   RGB Camera: Marker-Based Tracking and Augmented Reality

Augmented Reality (AR) is a technology that allows virtual objects to be overlaid on real-world [32]. Recent achievements in AR systems reveal several significant directions of current research, including tracking techniques, display technologies, mobile AR or interaction techniques. Augmented reality proves its utility, particularly in the medical field [33]. The most notable examples are deformable body atlases, AR surgical navigation systems, interfaces and visualization systems [34, 35]. AR aims at improving support for pre, intra and postoperative visualization of clinical data by presenting more informative and realistic three-dimensional visualizations [36]. One of the most difficult parts in building an AR system is to precisely align the virtual object with the "real world" image taking into account the position of the user who might look at the same object from different distances and angles. The algorithm has to be not only precise but also fast enough to support

(a)   **(b)**

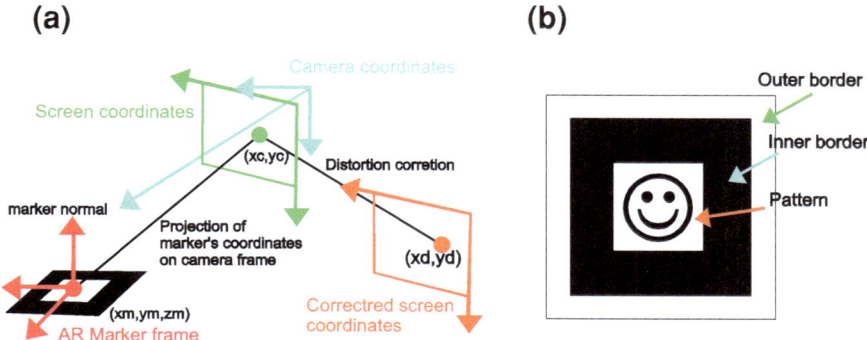

Fig. 5.9 *Left* the relationship between the marker position, the camera position and screen coordinates estimated by the ARToolkit algorithm. *Right* an example ArToolkit pattern. (*xm, ym, zm*) is the point in the center of the marker, (*xc, yc*) is the projection of this point onto the screen plane. (*xd, yd*) are the corrected screen coordinates. The outer border of pattern is used to give a good contrast to the inner border surrounding the pattern situated in the middle of the marker. **a** Pose and position estimation, **b** example ArToolkit marker

calculating virtual object orientation in real-time. In case of VUI approaches, when there is no additional data from other sensors (for example the gyroscope or the GPS), one of the most common approaches to solve this program is to use an RGB camera together with so-called AR markers. AR markers are most often size known square cards with some pattern drawn on them—see Fig. 5.9, right hand side. This approach is used, e.g., in the ARToolkit software [37] which still remains among the most popular AR software for RGB cameras. An RGB camera is used to capture a picture of the observed environment. Then, the image processing algorithm detects the square markers and uses their orientation (marker normal vector), the distance and the relative position of the camera are calculated. Additionally, the software can also correct screen distortions introduced by the camera leans. Figure 5.9 presents the relationship between the marker position, the camera position and the screen coordinates estimation by the ARToolkit algorithm.

The image processing and algebra methods used to calculate screen coordinate are detailed in [32]. Figure 5.10 presents the most important stages in the image processing procedure.

In paper [38], we reported our use of the AR marker technology to create a portable AR interface for visualizing volumetric medical data in a commercial OS that can be used with off-the-shelf hardware. The AR environment was used to visualize direct volume rendering visualizations of CT/CTA data onto which 2D brain perfusion maps were superimposed. The system is also capable of displaying additional information about potential lesions in CTP images. The medical data is visualized over AR markers. This enables a fast and intuitive navigation in a three-dimensional environment and exploring the visualized images from different angles and distances. For direct volume rendering and superimposing, we used algorithms previously described in Chap. 4. The CTP (Computed Tomography Perfusion)

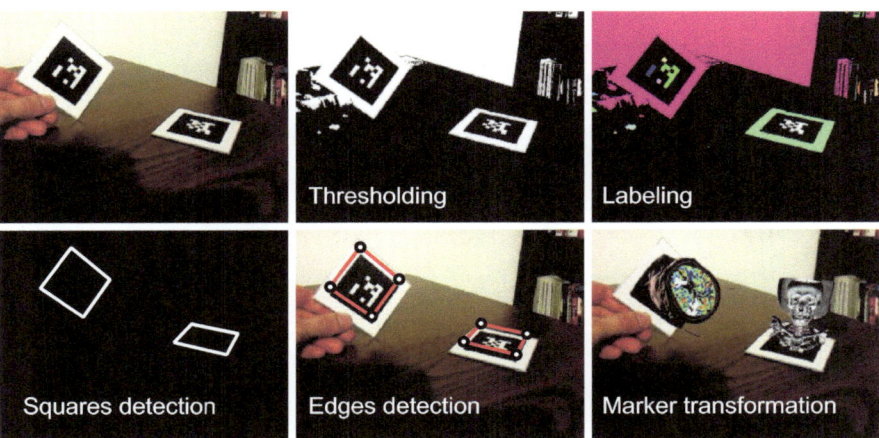

Fig. 5.10 This figure presents the most important stages of the image processing procedure in the ARToolkit software. These stages are ordered starting with the *top left image* and should be read row by row. The input image is thresholded, a *black and white image* is generated. In the next step, the *black and white image* is labelled in order to find potential regions of interest and speed up the remaining processing. At the square detection step, regions which outline the contour and can be fitted with *four line segments* are extracted. The parameters of these *four line segments* and the coordinates of the four vertices of the regions determined from the intersections of the line segments are stored for later processing (see [32]). The regions limited by squares are normalized and the subimage within the region is compared by template matching with predefined AR patterns. If the pattern matches, the detected edges are used to compute a transformation which is used to align the virtual object with the marker

image processing, analysis and potential perfusion lesions detection are done using algorithms described in Chap. 3 (the so-called DMD system). Figure 5.11 presents screenshots taken during the work on our system. One can see that our implementations of direct volume rendering algorithms are capable of visualizing many volumes at the same time.

5.2.2 Infrared Cameras and Markerless Tracking

In the last few years, more and more relatively low-priced multimedia controllers utilizing IR cameras have appeared on market. The most noteworthy from the point of view of their popularity—the commercial interest—were Leap Motion and Microsoft Kinect (lower down we will be referring to it as Kinect). What makes these devices so popular was (beside the big advertising campaign) their price, capabilities and SDK libraries making it possible to generate new projects based on the capabilities of those devices. The Leap Motion is a small box sized $8 \times 3 \times 1.1$ cm (length × depth × height) that weighs about 45 g. It uses USB 2.0 or 3.0 to connect to the computer. It uses two monochromatic IR cameras and

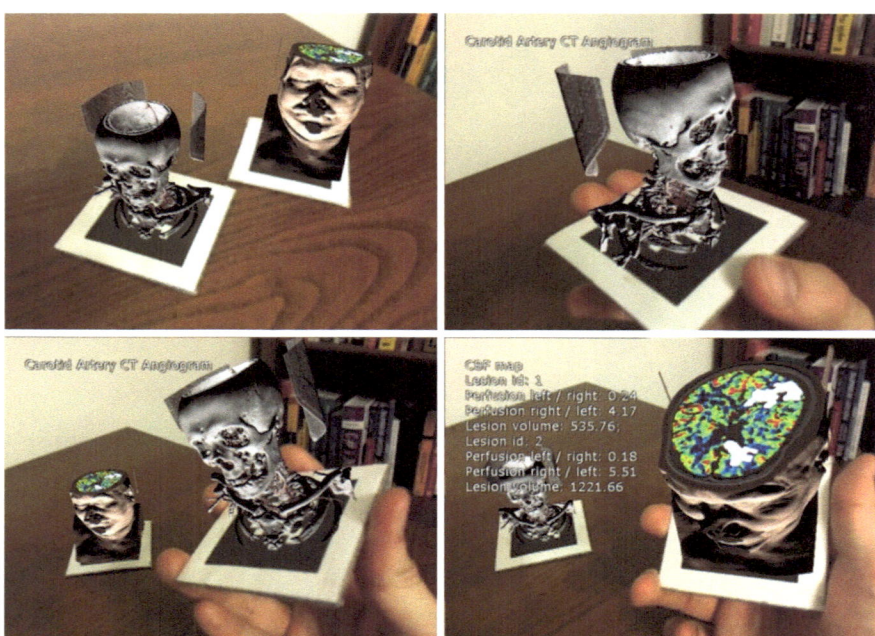

Fig. 5.11 The direct volume rendering visualization in an AR environment performed by our system. From left to right (row by row) visualization of the same volume, but with different transfer functions. Next two images close up of the CTA image, top left part of the screen—a system description of the image modality to the user. Last image—a close up of CTP data superimposed onto a volumetric image. The CTP image processing, analysis and potential perfusion lesions detection are done using algorithms described in Chap. 3 (the description of the image is an output of the DMD system)

three IR LEDs in order to observe a hemispherical area up to the distance of about 1 m. The data generated by the controller is sent to the computer for further calculation. Products libraries that must be installed on the host computer enable inter alia the detection and tracking of user's hands, fingers (their position, direction, velocity), tools (for example an ordinary pen) and identifying some basic gestures (for example a rapid finger, or tool movement, called a swipe gesture). No special hand-held markers are required for this process. The community of Leap Motion controller developers is constantly growing and there are more and more interesting applications of this technology serving many purposes. These include educational applications, contactless interfaces for well-know programs and services (Autodesk Maya, Google Earth), Games, Music and Entertainment applications. Figure 5.12 presents screenshots from two Cyber Science—Motion applications that allow a human skull and a tarantula to be explored, dissected, and assembled. The unparalleled interaction allows users to experience subtle and complex spatial relationships of the human and spider anatomy.

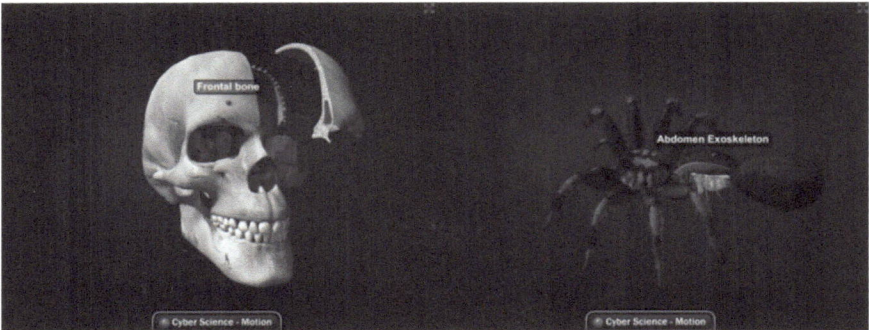

Fig. 5.12 The *left part* of the figure is screen shot from the application Cyber Science—Motion (*exploring a human head*) and on the *right*—a tarantula. Both interactions are controlled by hand or single finger movements

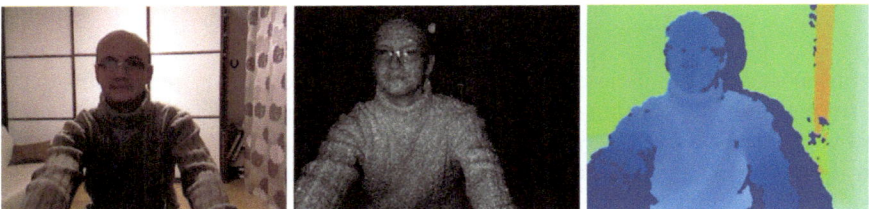

Fig. 5.13 Example RGB and IR images and a depth map generated by a Kinect controller

The next technology we will focus on in the rest of this chapter is Microsoft Kinect. Just like Leap Motion, the Kinect device is connected to the computer via USB 2.0 and can be utilized for markerless tracking interaction with computers, but the structure and the application of Kinect is a bit different. The Kinect head (the part with sensors) is sized $\sim28 \times \sim6 \times \sim3.5$ cm (length × depth × height). Kinect consists of several components (for details see [39]). The first is an RGB camera which records three channels, enabling color image capture. The second is an IR emitter and an IR depth sensor. The emitter emits IR light beams and the depth sensor reads the IR beams reflected back to the sensor. These reflected beams are converted into depth information measuring the distance between an object and the sensor. This makes capturing a depth image possible. The third element is a multiarray microphone made up of four microphones for capturing sound. Because there are four microphones, it is possible to record audio as well as to find the location of the sound source and the direction of the audio wave. The last part is a 3-axis accelerometer which can be used to determine the current orientation of Kinect. Example images taken by RGB and IR cameras together with a depth map are presented in Fig. 5.13.

The Kinect sensor was created for a different purpose than Leap Motion—it is used for full body tracking rather than hand tracking. It is also far less precise in

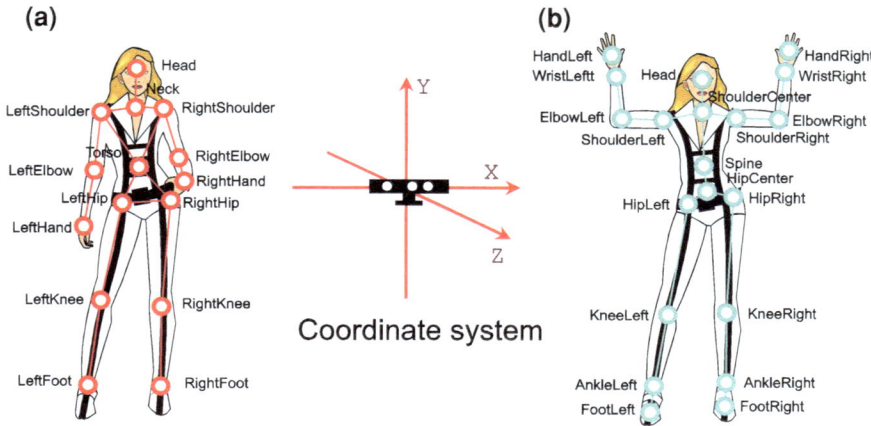

Fig. 5.14 Skeletons generated by the NITE 1.3 tracking (*left*) and Kinect SDK algorithms (*right*). **a** NITE skeleton, **b** Kinect SKD skeleton

terms of its distance measurement than Leap Motion (see [40, 41]). According to the documentation [39], within the default range mode, Kinect can see people standing between 0.8 and 4.0 m away. Full body tracking is utilizing a depth map generated by the device. At first, the potential user's body is segmented out of the map. Then, body feature points are detected (so called body joints). All joints together create a so-called skeleton. The segmentation of the human body from depth images and the skeleton tracking has been solved and reported in many papers [42–46] before. The joint video/depth rate allocation has also been researched [47]. Neither do these algorithms require any markers to be put around the tracked user's body. The number of tracked body parts and the information connected with body joints depends on the libraries that are used for tracking. In our further research, we will be using two types of tracking libraries: Prime Sensor NITE 1.3 [44] which tracks 15 body joints and Kinect SDK [43] tracking 20 joints. Figure 5.14 presents idealized skeletons generated by these two libraries together with predefined names of body joints. Both libraries use a right-handed coordinate systems where the beginning of Cartesian Frame is in the lens of the IR depth sensor and the Z axis is parallel to the observation direction. In both NITE and Kinect SDK, every joint has three coordinates describing its position in the right-handed coordinate system (note that the left and right side are mirrored in Fig. 5.14). In addition, both libraries enable skeleton data to be tracked in real-time. Real-time in this context means "with the same speed that data arrives from the hardware" approximately 30 fps.

This skeleton data stream is a crucial source of information for a vision-based user interface. Coupled with a proper pattern recognition method for natural gesture identification, it can be used to create a useful and intuitive NUI for medical purposes. In the rest of this chapter we will present state-of-the-art review of gestures recognition algorithms for VUIs. Then, we will describe our Gesture Description Language (GDL) classifier and its application in a prototype medical visualization system.

5.2.3 Application of IR-Based VUI in Medicine

It can be said that almost every day brings new information about a successful application of a VUI-based system prototype in medicine. Proposed applications are mostly touchless interfaces for the operating room, rehabilitation and postural control systems. Because of the great number of papers about that subject, we will only summarize one example paper for each subject mentioned.

Authors of [48] implemented a hand tracking and gesture recognition system based on the Kinect device that enables surgeons to successfully touchlessly navigate through the image in the intraoperative setting using a personal computer. In the operating room, a touchless interface is ideal because it does not demand any physical contact and can still provide the necessary control features in a cleansed and sterilized environment. The authors used the InVesalius software, which provides high-quality 3D reconstructions of medical images. This chapter (to our knowledge) is the first mention in the literature of a touchless user interface solution applying the Kinect device which proved to be very efficient in the intraoperative context. The proposed solution can be used with any mouse-controlled software, opening an avenue for potential applications in many other areas, such as data visualization, AR, accessibility, and robotics.

Study [49] assessed the possibility of rehabilitating two young adults with motor impairments using a Kinect-based system in a public school setting. This study was carried out according to an ABAB sequence in which A represented the baseline and B represented intervention phases. Data showed that the two participants significantly increased their motivation for physical rehabilitation, thus improving exercise performance during the intervention phases.

Study [50] assessed the concurrent validity of the Microsoft Kinect against a benchmark reference—a multiple-camera 3D motion analysis system—in 20 healthy subjects during postural control tests. Findings suggest that the Microsoft Kinect can validly assess kinematic strategies of postural control. Given the potential benefits it could therefore become a useful tool for assessing postural control in the clinical setting.

5.3 State of the Art of Gesture Recognition for VUI

Gestures recognition can be considered as a multidimensional signal identification task. Hence methods that are used for signal identification are often applied to human movement classification.

5.3.1 Probabilistic and Statistical Approach

Activity recognition is one of the most challenging problems in the video content analysis and high-level computer vision. Paper [51] proposes a novel activity recognition approach in which an activity is decomposed into multiple interactive stochastic processes, each corresponding to one scale of motion details. For modeling the interactive processes, authors present a hierarchical durational-state dynamic Bayesian network (HDS-DBN) to model two stochastic processes which are related to two appropriate scales in intelligent surveillance. The main objective of paper [52] is to introduce a Gaussian Process Dynamical Model as an alternative machine learning method for hand gesture interpretation in the Sign Language. In paper [53], authors present the framework and components of a real-time 3D conceptual generation and visualization system. Real-time hand gesture recognition was performed by a skeleton model-based template matching, and the use of hidden Markov models (HMMs). Paper [3] presents algorithms for reducing latency when recognizing actions. Authors use a latency-aware learning formulation to train a logistic regression-based classifier that automatically determines distinctive canonical poses from data and uses these to robustly recognize actions in the presence of ambiguous poses. paper [54] presents a human action recognition framework based on the theory of nonlinear dynamical systems. Authors propose a distance to compare trajectories within the reconstructed phase portraits. These distances are used to train Support Vector Machine (SVM) models for action recognition. In the method proposed in [55], after using local Gabor filters, the features are being reduced by Principal Component Analysis (PCA) to overcome the small sample size problem. The classification of the gestures to their classes was done with the help of a one against one multiclass SVM. Paper [56] addresses the multiview action recognition problem with a local segment similarity voting scheme, upon which authors build a novel multisensor fusion method. The random forests classifier is used to map the local segment features to their corresponding prediction histograms. Authors compare the results of their approach with those of the baseline Bag-of-Words (BoW) and the Naive–Bayes Nearest Neighbor (NBNN) methods on the multiview IXMAS dataset. It has also been proven that the proposed sensor fusion technique, coupled with the random forests classifier, is effective for multiple view human action recognition. Research work [57] focuses on developing an automated approach for posture estimation and classification using a range camera for posture analysis and categorizing it as ergonomic or nonergonomic with Linear discriminant analysis. In paper [58] authors propose using point cloud processing and the Viewpoint Feature Histogram (VFH) as the global descriptor of the scene. To empower the distinctiveness of the descriptor, a modification is proposed which consists in dividing the work space into smaller cells and calculating the VFH for each of them. The method is applied to chosen dynamic gestures of the Polish sign language. The classification of gestures is based on the nearest neighbor classifier using dynamic time warping to compare sequences. In paper [59], the authors describe a system for recognizing various human actions from compressed video based on motion history information. The notion of quantifying the motion involved, through the so-called Motion Flow History (MFH), is introduced. The encoded motion information, readily available in the compressed MPEG stream, is used to construct the coarse Motion History Image (MHI) and the corresponding MFH. The features extracted from the static MHI and MFH briefly characterize the spatiotemporal and motion vector information about the action. The extracted features are used to train the k-nearest neighbor (k-NN), Neural Network, SVM and Bayes classifiers to recognize a set of seven human actions.

5.3.2 Geometric Template Matching

An alternative approach was proposed in the Full Body Interaction Framework (FUBI) which is a framework for recognizing full body gestures and postures in real-time from a depth sensor (Microsoft Kinect) [60, 61]. FUBI recognizes four categories of posture and gestures: static postures, gestures with linear movements, a combination of postures and a linear movement and complex gestures. The fourth type of gestures are recognized using $1 recognizer algorithm which is a geometric template matcher [62].

5.3.3 Fuzzy Sets

Paper [63] presents an application of a fuzzy rule-based aggregation to a data glove for the recognition of gestures. The fuzzy glove is a data glove that has fuzzy sensor functionalities. The approach is used for the definition of the numerical to linguistic conversion, and for the definition of the sets of rules. The system [64] transforms the preprocessed data about the detected hand into a fuzzy hand-posture feature model by using fuzzy neural networks. Based on this model, the developed system determines the actual hand posture by applying fuzzy inference. Finally, from the sequence of detected hand postures, the system recognizes the hand gesture of the user.

5.3.4 Syntactic Descriptions, Semantic Analysis and Finite State Machines

Paper [65] proposes a two-level approach to solve the problem of the real-time vision-based hand gesture classification. The lower level of the approach recognizes posture using Haar-like features and the AdaBoost learning algorithm. This algorithm allows real-time performance and high-recognition accuracy to be obtained. The higher level linguistically recognizes hand gestures using a context-free grammar-based syntactic analysis, but the chapter does not give many details of how it was exactly done. Another system, very similar to paper [65] real-time one, for sign language recognition via hand gestures is proposed in paper [66]. Hands postures are detected and hand gestures are recognized based on features of the hand which are extracted using Haar-Like features. A k-means clustering algorithm is used to reduce the number of extracted features and hence the computational complexity. The hand is detected by the AdaBoost algorithm. The AdaBoost learning algorithm is used to choose a small number of weak classifiers and to combine them into a strong classifier which decides whether an image contains a hand or not and also classifies the hand posture. Then, by using a stochastic context free grammar (SCFG), a specific hand gesture is recognized. The production rule with the highest probability is used to identify the specific hand gesture. Paper [67] describes GestureLab, a tool designed for building domain-specific gesture recognizers, and its integration with Cider, a grammar engine that uses GestureLab recognizers and parses visual languages. Recognizers created with GestureLab perform probabilistic lexical recognition with disambiguation occurring during the parsing, based on contextual syntactic information. Creating domain-specific gesture recognizers requires significant amounts of experimentation and training with large gesture corpora to determine a suitable set of features and a classifier algorithm. In paper [68], authors propose a structured approach to studying patterns of a multimodal language in the context of a 2D-display control. They attempt to use syntactic methods to analyze gestures, starting from describing the observable kinematical primitives up to their holistic analysis. The proposed semantic classification of coverbal gestures distinguishes six categories based on their spatiotemporal deixis. In paper [69], the authors propose a vision-based system for automatically interpreting a limited set of dynamic hand gestures. This involves extracting the temporal signature of the hand motion from the performed gesture. The concept of motion energy is used to estimate the dominant motion from an image sequence. To achieve the desired result, the authors introduce the concept of modeling the dynamic hand gesture using a finite state machine. The temporal signature is subsequently analyzed by the finite state machine to automatically interpret the gesture made.

5.3.5 Rule-Based Approach

In paper [70], the Flexible Action and Articulated Skeleton Toolkit (FAAST), a middleware software framework for integrating full body interaction with virtual environments, video games, and other user interfaces, is presented. This toolkit provides a complete end-to-end solution including a graphical user interface for custom gesture creation, sensor configuration, skeletal tracking, action recognition, and a variety of output mechanisms to control third party applications, allowing virtually any PC application to be repurposed for gestural control even if it does not explicitly support input from motion sensors. To facilitate an intuitive and transparent gesture design, authors define syntax for representing human gestures using rule sets corresponding to the basic spatial and temporal components of an action. These individual rules form primitives which, although conceptually simple on their own, can be combined both simultaneously and sequentially to form sophisticated gestural interactions. This chapter was published independently of our initial work on the GDL [71, 72] (our work preceded it). It should be mentioned that compared to our GDL technique, the FAAST methodology is interesting, but highly constrained by the syntax limitation of defining features and rules.

5.4 Semantic Gesture Recognition with a Syntactic Description: Gesture Description Language

Gesture recognition with automatic computing of decision borders (training) for the classifier, which can be seen in the above state-of-the-art review, is a common approach. However, one should keep in mind that approaches utilizing fully automatized techniques of gesture classification either require very large training and validation sets (consisting of dozens or hundreds of cases) or have to be manually tuned, which might be very unintuitive even for a skilled system user [73]. What is more, it is impossible to add any new gesture to be recognized without intensive extra training of the classifier. What is more, the identification and the definition of proper features of body movements, which is often one of the most demanding activities before the training algorithm can even be run, depends greatly on the skills and intuition of a computer scientist. These four factors could significantly limit the potential application of these solutions in real-life development to institutions that are able to assemble very large pattern datasets. On the other hand, body gesture interpretation is completely natural to every person and—in our opinion—in many cases there is no need to employ a complex mathematical and statistical approach for the correct recognition. Based on those observations, we created the foundations of our Gesture Description Language (GDL) classifier which trades the automatics training of the method for the simplicity of feature and class definition and the intuitive interpretation of results. Our method utilizes a syntactic description of static body poses and body gestures making use of input features generated by the tracking software. These descriptions, coupled with input data, are interpreted by a special reasoning module. The first articles describing the basic functionalities of the GDL and its implementation prototype were published in international journals [71, 72]. Today, GDL is a well-established technology with an implementation as a dynamic linked library in the C# language both for NITE/OpenNI and Kinect SDK tracking libraries. Commercial licenses for products based on the GDL 1.0 specification described in paper [73] have already been granted to several companies around the world. Some implementations of this technology can also be used freely for scientific and educational purposes. To obtain the actual implementation of the GDL, visit its official website [74] or the

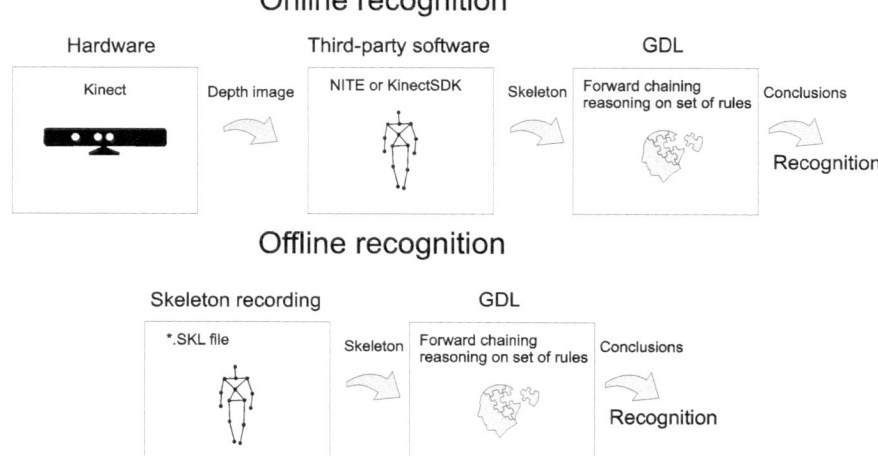

Fig. 5.15 The place of the GDL in the gesture recognition pipeline

website of the Laboratory of Cryptography and Cognitive Informatics [75]. In this and the following sections of this chapter, we present a specification of the new GDL edition, that is GDL version 1.1. In version 1.1, we introduced new syntactic elements, very useful when describing features of gestures to be recognized. We also defined a new function that can be used to check the persistence of gestures in the time domain. Sect. 5.9 contains the complete formal language definition and code examples of the GDL script 1.1. We are also presenting a method of overcoming the limitation of body joint tracking with a single Kinect by calibrating multikinect environment. Finally, we will discuss results of validating our proposed approach on a "natural gestures" dataset and a Shorin-ryu Karate dataset.

5.5 GDL Classifier Fundamentals

The GDL approach is based on the assumption that (almost) every person has broad experience in how real-life (natural) gestures are made by a typical person. Every individual gains this experience subconsciously over years of observation. The GDL classifier allows the user's knowledge to be defined with a formal grammar description. Of course, each practical implementation of a real-time recognition system has some assumptions about the input data processing model. In case of the GDL, we have made following assumption (see Fig. 5.15).

In case of online (real-time) recognition:

- Data is captured by a hardware device capable of working at a frame rate sufficient to track natural gestures (approximately 30 fps). In our experiments, we used a Kinect sensor.

- We have access to third-party software libraries which generate input data for the classifier, in case of GDL this is the set of body joints combined into a skeleton (see Sect. 5.2.2). For this task, we used the NITE/OpenNI library or the Kinect SDK library.

In case of offline recognition:

- Skeleton data was previously captured by the hardware device and third-party software and was stored in a file and used to generate a skeleton.

5.5.1 Relationship Between the GDL and Pattern Recognition Methods

The GDL approach uses a pattern recognition approach which could be defined as a multidimensional time-series recognition task. We are given:

$S = [S(0), S(1),..., S(n)]$—a series of skeletons where $S(0)$ is the first sample and $S(n)$ is the last sample of the recording made over time. The time spans between samples are not uniform.

$S(t) = [[x_{1t}, y_{1t}, z_{1t}], [x_{2t}, y_{2t}, z_{2t}], ..., [x_{mt}, y_{mt}, z_{mt}]]$—is a series of M body joints. The number of body joints depends on the third-party tracking library.

$C = \{c_1, c_2, ...c_k\}$—labels of classes.

Let S_i be the nonempty subset of S and C_i—a subset of C.

Our task is to find the following function:

$$R : S_i \rightarrow C_i$$

We are assuming that not every subset of S can be labeled with labels from C.

One possible solution for finding function R is to represent the signal S with the series of features derived from signal samples:

$F = [f_1, f_2, ...f_k], G : S_i \rightarrow F$

This is often done to reduce the dimensionality of the problem (because quite often m*n $\gg$ k). After applying function G to S_i, the signal becomes a series of k-dimensional points in the k-dimensional space. If we defined G correctly, points belonging to the same classes should be "close" to one another according to some metric in the obtained k-dimensional space. Knowing this, we can partition this k-dimensional space by a set of hyper planes H (so-called decision borders) in such a manner that these subspaces we obtained after the partitioning contain points belonging to the same class. $G(S_p) \in P_r \Rightarrow R(S_p) = C_t$

In other words, if feature vector $G(S_p)$ obtained from signal S_p belongs to subplane P_r, this means that signal S_p is of class C_t.

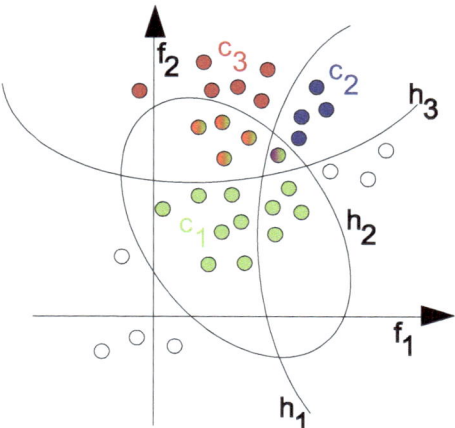

Fig. 5.16 An example two-dimensional feature space with three curves defining decision borders. There are three classes: the green c_1 class inside a region defined by h_2, the blue c_2 that is above h_3 and to the right of h_1 and c_3 located above h_3 and to the left of h_1. Points are colored according to the class they belong to. There are also points belonging to two classes at the same time (marked with mixed colors) and points belonging to neither of them (they are black circles with white interiors)

Summing up: to define a classifier we have to find following function:

$$R' : F \rightarrow C \cup \emptyset$$

An example graphical representation of a two-dimensional feature space with decision borders can be seen in Fig. 5.16.

The GDL classifier uses exactly this approach: it facilitates the manual definition of the set of features F, set of hyper-planes H and a mapping of F to $C \cup \emptyset$. All these definitions are stored in a special GDL script file written in a context-free grammar (the grammar defines the so-called GDL script, GDLs). Two types of GDL script construction are possible: a Feature definition (which defines the G function) and a Rule definition (which defines R'). An example feature definition is as follows:

FEATURE `Head.y[0] - HandRight.y[0]` **AS** `HeadMinusHand`

This feature computes the difference between the vertical position of the head and the right hand and stores the result into the variable "HeadMinusHand". The variable defined by this feature can also form a part of another feature:

FEATURE `ABS(HeadMinusHand)` **AS** `AbsoluteHeadMinusHand`

The variable "AbsoluteHeadMinusHand" contains the absolute value of the variable HeadMinusHand. If one feature uses the value of another feature or vice versa, both feature values will not be computed (in our approach it is impossible to use recursive definitions). An example rule that uses a previously defined feature is as follows:

RULE HeadMinusHand < 0 **THEN** HandOverHead

This rule checks if the variable value is lower than zero. If it is, its conclusion "HandOverHead" is satisfied (its value becomes true).

It is also possible to define G inside rules without using features:

RULE Head.y[0] - HandRight.y[0] < 0 **THEN** HandOverHead

In addition, the conclusion of the rule can form a part of another rule:

RULE Head.y[0] - HandLeft.y[0] < 0 & HandOverHead
THEN BothHandsOverHead

The conclusion "BothHandsOverHead" is satisfied if both hands are overhead. If one rule uses the conclusion of another feature and vice versa (recursive definition), the conclusions of both rules will always be false.

The difference between features and rules is that features define numerical values and it is always possible to compute values of variables they define. For rules: until the rule is satisfied its conclusion has the logical value of false. The rule becomes satisfied if the logical expression defined in it has the logical value of true. If the rule is satisfied, the logical value of its conclusion becomes true even if it was previously referenced as false.

Body joints change their value in time (for example if the tracked person is raising his or her hand, the y-parameter of the body joint representing this hand also rises). It is obviously impossible to define a class for each possible body joint position that can appear in the gesture and to manually track movement frame-by-frame. Because of that we have approached this differently: the gesture is partitioned into a set of key frames which should appear one by one in a defined order subject to the given time constraints. Each key frame is defined by at least one rule and the orders of rules are checked by a specially defined sequence-checking function. All rules in the GDL script together create a knowledge base concerning the gestures we want to recognize. With this in mind, we decided that the classification of the gestures will be overseen by a specially defined forward-chaining reasoning module that is described in following section.

5.5.2 Reasoning Module

The very heart of our method is an automated reasoning module. It carries out forward chaining reasoning (similar to that of a classic expert system) using a knowledge base and its inference engine every time a new portion of data arrives

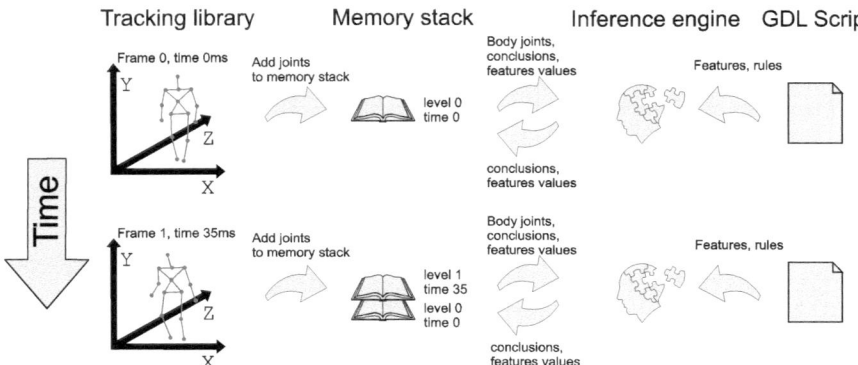

Fig. 5.17 Schema of an algorithm used by the reasoning module. The tracking library stores body joints on *top* of the memory stack. The inference engine uses the memory stack to retrieve body joints, names of conclusions and feature values. These variables are used to compute values of features and rules that are taken from the GDL script. The inference engine stores values of computed features and satisfied conclusion names in the current level of the memory stack

from the feature extraction library. All rules and features of the knowledge base are defined in the GDL script, i.e., written in the GDL script language. What is more, the reasoning module uses a special memory stack which stores all values of features, names of conclusions of satisfied rules, body joints, and the timestamp value. The timestamp value shows how much time passed between one body joint acquisition and another. Because the conclusion of one rule can form the premise of another one, the satisfaction of a rule does not necessarily mean recognizing a particular gesture. The interpretation of a conclusion appearance depends on the GDL script code. An algorithm that is used by the reasoning module goes as follows (see Fig. 5.17):

Repeat the instructions below until the application stops:

1. If new data (a set of body joints) arrives from the data tracking library, create a new level of memory stack on the top of the stack. Use this new level to store a new set of body joints. The new level of the memory stack receives the actual timestamp value. The size of the memory stack in our implementation is 256 layers (over 8.5 s of data capture at the frequency of 30 Hz). We did not find a "deeper" stack useful, but because data stored in the stack is not memory-consuming, the stack might be implemented as "virtually unlimited in depth".

2. Compute the values of features that had not yet been computed (are not present in the current top level of the memory stack), if any feature f_j uses the value of another feature f_i whose value has not yet been computed, skip the computing of f_j. Store values of newly computed features in the current level of the memory stack.

3. If in step 2 above any new feature value was added to the memory stack, return to step 2.

4. Check if any of the rules that had not yet been satisfied (its conclusion is not present in the current level of the memory stack) is now satisfied. If a rule becomes satisfied, store its conclusion in the current level of the memory stack.
5. If any new conclusion was added to the memory stack in step 4, return to step 4.
6. Go to step 1 and wait for new body joint data to arrive.

The next paragraph presents an application of the GDL script language for describing static body poses and gestures. The examples cited clarify most of the possible syntax structures and the GDL algorithm flow.

5.5.3 Static Body Pose and Gesture Description in the GDL Script Language

The GDL script contains a set of features and rules. The GDL script is written in the GDL script (GDLs) which is a formal, context-free grammar. GDLs is not case-sensitive. Each feature consists of a mathematical expression that returns either a single floating-point value (called a numeric rule) or a three-dimensional floating-point vector (called a numeric 3D rule). A rule (similarly to rules in expert systems) is made up of premises that are connected by conjunction or alternative operators. In GDL, premises are called logical rules. A logical rule can take two values: true or false. A numeric rule might become a logical rule after it is combined with another numeric rule by a relational operator. Brackets in logical and numeric 3D rules are used to change the order in which instructions are executed.

GDLs contains a set of predefined variables called Body parts and Body parts 3D that return the value of body joint coordinates. It is possible to take not only the current position of a joint but also the positions from prior captures that are stored in the memory stack. A GDLs programmer can refer to a particular level of memory stack by giving the stack level index (0 is the top of the stack, 1 is one level below the top, etc.) during a call of the Body parts variable. There is also a set of functions which return either numerical or logical values. For example, the following function checks if the Euclidean distance between the current position of the HipCenter (x, y, and z coordinate) and the previous position stored one stack level below is greater than 10 mm. If it is, the rule is satisfied and the conclusion 'Moving' is added to the memory stack at level 0. This means that the GDL recognized the movement of the observed user.

RULE
```
Distance(HipCenter.xyz[0], HipCenter.xyz[1]) > 10
THEN Moving
```

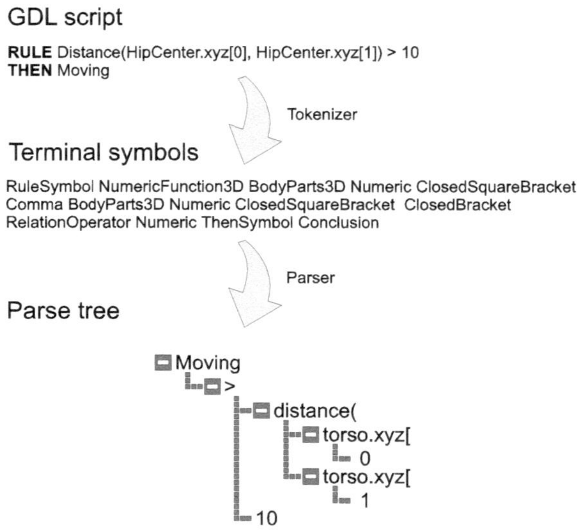

GDL script

RULE Distance(HipCenter.xyz[0], HipCenter.xyz[1]) > 10
THEN Moving

Tokenizer

Terminal symbols

RuleSymbol NumericFunction3D BodyParts3D Numeric ClosedSquareBracket
Comma BodyParts3D Numeric ClosedSquareBracket ClosedBracket
RelationOperator Numeric ThenSymbol Conclusion

Parser

Parse tree

```
☐ Moving
 └─☐ >
     ├─☐ distance(
     │    ├─☐ torso.xyz[
     │    │   └─ 0
     │    └─☐ torso.xyz[
     │        └─ 1
     └─ 10
```

Fig. 5.18 An example parsing result of a script with the conclusion 'Moving'. At first, the lexical analyzer generates a set of terminal symbols. These symbols are then parsed (*for a formal definition of the GDLs* 1.1 *grammar* see Sect. 5.9). As a result, a parse tree is obtained. The last step is to replace the tags linked to rule keywords (*RuleSymbol and ThenSymbol*) with the name of the conclusion. This replacement simplifies the processing with the GDLs interpreter

It can be also rewritten as:

FEATURE Distance(HipCenter.xyz[0], HipCenter.xyz[1])
AS Distance
RULE Distance > 10 **THEN** Moving

For simplicity's sake, the following examples of GDLs in this chapter will be defined by rules only.

After the parsing is finished (for the formal definition of the GDLs 1.1 grammar see Sect. 5.9) and no reduction error has appeared, the tree structure is generated—see Fig. 5.18. The only case of a reduction error could be a syntax error in the GDL script file.

The previous rule can be also rewritten as:

RULE sqrt((HipCenter.x[0] - HipCenter.x[1])^2
+ (HipCenter.y[0] - HipCenter.y[1])^2
+ (HipCenter.z[0] - HipCenter z[1])^2) > 10
THEN Moving

More complex gestures can be partitioned into several subrules. The following GDL script describes a so-called PSI-pose that is often used for calibration purposes (see Fig. 5.19).

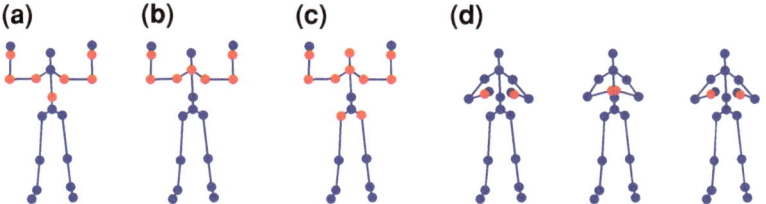

Fig. 5.19 This figure presents key frames described by four examples of GDLs in this chapter. Body joints are taken from the Kinect SDK. Red marks body joints that are used in the GDLs description, *blue*—joints that are not used. **a** PSI, **b** psiInsensitive, **c** psiInsensitive2, **d** clapping

```
RULE ElbowRight.x[0] > Spine.x[0]
& WristRight.x[0] > Spine.x[0]
& WristRight.y[0] > ElbowRight.y[0]
& abs(WristRight.x[0] - ElbowRight.x[0]) < 50
& abs(ShoulderRight.y[0] - ElbowRight.y[0]) < 50
THEN RightHandPsi
RULE ElbowLeft.x[0] < Spine.x[0]
& WristLeft.x[0] < Spine.x[0]
& WristLeft.y[0] > ElbowLeft.y[0]
& abs(WristLeft.x[0] - ElbowLeft.x[0]) < 50
& abs(ShoulderLeft.y[0] - ElbowLeft.y[0]) < 50
THEN LeftHandPsi
RULE RightHandPsi & LeftHandPsi THEN Psi
```

The first rule checks if the right elbow and the right wrist are situated to the right of the torso (spine joint), if the wrist is above the right elbow and if the vertical coordinates of the right wrist and the right elbow are no more than 50 mm different. The last part of the rule is the premise that checks if the horizontal coordinates of the right shoulder and the right elbow are no more than 50 mm different. The second rule is similar to the first, but it describes the left wrist, shoulder and elbow. The last rule checks if both previous rules are satisfied. This is done by checking the logical conjunction of both previous conclusions.

The above approach works fine when the user is standing perpendicular to the camera plane facing it, but it is possible to redefine this set of rules to make the right prediction when the camera is at an angle. In order to do so, the GDL script introduces the ability to compute the angle between two given vectors in a three-dimensional space using the angle() function. The function takes two parameters that are vector coordinates and computes the angle between them within the range of [0, 180] degrees (see a detailed explanation in Sect. 5.9). Using this approach, we can rewrite the "PSI pose" formula to be independent of the camera position rotation around the y-axis (up axis).

```
RULE abs(angle(ShoulderCenter.xyz[0]
- ShoulderRight.xyz[0],
ElbowRight.xyz[0] - ShoulderRight.xyz[0]) - 140) < 20
& abs(angle(ElbowRight.xyz[0] - ShoulderRight.xyz[0],
ElbowRight.xyz[0] - WristRight.xyz[0]) -90) < 20
& WristRight.y[0] - ElbowRight.y[0] > 0
THEN RightHandPsi_in
RULE abs(angle(ShoulderCenter.xyz[0]
- ShoulderLeft.xyz[0],
ElbowLeft.xyz[0] - ShoulderLeft.xyz[0]) -140) < 20
& abs(angle(ElbowLeft.xyz[0] - ShoulderLeft.xyz[0],
ElbowLeft.xyz[0] - WristLeft.xyz[0]) -90) < 20
& WristLeft.y[0] - ElbowLeft.y[0] > 0
THEN LeftHandPsi_in
RULE RightHandPsi_in & LeftHandPsi_in
THEN PsiInsensitive
```

The first rule checks if the angle between the vector defined by the Shoulder-Center (places near neck) and the right shoulder and the vector defined by the right elbow and the right shoulder is $140 \pm 20°$. The second part of the rule checks if the vector defined by the right elbow and the right shoulder and the vector defined by the right elbow and the right wrist are perpendicular ($\pm 20°$). This rule also checks if the right wrist is above the elbow. The second rule is similar to the first but it applies to the left hand. The last rule is true if both previous rules are satisfied. If the conclusion PsiInsensitive is true, this means that the gesture was classified.

It is also possible to write a GDL script that describes the PSI pose and is insensitive to the rotation around any axis. In the example below, instead of checking if both the left and right wrists are above the elbows, the GDL script examines if the distance between the right wrist and the head is smaller than distance between the right wrist and the right hip (similarly for the left wrist and the left hip). If this is true, we know from two possible hands orientations that satisfy previous conditions that the hands are above (and not below) the elbows.

```
RULE abs(angle(ShoulderCenter.xyz[0]
- ShoulderRight.xyz[0],
ElbowRight.xyz[0] - ShoulderRight.xyz[0]) - 140) < 20
& abs(angle(ElbowRight.xyz[0] - ShoulderRight.xyz[0],
ElbowRight.xyz[0] - WristRight.xyz[0]) -90) < 20
& distance(WristRight.xyz[0], Head.xyz[0]) <
distance(WristRight.xyz[0], HipRight.xyz[0])
THEN RightHandPsiIn2
RULE abs(angle(ShoulderCenter.xyz[0]
- ShoulderLeft.xyz[0],
ElbowLeft.xyz[0] - ShoulderLeft.xyz[0]) - 140) < 20
& abs(angle(ElbowLeft.xyz[0] - ShoulderLeft.xyz[0],
ElbowLeft.xyz[0] - WristLeft.xyz[0]) -90) < 20
& distance(WristLeft.xyz[0], Head.xyz[0]) <
distance(WristLeft.xyz[0], HipLeft.xyz[0])
THEN LeftHandPsiIn2
RULE RightHandPsiIn2 & LeftHandPsiIn2
THEN PsiInsensitive2
```

The majority of the following GDL scripts introduced in this book are designed to be insensitive to the y-axis rotation. If the camera up-vector rotates around the x- and/or z- axis and the angles of rotation are known, it is easy to use the linear transformation to recalculate the coordinates of observed points to the Cartesian frame, in which the camera up-vector is perpendicular to the ground plane. For this reason, we did not consider any rotation other than y-axis rotation in the proposed descriptions.

GDLs can check if particular sequences of key frames appeared in a constrained time range. Because a gesture is modeled in GDL as a sequence of key frames, detecting this sequence means recognizing the gesture. The example below checks if the tracked user is clapping his/her hands:

```
Rule Distance(WristLeft.xyz[0], WristRight.xyz[0]) < 100
THEN ClappingTogether
Rule Distance(WristLeft.xyz[0], WristRight.xyz[0]) >= 100
THEN ClappingSeparate
RULE (ClappingSeparate &
Sequenceexists("[ClappingTogether,0.5][ClappingSeparate,0.5]"))
| (ClappingTogether &
Sequenceexists("[ClappingSeparate,0.5][ClappingTogether,0.5]"))
THEN Clapping
```

The first rule checks if the distance between the wrists is shorter than 10 cm, the second rule checks if it is greater than 10 cm. The last rule checks if the observed person is striking the ClappingSeparate pose and if the following sequence of conclusion names is present in the memory stack: the ClappingTogether pose has to be found in the stack no later than half a second ago, then the time between the ClappingTogether and the ClappingSeparate (the ClappingSeparate had to appear before the ClappingTogether) does not exceed half a second. The second part of the rule is connected with the "or" conjunction and checks the opposite order of conclusions (a ClappingTogether after a ClappingSeparate after a ClappingTo-gether). One can see that the sequence of gestures is described from the one that should appear most recently to the one that should have happened at the beginning of the sequence. That is because the sequence describes the order of conclusions on the memory stack starting from the top and going into lower layers. The sequence exists function returns the logical value true if all conditions are satisfied and the false value if any of the conditions in the time sequence is not satisfied. If the conclusion name Clapping appears in the memory stack, this means that the gesture was identified.

The last useful construction in GDLs that we discuss in this section allows one to check how long a particular conclusion persist in the memory stack. In other words, how long did the observed person keep on making a particular gesture (or remained in the same position).

```
RULE HandRight.y[0] > Head.y[0] THEN HandOverHead
RULE rulepersists(HandOverHead, 5, 0.92)
THEN HandOverHeadPersists
```

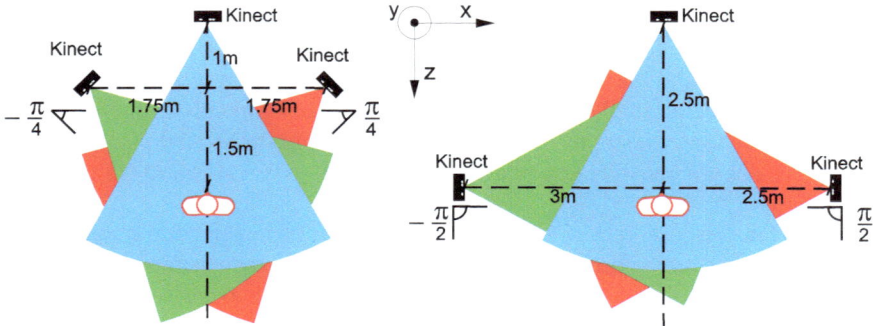

Fig. 5.20 Two multi-Kinect environments used in our experiments. The *colored triangles* in the picture show the view cone of each Kinect. The Kinect view cone is 4 m long

The first rule checks if the right hand is situated overhead. The second checks if the conclusion HandOverHead is present in at least 92 % of memory stack levels for the last 5 s.

GDLs puts the burden of feature and rule definition on the computer scientist or expert who tailors them. Hence, when there are many similar gestures, the recognition efficiency is based on the way the rule is written. Overlapping rules introduce a new challenge and an incorrect handling could result in the recognition (efficiency) slowing down to the rate of the longest gesture, but the effectiveness of the GDL will remain at the same level as it would were the GDLs written optimally. The recommended way of building GDLs descriptions is to create a hierarchical structure for features and rules that optimally exploits dependences between gestures [73]. Like in any programming language, the ability to create these kinds of descriptions is a matter of experience.

5.6 Multikinect Environment: Setup and Calibration

The Kinect controller supports computer applications with a two-dimensional depth map of points in the image. The tracking software that generates the three-dimensional skeleton suffers from a very important limitation: it does not allow every possible body pose of the observed user to be tracked. If, for example, one part of the body represented by a joint is covered by another body part and Kinect cannot "see" it, this joint cannot be directly tracked and its position is estimated by software. However, our experience shows that the estimation rarely predicts the correct position of the missing body part. In order to overcome this problem, we are proposing a multikinect environment for user tracking [76]. Figure 5.20 presents two multikinect environment configurations that we used in our experiments. Each Kinect uses its own tracking module that segments and tracks the user's skeleton in real-time.

Our solution utilizes standard body tracking libraries and the following algorithm to integrate separate joint recordings into a single one:

- All Kinect devices work at the same time and supply tracking libraries with depth data. Each instance of tracking library segments body joints.
- One of the Kinect devices is chosen to be a "master", the rest are "slaves." The skeleton data for gesture recognition is taken from the "master" Kinect.
- If the "master" Kinect cannot "see" a particular body joint (its position was estimated), the system checks if this joint is visible to another device. If it is, our software takes coordinates measured by that assistant device. If more than two devices have detected the same joint, coordinates are taken from the camera closest to the observed point.

Each Kinect measures the distance to the observed point in its own right-handed Cartesian frame situated relatively to the sensor orientation. Consequently, the same point V has different coordinates $\overline{v'} = [x', y', z', 1]$ and $\overline{v} = [x, y, z, 1]$ for each pair of devices. For this reason, we need to find a transformation that would map all of these points to the same coordinate system. This process is called the multikinect environment calibration. Let us assume that a Cartesian frame representing the orientation of each Kinect was translated along the X, Y, and Z axes and rotated around the Y (vertical) axis relative to the "master" device frame. This means that there are four degrees of freedom (three for the translation, one for the rotation). Knowing that the linear transformation mapping the coordinates of a point represented by vector $\overline{v'}$ in one coordinate system to the coordinates $\overline{v}$ in another one has the form of the following matrix:

$$\overline{v'} \cdot \begin{bmatrix} \cos(\beta) & 0 & -\sin(\beta) & 0 \\ 0 & 1 & 0 & 0 \\ \sin(\beta) & 0 & \cos(\beta) & 0 \\ t_x & t_y & t_z & 1 \end{bmatrix} = \overline{v} \qquad (5.2)$$

By multiplying the vector and the matrix, we obtain the following linear system:

$$\begin{cases} x' \cdot \cos(\beta) + z' \cdot \sin(\beta) + t_x = x \\ y' + t_y = y \\ -x' \cdot \sin(\beta) + z' \cdot \cos(\beta) + t_z = z \\ 1 = 1 \end{cases}$$

From the second equation we can directly compute t_y if y' and y are known.

$$t_y = y - y'$$

Let us reorder the first and third equation and skip the second and fourth:

$$\begin{cases} x' \cdot \cos(\beta) + z' \cdot \sin(\beta) + t_x + 0 = x \\ z' \cdot \cos(\beta) - x' \cdot \sin(\beta) + 0 + t_z = z \end{cases} \qquad (5.3)$$

Now let us assume that we have two points whose coordinates are known in both Cartesian frames $\overline{v_1} = [x_1, y_1, z_1, 1]$, $\overline{v_2} = [x_2, y_2, z_2, 1]$, $\overline{v_1'} = [x_1', y_1', z_1', 1]$, $\overline{v_2'} = [x_2', y_2', z_2', 1]$.

(5.3) can now be rewritten as:

$$
\begin{cases}
x_1' \cdot \cos(\beta) + z_1' \cdot \sin(\beta) + t_x + 0 = x_1 \\
z_1' \cdot \cos(\beta) - x_1' \cdot \sin(\beta) + 0 + t_z = z_1 \\
x_2' \cdot \cos(\beta) + z_2' \cdot \sin(\beta) + t_x + 0 = x_2 \\
z_2' \cdot \cos(\beta) - x_2' \cdot \sin(\beta) + 0 + t_z = z_2
\end{cases}
\tag{5.4}
$$

And after representing (5.4) with matrices we get:

$$
\begin{cases}
\begin{bmatrix}
x_1' & z_1' & 1 & 0 \\
z_1' & -x_1' & 0 & 1 \\
x_2' & z_2' & 1 & 0 \\
z_2' & -x_2' & 0 & 1
\end{bmatrix}
\cdot
\begin{bmatrix}
\cos(\beta) \\
\sin(\beta) \\
t_x \\
t_z
\end{bmatrix}
=
\begin{bmatrix}
x_1 \\
z_1 \\
x_2 \\
z_2
\end{bmatrix} \\
t_y = y_1 - y_1'
\end{cases}
\tag{5.5}
$$

Summing up: in order to find unknown matrix coefficients in (5.2), linear system (5.5) has to be solved. What is important, we only need a pair of points with known coordinates in both Cartesian frames to solve this equation.

During the multikinect environment calibration procedure we need to solve (5.5) for each pair of the "master" Kinect and its "slaves." For example, if we have three Kinects, we have to find two linear transform matrices (solve two linear equation systems) between the "master" Kinect and assistance Kinects. If there are be four Kinect, we have to find three linear transform matrices, if five–four etc.

5.7 Applying a Gestures-Based Interface in Medical Systems

A touchless interface could be applied in medical systems in which direct contact with a standard interface like a keyboard or a mouse is not allowed. It might happen, e.g., during a surgical intervention when the physician's hands must be sterile and they want to control the displayed image on their own (without any assistant's help). Because most up-to-date computer applications use mouse to control the interface, contemporary gesture-based interfaces also frequently offer a mouse-like indicator, often controlled by the user with one hand. If we intend to use the Kinect controller to capture data, the most obvious approach is to utilize, e.g., hand or wrist joints as the remote cursor. With this in mind we have developed a prototype application that uses a Kinect-based VUI with GDL and a NITE tracking driver. This application is a three-dimensional desktop that supports displaying and exploring 3D volumetric data. The visualization module is based on algorithms described in Chap. 4. Our application supports:

- Visualising multiple volumetric images at the same time.
- Selecting a particular volume and rotating or translating it, or changing its transfer function to one of three predefined functions.

The right hand is used for data selection and navigation, the left to activate the navigation and to switch between the rotation and the translation mode. The right hand selects the particular volume we want to navigate. In order to check if we are "touching" this volume, we need to find out if our cursor is in the 2D region that contains the projected 3D volume. To solve this problem for each volume we visualize, a bounding sphere is defined. A bounding sphere is a 3D spherical structure containing another 3D object inside it. It is a common approach in 3D graphics to, instead of checking if the mouse cursor is "touching" the projection of a particular object, check if it is "touching" the projection of its bounding sphere. An algorithm that checks this condition proceeds as follows:

1. We are given coordinates of the mouse (or VUI mouse) cursor $\overline{m} = [m_x, m_y]$, the position of the center of the bounding sphere $\overline{v_c} = [b_x, b_y, b_z]$, its radius b_r and the matrices that are necessary for 3D rendering (projection, view and world).
2. Having a known projection, the view and world matrices, we compute the projection of $\overline{v_c}$ onto the projection plane. The new vector is $\overline{v_{cP}} = [v_x, v_y]$.
3. We compute the radius length of the projected bounding sphere:

   - We create vector $\overline{v_r} = [b_r, 0, 0]$ and we compute the projection of $\overline{v_r}$, but instead of the given world matrix, we use a new world matrix that only translates the vector. We create it in order not to rotate $\overline{v_r}$, just to rescale it according to how far/near the projection plane the boundary sphere is located. The new vector is $\overline{v_{rP}}$.
   - We compute $r = \|\overline{v_{rP}} - \overline{v_{cP}}\|$, which is the bounding sphere radius.

4. We check if $(m_x - v_x)^2 + (m_y - v_y)^2 < r^2$. If this is true, the mouse cursor is inside the projected bounding box.

We have defined the following GDL script:

```
RULE LeftHand.y[0] > LeftElbow.y[0] & LeftHand.x[0]
- LeftElbow.x[0] <= -20 THEN WavingGestureLeft
RULE LeftHand.y[0] > LeftElbow.y[0] & LeftHand.x[0]
- LeftElbow.x[0] >= 20 THEN WavingGestureRight
RULE distance(RightHand.xyz[0], LeftHand.xyz[0])
< 100 THEN HandsTog
RULE distance(RightHand.xyz[0], LeftHand.xyz[0])
>= 100 THEN HandsSep
RULE sequenceexists("[HandsSep,0.5][HandsTog,0.5][HandsSep,0.5]")
THEN Clapping
RULE distance(LeftHand.xyz[0], RightElbow.xyz[0]) < 150
THEN TouchingElbow
RULE TouchingElbow
& sequenceexists("[!TouchingElbow,1]")
THEN ChangeTransfer
```

Our visualization application is governed by the following logic:

1. If `WavingGestureLeft` is satisfied, the data navigation is switched to the translation mode. In this mode, if the right hand is "touching" a visualized object, we translate this volume according to the difference between the current and previous x, y, z coordinates of the body joint representing the right hand multiplied by the scaling factor proportional to the distance between the user and the Kinect device.
2. If `WavingGestureRight` is satisfied, the data navigation is switched to the rotation mode. In this mode if the right hand is "touching" a visualized object, we perform a rotation of this volume according to the difference between the current and the former x,y coordinates of the body joint representing the right hand multiplied by a scaling factor proportional to the distance from the user to the Kinect device.
3. In order to change the transfer function, the user has to touch their right elbow with their left hand. If `ChangeTransfer` is satisfied, the transfer function in the "touched" volume is changed to the next one from the list of predefined functions. The `ChangeTransfer` function can be true only once a second because of the `sequenceexists('`[!TouchingElbow,1]'`)` condition. The reason is that when the transfer function changed each time `TouchingElbow` is true, the transfer function would be changed at a frequency of data capture (about 30 Hz) which is way too fast for the user.
4. If `Clapping` is satisfied, all volumes are distributed evenly on the 3D desktop.

The hardware setup of a prototype application of our design is presented in Fig. 5.21, while Fig. 5.22. shows pictures taken during tests of our application. It uses a single Kinect controller, a PC running the volume rendering application written in the XNA framework, a GDL interpreter and a program that implements the above application logic. We used NITE library to track body joints. Visualizations are displayed by a multimedia projector onto a screen. Our prototype also uses an LCD monitor for debugging purposes. The performance speed of this interface is limited by the data acquisition frequency of the Kinect (approximately 30 fps). Navigation precision depends on the pose estimation accuracy of the device and its tracking software (see [40, 41, 43, 77])

5.8 GDL Approach Validation

In order to evaluate the accuracy of the GDL classifier, we have performed tests on two datasets. The first consisted of recordings of 20 people making everyday life (natural) gestures that might appear in a typical NUI interface system. The second test set consisted of various Okinawa Shorin-ryu Karate techniques performed by a black-belt instructor. In the validation on the Karate dataset we also checked the utility of multikinect data tracking systems.

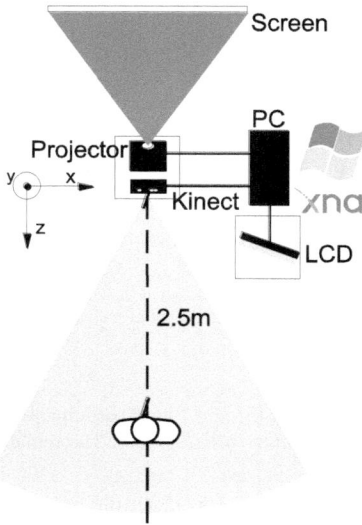

Fig. 5.21 The hardware setup of a prototype application using a Kinect-based NUI with GDL and a NITE tracking driver

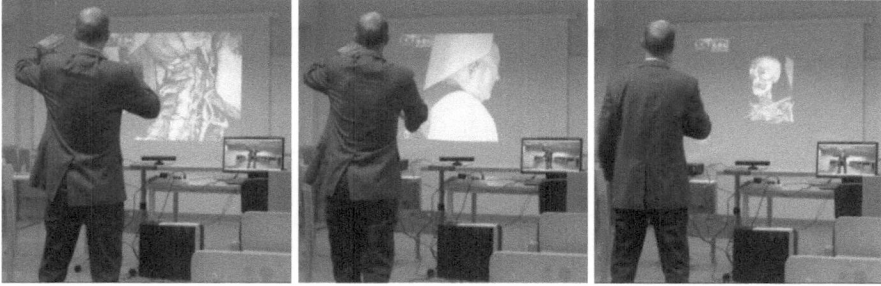

Fig. 5.22 Pictures taken during tests of the three-dimensional desktop described in this paragraph. The analyzed data is observed at various magnifications, angles and with different transfer functions

5.8.1 Validation on the Natural Gesture Dataset

We have described the results of a GDL classifier test on this dataset in our paper [73], but we decided to include a part of this evaluation here to provide a robust evaluation of the GDL approach.

We collected a large dataset of NITE skeleton recordings of 20 people (13 men and 7 women). Individuals taking part in the experiment declared that they had no previous experience with this kind of technology. All experiment participants were adults of different ages, postures (body proportions) and fitness levels (the test set

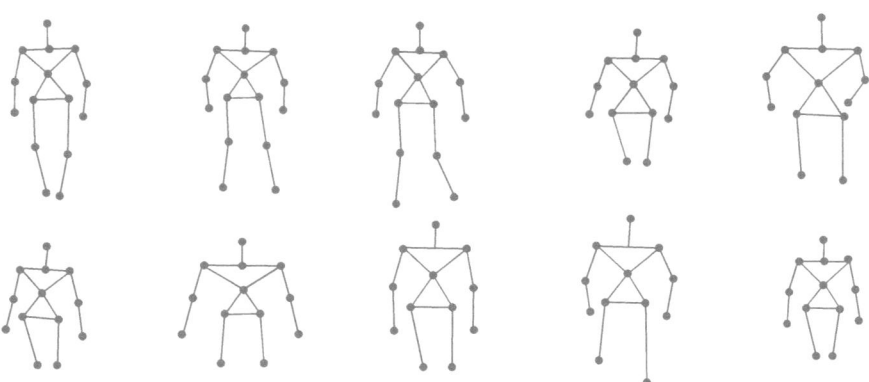

Fig. 5.23 Example skeleton frames of the first 10 test participants. One can see that only the first three NITE skeletons are complete (*have all 15 joints*). The remaining seven lack foot joints

consisted of both active athletes—for example a karate trainer—and persons declaring they had not done any physical exercises from a long time). Figure 5.23 presents example skeleton frames of the first 10 participants in the test. It can be noted that only the first three NITE skeletons are complete (have all 15 joints). The remaining seven lack foot joints. This is because the only requirement concerning the distance from experiment participants to the Kinect device was that the body parts above the knee had to be captured by the device. This condition, however, does not affect overall results because feet were irrelevant in the gestures we wanted to detect.

The test set consisted of a recording of 10 people (8 men and 2 women) who made four types of gestures (hands clapping—"Clapping", raising both hands simultaneously—"Not me!", waving with both hands over the head—"Jester"— see Fig. 5.24, and waving with the right hand) and another 5 men and 5 women who made another four types of gestures (touching the head with the left hand— "Head", touching hips with both hands—"Hips", rotating the right hand clockwise—"Rotation clockwise" and rotating the right hand anti-clockwise—"Rotation anti-clockwise"). These particular gestures have been chosen because some movements have similar joint trajectories (for example the middle part of the Jester could be recognized as clapping, also the Waving could be a part of the Jester—see Sect. 5.10 for explanations) which makes it more difficult to recognize them unambiguously. What is more, all gestures are based on arm movements, which makes these gestures easier to make for test participants, as a result of which the latter may be more relaxed and make the gestures naturally. We have observed that this relaxation makes people start performing these gestures in harmony with their body language and the details of recordings differ significantly between participants.

Each person made each gesture 20 times, which means the whole database contains 1,600 movement samples. The samples were not filtered (normalized or smoothed) with any preprocessing procedure.

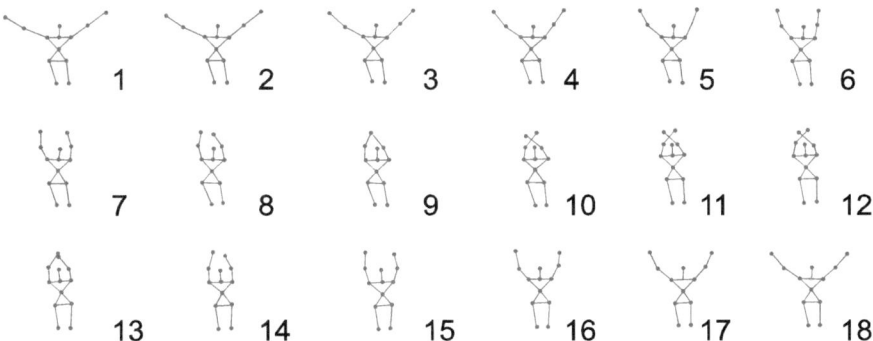

Fig. 5.24 A sequence of skeleton frames captured for a person that made "Jester" gestures. Numbers in the picture shows the order of the frames

Table 5.5 Characteristics of the dataset containing natural gestures recordings

Number of participants	20 (13 men, 7 women)
Number of samples	1,600
Number of classes (gestures types)	8 (200 samples per class)
Recording speed	Low frame rate acquisition (7–13 fps) for 480 samples. High frame rate acquisition (19–21) for 1,120 samples.
Error of data acquisition hardware	[40, 41]
Error of tracking software accuracy	[43, 77]

GDLs rules are time-dependent. That is because the 'sequence exists' function, which checks the order of rules that were satisfied, requires the maximum time span that can pass between key frames of gestures to be written explicitly. In order to check the extent to which these time constraints affect the final results, skeleton recordings were made at two speeds: a low-frame rate acquisition speed (from 7 to 13 fps for 6 persons in the test set) and a high frame rate acquisition speed (19–21 fps for 14 persons in the test set). The recording speed limitation was due to the performance of the NITE library we used. The next training dataset tracked with Kinect SDK was acquired at the speed of 30 fps (so it was limited by the Kinect capture rate). The random error of the depth measurement by our recording hardware (Kinect) increases along with the increasing distance from the sensor, and ranges from a few millimeters up to about 4 cm at the maximum range of the sensor [40, 41]. This error affects the accuracy of the joint segmentation algorithm, causing the constant body point distance to fluctuate over time. Because of the presence of this random error, we did not consider adding other noise to the recorded dataset. Table 5.5 presents the summary of our first dataset characteristics.

The GDLs scripts we used to describe classes from the natural gesture dataset can be found in Sect. 5.10.1. There, we also added figures showing the key frames of GDL description and short commentaries. Tables 5.6, 5.7 and 5.8 present results of the GDL classifier validation on a dataset containing natural gestures. Figures 5.25, 5.26 and 5.27 graphically represent results from those tables.

Table 5.6 Results of the GDL approach validation on a dataset containing natural gestures

	Clapping	"Not me!"	"Jester"	Waving	Head	Hips	Rotation anti-clockwise	Rotation clockwise	No recognition
Clapping	90.0±1.6%	0	0	0	1.0%	0	0	0	9.0±1.8%
"Not me!"	2.0%	93.5±1.1%	0	1.5±0.4%	2.5±1.1%	0	0	0	2.0%
"Jester"	3.5±0.3%	0	92.0±0.6%	0	0	0	0	0	4.5±0.4%
Waving	0	0	0	93.0±2.2%	0	0	2.5±1.1%	0.5%	7.0%
Head	0	0	0	0	98.5±0.5%	0	0	0	1.5%
Hips	0	0	0	0	0	95.5±1.0%	0	0	4.5±0.4%
Rotation anti-clockwise	0	0.5%	0	2.0%	0	0	87.5±1.7%	0	11.0±1.4%
Rotation clockwise	0.5%	0	0	2.0%	0	0	0	80.5±1.8%	18.5±1.5%

The table presents numbers of samples classified to particular classes divided by the numbers of samples actually belonging to the specific class multiplied by 100 %. The plus/minus sign precedes the standard deviation in recognition between recordings of different participants. Each class consists of 200 samples. In this table columns represent recognition result and rows represent actual condition

Values in Tables 5.6, 5.7 and 5.8 are numbers of samples that were classified to a particular class divided by the number of samples that actually belong to that class and multiplied by 100 %. A value above zero in the blue fields "no recognition" (NR %) means that in response to a particular signal that should be classified, the GDL classifier did not return any class label. Values in yellow fields are cases in which the GDL classifier returned a label of the class that appeared in the recording (the correct recognition percentage—CR %). Values in orange fields mean that the classifier returned the wrong class label (the incorrect recognition percentage—IR %). Fields with white background represent cases which do not belong to any class, in which a particular gesture was not detected in a sequence that did not contain this gesture. We presented recognition results in percentages to show the proportion of each right and wrong recognition case to the overall number of class exemplars.

As a result of these definitions of the NR, CR and IR %, the sum of values in each row can exceed 100 %. This is because the GDL classifier is able to return multiple class labels for each recording sample (to recognize two or more different gestures in one recording): the GDL is not a binary classifier. This is a very important feature of our classifier, but in a natural gesture dataset we do not have

Table 5.7 Results of the GDL approach validation on a low frame rate sample set

	Clapping	"Not me!"	"Jester"	Waving	Head	Hips	Rotation anti-clockwise	Rotation clockwise	No recognition
Clapping	78.8±5.4%	0	0	0	2.5%	0	0	0	18.8±5.5%
"Not me!"	5.0%	83.8±3.3%	0	3.8±0.9%	6.3±2.7%	0	0	0	5.0%
"Jester"	2.5%	0	91.3±1.2%	0	0	0	0	0	6.3±1.4%
Waving	0	0	0	82.5±8.8%	0	0	0	0	17.5%
Head	0	0	0	0	100.0%	0	0	0	0
Hips	0	0	0	0	0	77.5±1.8%	0	0	22.5±1.8%
Rotation anti-clockwise	0	2.5%	0	0	0	0	72.5±5.3%	0	25.0±3.5%
Rotation clockwise	0	0	0	5.0%	0	0	0	92.5±5.3%	7.5%

The table presents numbers of samples assigned to a particular class divided by numbers of samples that actually belong to that class and multiplied by 100 %. The plus/minus sign is followed by the standard deviation in the recognition between recordings of different participants. In this table columns represent recognition result and rows represent actual condition

such types of multitype gestures. Thus all these cases were errors—the so-called excessive misclassification. Excessive misclassifications are evaluated as a component of the IR % coefficient. The number of excessive misclassification cases is 14 for 1,600 recordings samples. In the analyzed datasets, excessive misclassifications never exceeded 5 % of overall result in any class evaluated in Tables 5.6, 5.7, 5.8. The source data from which the percentage data was generated can be found in paper [73].

Table 5.6 and Fig. 5.25 substantiate the claim that the GDL classifier achieved quite rewarding results on the test dataset. The CR % falls below 90 % only for two classes (i.e. for the right hand rotation clockwise and anticlockwise). What is more, the standard deviation of the CR % between experiment participants is low—only in one case (waving) does it exceed 2 %. This means that the classification of a particular gesture class is stable between different users. The most difficult groups of movements to be recognized by the GDL classifier are those that require complex paths, for example circles, to be analyzed. Consequently, both movement classes that represent movements with circular paths are characterized by the lowest recognition rate.

Table 5.8 Results of the GDL approach validation on a set of high-frame-rate samples

	Clapping	"Not me!"	"Jester"	Waving	Head	Hips	Rotation anti-clockwise	Rotation clockwise	No recognition
Clapping	97.5±0.7%	0	0	0	0	0	0	0	2.5±0.6%
"Not me!"	0	100.0%	0	0	0	0	0	0	0
"Jester"	4.2±0.7%	0	92.5±1.9%	0	0	0	0	0	3.3±0.7%
Waving	0	0	0	100.0%	0	0	4.2.0±2.7%	0.8±%	0
Head	0	0	0	0	98.1±0.7%	0	0	0	1.9±%
Hips	0	0	0	0	0	100.0%	0	0	0
Rotation anti-clockwise	0	0	0	2.5%	0	0	91.3±2.1%	0	7.5±2.1%
Rotation clockwise	0.6%	0	0	1.3%	0	0	0	77.5±2.3%	21.3±1.9%

The table presents numbers of samples assigned to a particular class divided by numbers of samples actually belonging to that class and multiplied by 100 %. The plus/minus sign is followed by the standard deviation in the recognition between recordings of different participants. In this table columns represent recognition result and rows represent actual condition

We also inspected how the recording speed influences the performance of the proposed classification method. In order to do that, we generated Table 5.7 for recordings made at 7 fps and 13 fps speeds, and Table 5.8 for recordings at 19 fps and 21 fps. These tables should be read in the same way as Table 5.6. It is apparent that all type of errors (NR and IR %) are present in both datasets. Our previous conclusions about the excessive misclassification error also hold true in low- and high-speed datasets.

As GDL is not a binary classifier, we cannot analyze errors using a confusion matrix. Instead of that, we made a comparison based on the CR % (see Table 5.9 and Fig. 5.28). This particular comparison checks how well the classifier identifies exemplars of a particular class so its meaning is similar to the sensitivity of a binary classifier. In all classes IR << CR %, which means that our classifier rarely confuses one class with another. This ability, talking in the language of a binary classifier, means that the GDL approach is of high specificity (the ability to identify negative results).

We can see that the tracking speed strongly affects the CR %. High-speed recordings give a higher CR % more frequently than low-speed recordings. This is apparent in case of the clapping gesture, where the CR % is 18.7 % higher in the high-speed recording set than in the low-speed one. The only remarkable

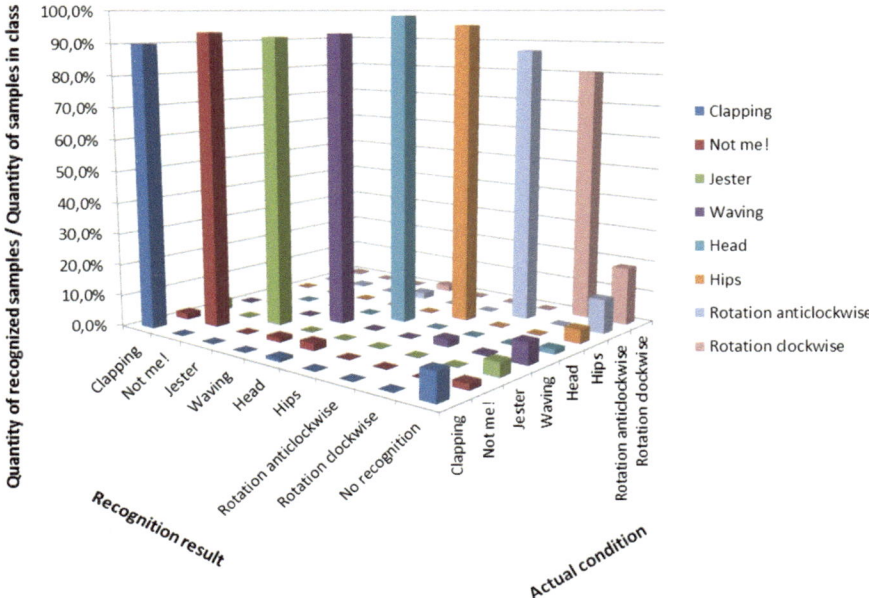

Fig. 5.25 Visualization of Table 5.6 results

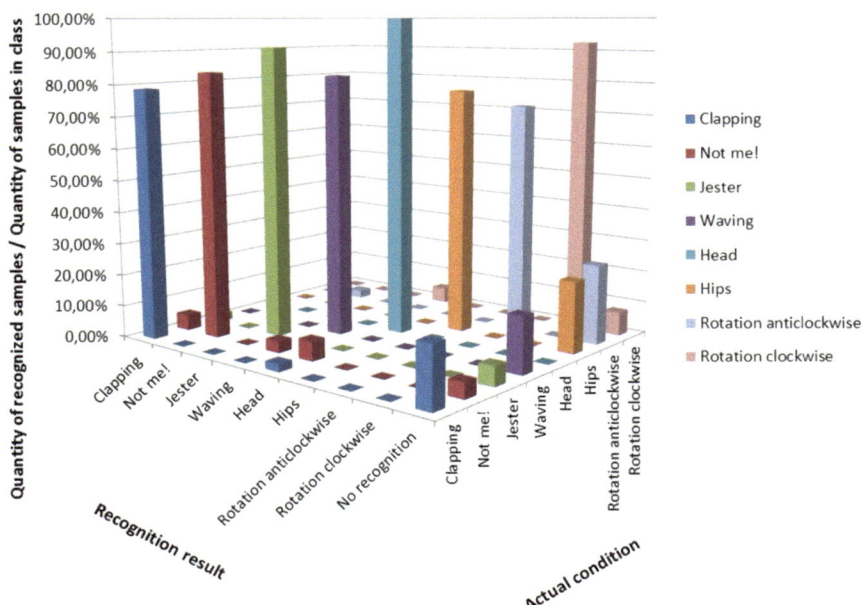

Fig. 5.26 Visualization of Table 5.7 results

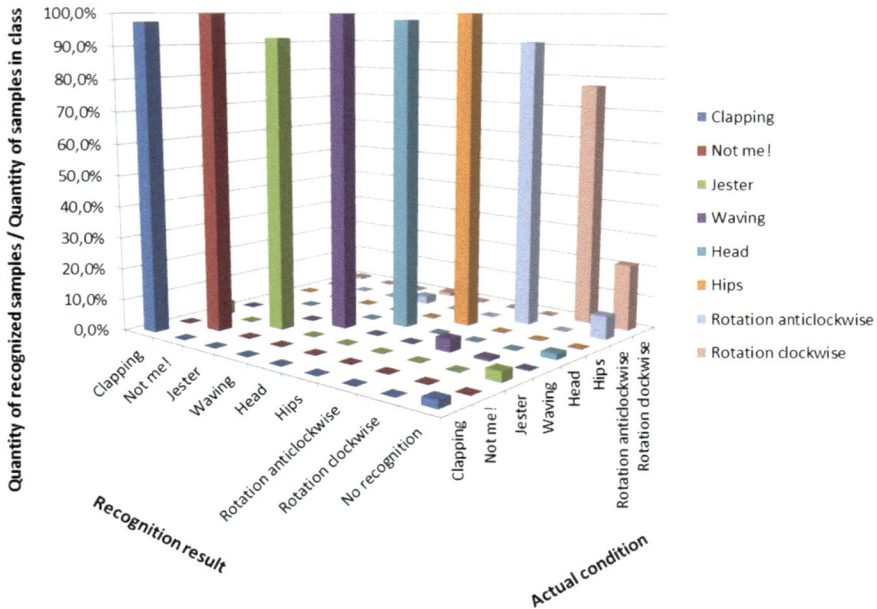

Fig. 5.27 Visualization of Table 5.8 results

Table 5.9 GDL CR % evaluated on a natural gesture data set and its subsets grouped by tracking speed

	Clapping (%)	Not me(%)	Jester (%)	Waving (%)	Head (%)	Hips (%)	Rotation anticlockwise (%)	Rotation clockwise (%)
7–13 fps	78.8	83.8	91.3	82.5	100.0	77.5	72.5	92.5
19–21 fps	97.5	100.0	92.5	100.0	98.1	100.0	91.3	77.5
7-21 fps	90.0	93.5	92.0	93.0	98.5	95.5	87.5	80.5

exception is the clockwise rotation of the right hand, where the recognition rate of low-speed samples was 92.5 ± 5.3 %, while that of high-speed samples was 77.5 ± 2.3 %. This result was caused by two participants in the low-speed sample who were performing their gestures very precisely and carefully. What is interesting is that they had greater difficulty with the anti-clockwise rotation than participants from the high-speed dataset. What is very important is that—according to our observations—all errors were caused by inaccuracies of the tracking software. Even though all participants were making the gestures as we expected them to, the key frames did not appear in the memory stack. Situations like these are, of course, unavoidable.

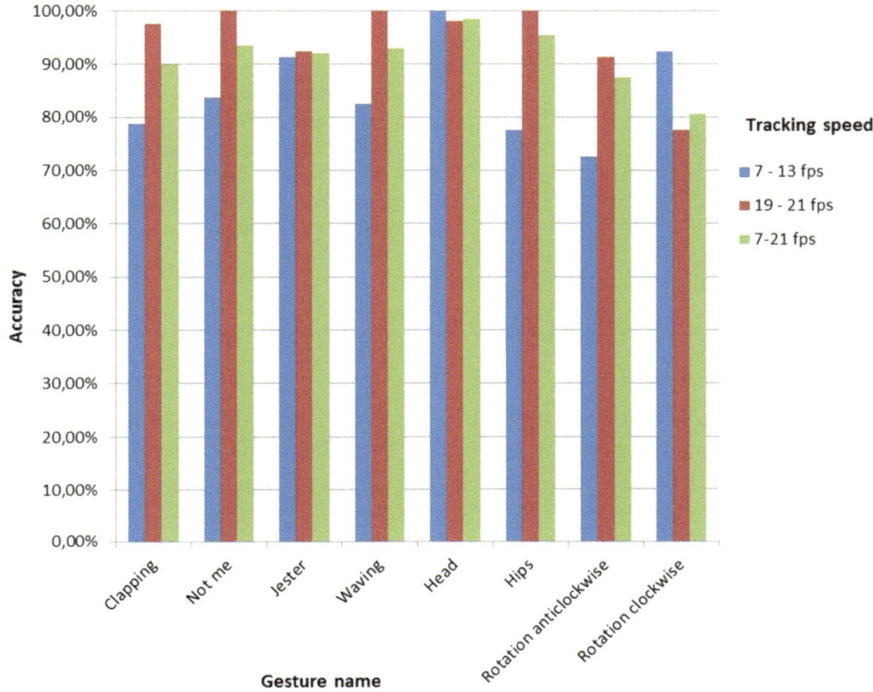

Fig. 5.28 Visualization of Table 5.9 resultsVisualization of Table

The CR % coefficient for the whole natural gesture set (tracking speed between 7 and 21 fps) varies from 98.5 to 80.5 %. These are quite rewarding results, particularly as these participants had no time to train their gesticulation and did not get any feedback from the gesture tracking application. We suppose that after a user gets accustomed to this type of interface and gets to know how to behave before the sensor, the results might be even better. This experiment showed that the main limitation of GDL approach lies in identifying gestures that are based on tracking trajectories, e.g. circular or linear. For this reasons clockwise and anti-clockwise hand rotations are the only gestures for which the CR % fell below 90 %. Apart from this problem, our approach based on a time-dependent definition of gestures as sequences of key frames has proven to be sufficient for the natural gesture classification problem. Using key frames instead of continuous trajectories is one of the biggest advantages of GDL, as it makes the recognition more resistant to body joint tracking noises which are a common problem in Kinect-based software. The next factor that might be critical for the correct identification of gestures is the tracking speed. The experiment showed that if this speed decreases, so does the CR %. The solution to this problem is to use hardware and tracking libraries which generate skeletons fast enough for the particular requirement. What

Table 5.10 Characteristics of the subset of Okinawa Shorin-ryu Karate recordings

Number of participants	1 man, black belt instructor (3 dan) of Shorin-Ryu Karate
Number of samples	150 samples for the multiple Kinect configuration shown on the left in Fig. 5.20
	150 samples for the multiple Kinect configuration shown on the right in Fig. 5.20
Number of classes (gesture types)	3 (50 samples for two classes, 100 samples for one in each multi-Kinect configuration)
Recording speed	30 fps
Error of data acquisition hardware	[40, 41]
Error of tracking software accuracy	[43, 77]

is very promising is that even during low-speed data acquisition (13 fps and less), the GDL still remains functional and the CR % coefficient in our experiment never dropped under 70 %.

5.8.2 Validation on a Okinawa Shorin-ryu Karate Dataset

The experiment which was the source of our data was a part of a dataset on which the GDL classifier was evaluated in [76, 78, 79]. The dataset was collected during a training session of a black belt instructor (3 dan) of Shorin-Ryu Karate. We have taken only a subset of the Shorin-ryu Karate dataset in which we can observe the improvement of the CR % after applying multikinect tracking. In the remaining set the CR % did not improve because single tracking devices were sufficient to gather all joint data. We decided to do this because there was no point in evaluating all GDLs descriptions of all Karate movements considered in our previous experiments, as this exceeds the scope of this book. The aim of validating using the subset of Okinawa Shorin-ryu Karate dataset was to test whether the GDL classifier is capable of recognizing rapid movement sequences characteristic for martial arts. The set consists of one stance (Moto-dachi), one block (Age-uke) in which the head joint is covered with a hand and wrist body joint and one kick (Mae-geri). The GDLs descriptions of those gestures and key frame pictures can be found in Sect. 5.10.2. Because of the movement speed and gesture complexity, this dataset can be considered to be more difficult to recognize than the previous one. The characteristics of our dataset are presented in Table 5.10. It should be noted that when our trainer does the Age-uke, he also takes the Moto-dachi stance. For this reason we have twice as many samples of Moto-dachi as of other classes.

We evaluated GDL classification results in two experiments. The experiment participant was always situated in front of the central IR sensor facing it. In the first configuration (see Fig. 5.20, right side) the two additional "slave" Kinects were put on the sides of user and were rotated around the y (vertical) axis by the

Table 5.11 Results of the GDL approach validation on a dataset where the "slaves" were rotated by $\frac{\pi}{2}$ and $-\frac{\pi}{2}$ angles, but only tracking data from the "master" was used

	Moto-dachi	Age-uke + Moto-dachi	Mae-geri	Not classified
Moto-dachi	100,0%	0	0	0
Age-uke + Moto-dachi	100,0%	44,0%	0	28,0%
Mae-geri	8,0%	0	26,0%	74,0%

The table presents numbers of samples that were assigned to a particular class divided by numbers of samples actually belonging to that class and multiplied by 100 %. In this table columns represent recognition result and rows represent actual condition

Table 5.12 Results of the GDL approach validation on a dataset where the "slaves" were rotated by $\frac{\pi}{2}$ and $-\frac{\pi}{2}$ angles using integrated recordings from "master" and "slave" devices

	Moto-dachi	Age-uke + Moto-dachi	Mae-geri	Not classified
Moto-dachi	100,0%	0	0	0
Age-uke + Moto-dachi	100,0%	86,0%	0	7,0%
Mae-geri	8,0%	0	68,0%	32,0%

The table presents numbers of samples that were assigned to a particular class divided by numbers of samples actually belonging to that class and multiplied by 100 %. In this table columns represent recognition result and rows represent actual condition

angle $\frac{\pi}{2}$ and $-\frac{\pi}{2}$. In the second, the "master" Kinect was also in front of the user but "slaves" were rotated around the y (vertical) axis by the angle $\frac{\pi}{4}$ and $-\frac{\pi}{4}$. Each configuration was tested in order to determine how using an additional Kinect improves overall recognition. In order to do this, we first examine the NR %, CR % and IR % while the gesture is tracked by the central "master" device only (we did not combine the "slave" recordings into a single one). Then, we find matrices (5.2) by solving linear systems (5.5) and we create the single recording as described in Sect. 5.6. The results for the $\frac{\pi}{2}$ / $-\frac{\pi}{2}$ data set are presented in Tables 5.11 and 5.12, and then visualized in Figs. 5.29 and 5.30 We used the same color designations in these tables as in the experiment with the natural gesture dataset.

The results for the $\frac{\pi}{4}$ / $-\frac{\pi}{4}$ data set are presented in Tables 5.13 and 5.14, and then visualized in Figs. 5.31 and 5.32.

In all experiments, the Moto-dachi was the easiest class to recognize. Practically all gestures of this type were recognized regardless of whether they were performed alone or together with the Age-uke. In the second dataset (Tables 5.13, 5.14), only one Moto-dachi done together with an Age-uke was not correctly classified (that is its CR % was 98 %). The stance was also the source of the only IR % of the GDL in this experiment when it was detected in Mae-geri recordings. This happened because at the beginning of the kick, the trainer's position was similar enough to be considered to constitute a Moto-dachi even though he did not

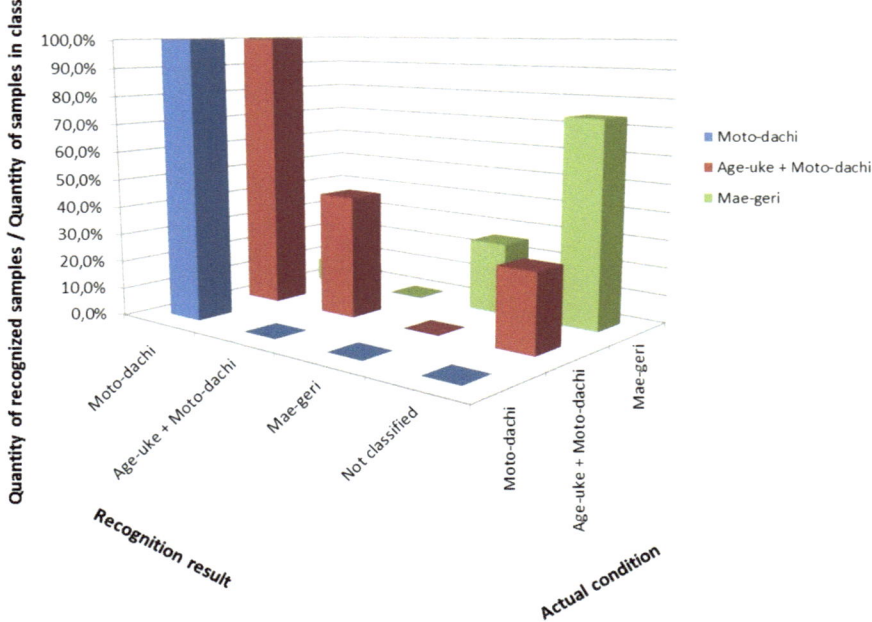

Fig. 5.29 Visualization of Table 5.11 results

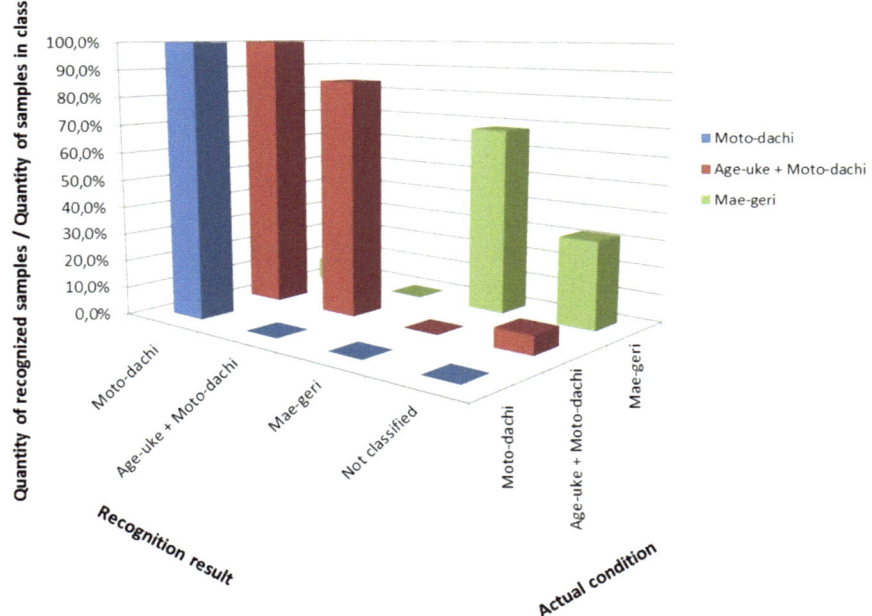

Fig. 5.30 Visualization of Table 5.12 results

Table 5.13 Results of the GDL approach validation on a dataset where the "slaves" were rotated by the $\frac{\pi}{4}$ and $-\frac{\pi}{4}$ angle, but only tracking data from the "master" was used

	Moto-dachi	Age-uke + Moto-dachi	Mae-geri	Not classified
Moto-dachi	100,0%	0	0	0
Age-uke + Moto-dachi	98,0%	42,0%	0	30,0%
Mae-geri	0	0	2,0%	98,0%

The table presents numbers of samples that were assigned to a particular class divided by numbers of samples actually belonging to that class and multiplied by 100 %. In this table columns represent recognition result and rows represent actual condition

Table 5.14 Results of the GDL approach validation on a dataset where the "slaves" were rotated by the $\frac{\pi}{4}$ and $-\frac{\pi}{4}$ angles and integrated recordings from "master" and "slave" devices were used

	Moto-dachi	Age-uke + Moto-dachi	Mae-geri	Not classified
Moto-dachi	100,0%	0	0	0
Age-uke + Moto-dachi	98,0%	84,0%	0	9,0%
Mae-geri	0	0	64,0%	36,0%

The table presents numbers of samples that were assigned to a particular class divided by numbers of samples actually belonging to that class and multiplied by 100 %. In this table columns represent recognition result and rows represent actual condition

do that intentionally. Blocks and kicks were harder to recognize. Because of the two gestures for which the IR % equals zero it will be easier to use Table 5.15 for the remaining GDL evaluation.

Table 5.15 and Fig. 5.33 present a comparison based on CR %. This particular comparison checks how well the classifier identifies exemplars of a particular class so its meaning is similar to that of the sensitivity of a binary classifier. In the case of Age-uke, one tracking device is often insufficient to classify the movement. This is because the tracking software often loses track of particular joints covered one by another and their positions must be estimated by the Kinect SDK library. This estimation introduces noise which cannot be compensated by the GDLs description. Nearly twice as many Age-uke blocks were correctly classified when a multikinect recording was used. The improvement was even better for Mae-geri. In the first case, the CR % was 2.6 times higher than for a single Kinect recording, while in the second it was 32 times higher (!). The reason was that front kicks are a major challenge for the tracking software. The feet are moving at a relatively high speed with a long radius of the path and, at the last stage of Mae-geri, the feet are situated nearly at the same horizontal position as the hip and knee. If the sportsman is filmed only in the frontal view, the knee and hip body joints are obstructed by the feet and the proper position of these joints has to be approximated by the software, which, in practice, generates serious positioning errors. In this dataset, too, (same as in natural gestures dataset), IR $\ll$ CR % in all classes which means

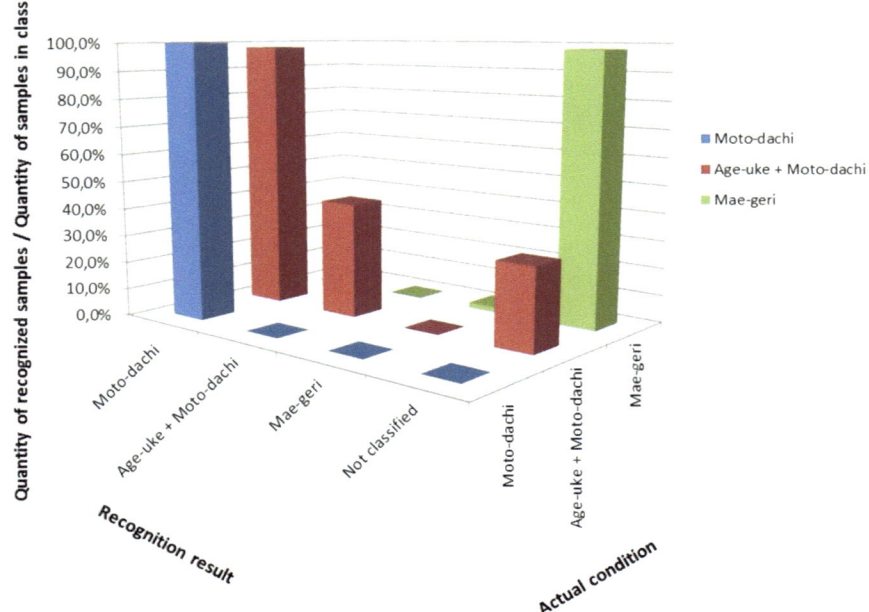

Fig. 5.31 Visualization of Table 5.13 results

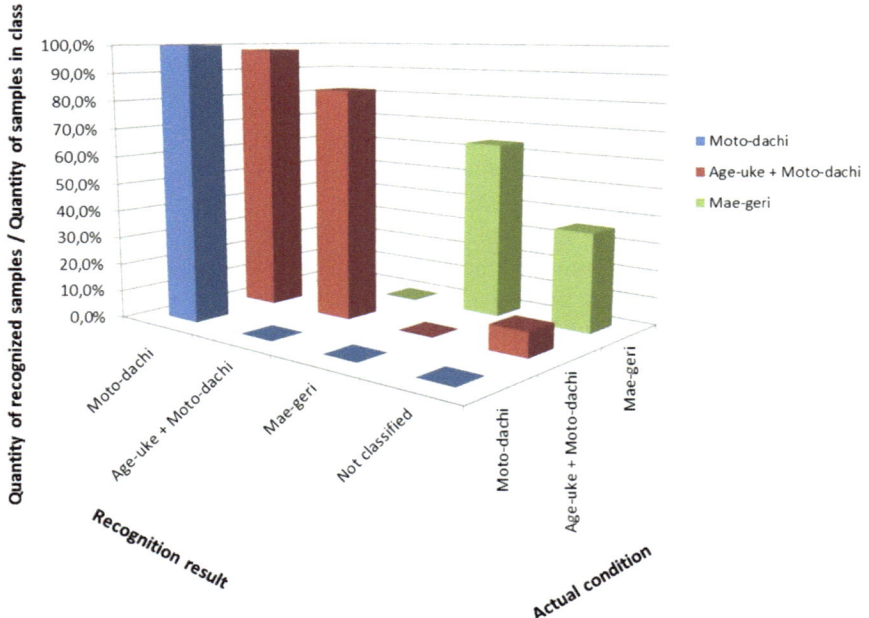

Fig. 5.32 Visualization of results from Table 5.14

Table 5.15 GDL CR % tested on a subset of the Okinawa Shorin-ryu Karate set

Tracking configuration	Moto-dachi (%)	Age-uke (%)	Mae-geri (%)
Only "master" Kinect tracking, slaves rotated by $\pm\frac{\pi}{2}$ (Single 90)	100, 0	44, 0	26, 0
"Master" and "slaves" tracking, slaves rotated by $\pm\frac{\pi}{2}$ (Triple 90)	100, 0	86, 0	68, 0
Only "master" Kinect tracking, slaves rotated by $\pm\frac{\pi}{4}$ (Single 45)	99, 0	42, 0	2, 0
"Master" and "slaves" tracking, slaves rotated by $\pm\frac{\pi}{4}$ (Triple 45)	99, 0	84, 0	64, 0

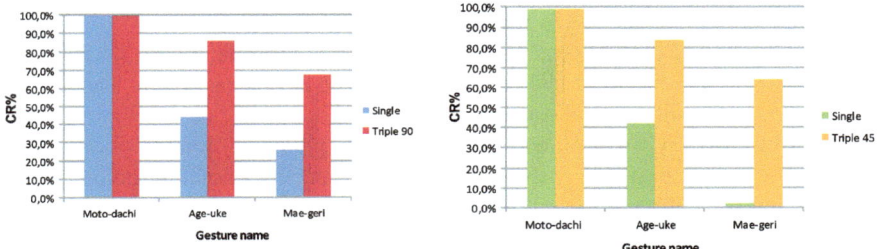

Fig. 5.33 Visualization of results from Table 5.15

that our classifier rarely confuses one class with another. This is another proof that, using the language of a binary classifier, that GDL approach exhibits a high specificity (the ability to identify negative results). In conclusion, a multikinect setup for data tracking and our algorithm for calibration and integration greatly increase the CR % of the GDL method. The method described in paragraph 5.6 is independent of the gestures classifier used and we suppose it could also be very useful as a general approach to improving the tracking accuracy.

Based on our theoretical description and the results from the evaluation procedure, we can summarize GDL classifier features in a way similar to that in [76]:

- GDL is capable of classifying human body movements in real-time.
- It can classify not only simple, real life gestures but also complicated movements like Karate techniques.
- It does not require a large training dataset. Gestures are defined in GDLs by the user (an expert in a particular field of physical activity). The user can utilize as many body features as they needs in each rule definition.
- Gestures are split into key frames that appear in some order subject to a given time restriction.
- The input data for the classifier consists of a set of body joints fed by the tracking software in real-time (at the approximate frequency of 30 Hz).

- Our notation is invariant to the user rotation around the camera viewport, because it can generate features concerning angles measured between vectors defined by pairs of body joints. These angles are defined dynamically while tailoring the GDL script description.

5.9 GDL Script Language 1.1 Specifications

GDL 1.1 is a context-free grammar.

$$GDL = \{V_N, V_T, SP, STS\} \tag{5.6}$$

Where V_N is a set of nonterminal symbols, V_T is a set of terminal symbols, SP is a set of productions and STS is the start symbol of the grammar.

Basically, an LR parser is sufficient to parse GDL script language 1.1 (GDLs), but some ambiguity has to be solved after the parsing tree is generated. The way of solving this ambiguity is described in Sect. 5.9.5.5

GDLs has three types of numeric values: double precision floating point values (signed), three-dimensional vectors of double precision floating point values (signed) and logical values (binary).

5.9.1 Nonterminal Symbols

Nonterminal symbols, or nonterminals in short, are the symbols which can be replaced; thus there are strings composed of some combination of terminal and nonterminal symbols.

```
V_N={NumericRule,    NumericRule3D,    LogicalRule,    Rule,
GDLScript, Sequence, FeatureNumeric, FeatureNumeric3D}
```

5.9.2 Terminal Symbols

Terminal symbols are literal characters that can appear in the inputs to or outputs from the production rules of a formal grammar and cannot be broken down into "smaller" units.

```
V_T={LogicalOperator,        NumericOperator,        Rela-
tionalOperator, OpenBracket, ClosedBracket, OpenSquare-
Bracket,  ClosedSquarebracket,  LogicalFunction,  Numer-
icFunction,   SequentialFunction,   RulePersistsFunction,
NumericFunction3D, NumericOperator3D, RuleSymbol, Then-
Symbol, Sequence, BodyPart, BodyPart3D, Conclusion, Nu-
meric,  Comma,  Quotation,    Excalamation,  FeatureNumer-
icName, FeatureNumeric3DName, FeatureSymbol, AsSymbol}
```

5.9.3 Grammar Start Symbol

The start symbol of the grammar is:
  STS = GDLScript
  When the GDL script file is parsed, the code has to be reduced to STS. If this is impossible, this means that the script file is not in GDL 1.1 grammar. This means it contains an error.

5.9.4 Grammar Productions

All productions that exist in the GDL script are listed in Table 5.16.

5.9.5 Terminal Symbol Definition for the Lexical Analyzer

This section defines terminal symbols that can appear in a GDL script file. If necessary, we will also show examples illustrating how to use particular symbols.

5.9.5.1 Numeric Values (Constants and Variables)

Numeric = *{number|number.number|.number}*—defines double precision floating point values, for example: 16, 17.456, .34345. Production 12 defines negative values of Numeric.

  Numeric3DRule—defines three-dimensional vectors of double precision floating point values, for example: [45.45, -.345, 34.789]

  Conclusion—Any string after ThenSymbol is a conclusion. Any unrecognized string is hypothetically a conclusion. Because rules can appear in any order (the previous declaration of a Conclusion after the ThenSymbol is not required), at the end of the parsing, the parser checks if all unrecognized strings appear after ThenSymbol. If not, the GDL script contains an error. If a conclusion appears as the premise of a rule, it returns a logical value. It equals true if the rule is satisfied at a given moment in time (the conclusion of the rule is present in a particular level of the memory stack) and false if it is not satisfied (the conclusion of the rule is not present in a particular level of the memory stack).

  For example:

RULE 12<14 **THEN** MyConclusion
RULE MyConclusion **THEN** MyConclusion2

  In this case MyConclusion and MyConclusion2 are always true (are always satisfied).

  FeatureNumericName, FeatureNumeric3DName—Any string after the AsSymbol is a FeatureName or a FeatureName3D. Any unrecognized string is

Table 5.16 Productions of GDL

No	Production
1	GDLScript → Rule
2	Rule → Rule Rule
3	Rule → FeatureNumeric
4	Rule → FeatureNumeric3D
5	Rule → RuleSymbol LogicalRule ThenSymbol Conclusion
6	NumericRule → Numeric
7	LogicalRule → Conclusion
8	FeatureNumeric → FeatureSumbol NumericRule AsSymbol FeatureNumericName
9	FeatureNumeric3D → FeatureSumbol Numeric3DRule AsSymbol FeatureNumeric3DName
10	NumericRule → FeatureNumericName
11	Numeric3DRule → FeatureNumeric3DName
12	NumericRule → NumericOperator("-") NumericRule
13	Numeric3DRule → NumericOperator3D("-") Numeric3DRule
14	NumericRule → NumericRule NumericOperator NumericRule
15	Numeric3DRule → Numeric3DRule NumericOperator3D Numeric3DRule
16	NumericRule → OpenBracket NumericRule ClosedBracket
17	Numeric3DRule → OpenBracket Numeric3DRule ClosedBracket
18	NumericRule → NumericFunction NumericRule ClosedBracket
19	NumericRule → BodyPart NumericRule ClosedSquareBracket
20	Numeric3DRule → BodyPart3D NumericRule ClosedSquareBracket
21	NumericRule → NumericFunction3D Numeric3DRule Comma Numeric3DRule ClosedBracket
22	Numeric3DRule → OpenSquareBracket NumericRule Comma NumericRule Comma NumericRule ClosedSquareBracket
23	LogicalRule → NumericRule RelationalOperator NumericRule
24	LogicalRule → LogicalRule LogicalOperator LogicalRule
25	LogicalRule → OpenBracket LogicalRule ClosedBracket
26	LogicalRule → LogicalFunction LogicalRule ClosedBracket
27	LogicalRule → SequentialFunction Sequence ClosedBracket
28	Sequence → Quotation SequencePart Quotation
29	SequencePart → SequencePart SequencePart
30	SequencePart → OpenSquareBracket Conclusion Comma Numeric ClosedSquareBracket
31	SequencePart → OpenSquareBracket Exclamation Conclusion Comma Numeric ClosedSquareBracket
32	LogicalRule → RulePersistsFunction Conclusion Comma NumericRule Comma NumericRule ClosedBracket

hypothetically one of these two. Because rules and features can appear in any order, at the end of the parsing, the parser checks if all unrecognized strings appear after the AsSymbol and if it forms a part of a FeatureNumeric or a FeatureNumeric3D. If not, the GDL script contains an error. Features are parsed before rules.

For example:

```
FEATURE 24 - 15.5 AS MyFeature
FEATURE [10,1,34] - [1,1,1] AS MyFeature2
```

In this case MyFeature equals 8.5 and MyFeature2 equals [9, 0, 33].

Conclusion, FeatureNumericName and FeatureNumeric3DName should consist of alphanumeric characters ([a–z], [A–Z], [0–9]) and can also contain "_" or "-"or "!" but the exclamation cannot constitute the first letter.

5.9.5.2 Operators

NumericOperator = *{+,-,*,/,%,^}*—the sum, difference, multiplication, division, modulo, and power of floating point numbers. For example the square root of 2 ($\sqrt{2}$) is 2^0.5.

NumericOperator3D = *{+,-}*—the sum and difference of three-dimensional floating point vectors.

RelationOperator = *{<, > ,=, <=, >=,! =}*—compares two floating point numbers: smaller than, greater than, equal, smaller or equal, greater or equal, not equal.

LogicalOperator = *{&,/}*—logical operators "and", "or" for logical values.

Exclamation = *{!}*—the exclamation mark is used as a negation in sequence strings for the sequenceexists function (see Sect. 5.9.5.3 for more details).

OpenBracket = *{(}, ClosedBracket* = *{)}*—brackets are used to specify the order of operations in an expression.

OpenSquareBracket = *{[}, ClosedSquareBracket* = *{]}*— square brackets are used to define three-dimensional floating point vectors. They are also present in sequence strings (see Sect. 5.9.5.3 for more details), where they define components of sequences, and in references to body joint values (see Sect. 5.9.5.4).

Comma = *{,}*—the comma is mainly used as the separator of parameters in function calls and in sequence strings.

Quotation = *{''}*—the quotation mark denotes the beginning and the end of sequence strings.

5.9.5.3 Functions

LogicalFunction = *{not(}*—the function returns a negation of its logical argument (for example not(12 < 14) returns false).

NumericFunction = *{abs(,sqrt(}*—the function abs returns an absolute value of its floating point argument (for example abs(−12) returns 12). sqrt returns the square root of its argument.

SequentialFunction = *{sequenceexists(}*—the function returns true if the sequence of conclusions defined in its sequence parameter has appeared within a given time period in the memory stack. The function returns false in other cases.

For example:

RULE
```
sequenceexists("[clappingT,0.5][clappingS,1.5][!notIn,2]")
```
THEN clapping

This sequence consists of three sequence parts: the first means that the conclusion clappingT should appear in any level of the memory stack no later than 0.5 s before now. The second part means that the conclusion clappingS has to appear within the time period starting from the first detection of the clappingT and no later than 1.5 after that. The third has a prefix "!" and means that the conclusion notIn should <u>not</u> be present within the time period starting from the first detection of the clappingS and lasting the entire following 2 s.

Summing up, presence of each conclusion in the sequence part is checked in the time period of the memory stack starting from the first appearance of the previous one (or from the "top level" of the stack, if it is the first sequence part) and down for a defined number of seconds. However, if a conclusion is preceded by a negation (exclamation mark), the conclusion must not be present in the whole defined time period and the check for the presence of the next conclusion in the sequence part starts after the expiry of this entire time period.

RulePersistsFunction **=** *{rulepersists()*—this function returns true if a given conclusion is present in the last x seconds in at least y percent of memory stack levels. This function returns false in other cases.

For example:

`rulepersists(gesture, 4.5, 0.92)`—returns true if the conclusion "gesture" is present in at least 92 % of memory stack levels over the last 4.5 s.

NumericFunction3D **=** *{distance(,angle()*—the distance function returns a floating point value which represents the Euclidean distance between two three-dimensional floating point vectors.

$$\text{distance}([x_1, y_1, z_1], [x_2, y_2, z_2]) = \sqrt{(x_1 - x_2)^2 + (y_1 - y_2)^2 + (z_1 - z_2)^2}$$

The function angle returns a floating point value that represents the angle between two three-dimensional floating point vectors. The angle belongs to the range [0,180]. Let us assume that vectors $\overline{X'}, \overline{Y'}$ are normalized vectors $\overline{X}, \overline{Y}$:

$$\overline{X'} = \frac{\overline{X}}{\|\overline{X}\|} \text{ and } \overline{Y'} = \frac{\overline{Y}}{\|\overline{Y}\|}$$

Angles are ultimately recalculated into degrees. The graphical illustration of (5.7) is shown in Fig. (5.34).

If $\theta \in \left[0, \frac{\pi}{2}\right]$ then $\sin\frac{\theta}{2} = \frac{\frac{\|\overline{X'}-\overline{Y'}\|}{2}}{1}$

If $\theta \in \left(\frac{\pi}{2}, \pi\right]$ then $\sin\frac{\pi-\theta}{2} = \frac{\frac{\|-\overline{X'}-\overline{Y'}\|}{2}}{1}$

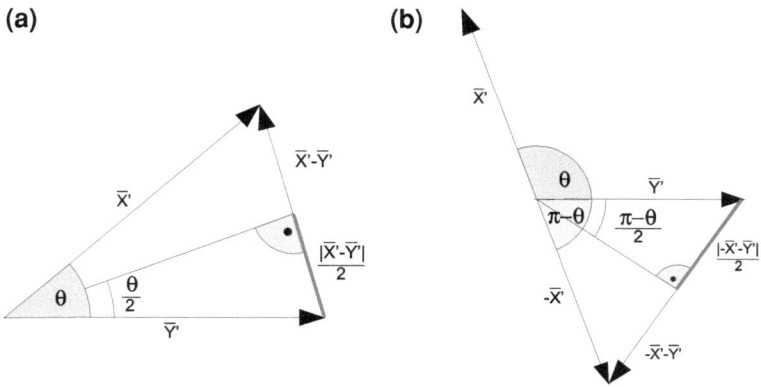

Fig. 5.34 This figure is a graphic illustration of the procedure of computing degrees between two normalized vectors. In case **a** angle $\theta \in \left[0, \frac{\pi}{2}\right]$, in case **b** $\theta \in \left(\frac{\pi}{2}, \pi\right]$

And eventually:

$$
\angle \overline{X}, \overline{Y} = \theta = \begin{cases} 2 \cdot \arcsin\left(\frac{\|\overline{X'} - \overline{Y'}\|}{2}\right) & if \quad \overline{X'} \circ \overline{Y'} \geq 0 \\ \pi - 2 \cdot \arcsin\left(\frac{\|-\overline{X'} - \overline{Y'}\|}{2}\right) & if \quad \overline{X'} \circ \overline{Y'} < 0 \end{cases} \tag{5.7}
$$

5.9.5.4 Body joints

Body joint sets supplied by the third-party tracking library are mapped to NumericRule and Numeric3DRule terminal symbols. Depending on the implementation of GDL script 1.1, the possible string set that represents these symbols can differ. For **NITE 1.3**, the joint set equals:

```
BodyParts={Head, Neck, LeftShoulder, RightShoulder,
Torso, LeftElbow, LeftHand, RightElbow, RightHand,
LeftHip, RightHip,LeftKnee, RightKnee, LeftFoot, Right-
Foot} + {.x|.y|.z} + {[]}
BodyParts3D={Head, Neck, LeftShoulder, RightShoulder,
Torso, LeftElbow, LeftHand, RightElbow, RightHand,
LeftHip, RightHip,LeftKnee, RightKnee, LeftFoot, Right-
Foot} + {.xyz[]}
```

For **Kinect SDK 1.7/1.8** it becomes:

```
BodyParts={HipCenter, Spine, ShoulderCenter, Head,
ShoulderLeft, ElbowLeft, WristLeft, HandLeft, Shoulder-
Right, ElbowRight, WristRight, HandRight, HipLeft,
KneeLeft, AnkleLeft, FootLeft, HipRight, KneeRight, An-
kleRight, FootRight} + {.x|.y|.z} + {[]}
```

BodyParts3D={HipCenter, Spine, ShoulderCenter, Head, ShoulderLeft, ElbowLeft, WristLeft, HandLeft, Shoulder-Right, ElbowRight, WristRight, HandRight, HipLeft, KneeLeft, AnkleLeft, FootLeft, HipRight, KneeRight, An-kleRight, FootRight} + {.xyz[}

For example:

`HipCenter.xyz[0]`—returns a three-dimensional vector with the present xyz coordinates of the HipCenter body joint (in right handed Kinect Cartesian frame). This call is valid if the Kinect SDK library is used to track the body.

`LeftHip.y[1]`—returns the floating point value of the y coordinate of the LeftHip body joint which was returned in the previous (one before present) capture. This call is valid if the NITE library is used to track the body.

`HandRight.z[3]`—returns the floating point value of the z coordinate of the HandRight body joint that was returned three captures before the present one (this body joint remains in the fourth level of the memory stack counting from the top). This call is valid if the Kinect SDK library is used to track the body.

5.9.5.5 Rule and feature definitions

RuleSymbol = *{Rule}*, *ThenSymbol* = *{Then}*—these keywords are used to define a rule. Each rule begins with the RULE keyword, and then contains an expression which must be reduced to a logical value. The expression is followed by the THEN keyword. The last part of the rule is its conclusion, i.e. a string.

For example:

RULE `angle(ShoulderRight.xyz[0] - ElbowRight.xyz[0],`
`WristRight.xyz[0] - ElbowRight.xyz[0]) < 90`
THEN `AngleElbowRight`

If the logical expression defined inside the rule is true, the rule is satisfied and its conclusion is true (the conclusion is added to the current top level of the memory stack).

FeatureSymbol = *{Feature}*, *AsSymbol* = *{As}*—these keywords are used to define features (both numeric and numeric3D features). Each feature begins with the FEATURE keyword, followed by the expression that must be reduced to a floating point value (in case of a featureNumeric) or a three-dimensional vector value (in case of a featureNumeric3D). The expression is followed by the AS keyword. The last part of the rule is a feature name, i.e. a string. For example:

FEATURE `Head.y[0] - HandRight.y[0]` **AS** `Difference`
FEATURE `HandRight.xyz[0]` **AS** `ActualRightHand`

Every feature name represents either a floating point or a three-dimensional vector floating point value. Features are computed prior to rules.

5.9.5.6 Commentaries

Commentaries are very useful for documenting the code and also during its debugging.

The GDL Script allows both one line and multiline commentaries:

A one line commentary—a one line commentary begins with the "//" characters. It excludes these characters and the rest of the line from the GDL script file parsing process. For example:

```
FEATURE Head.y[0] - HandRight.y[0] AS Difference
//computes distance
```

A multiline Commentary—begins with the "/*" chars and ends with "*/". It excludes these chars and all symbols between them from the GDL script data parsing process. If "*/" is not present in a file, the lexical analyzer returns an error.

For example:

```
FEATURE Head.y[0] - HandRight.y[0] AS Difference
/* This and next line of code will not be parsed
FEATURE HandLeft.y[0] - HandRight.y[0] AS Difference
*/
RULE angle(ShoulderRight.xyz[0] - ElbowRight.xyz[0],
WristRight.xyz[0] - ElbowRight.xyz[0]) < 90
THEN AngleElbowRight
```

5.10 Implementations

This section presents example implementations of gestures in the GDL 1.1 specification.

5.10.1 GDL Scripts for a Natural Gesture Dataset

This section presents the GDL script for the NITE set of joints that we used to classify everyday life (natural) gestures. We also added short descriptions that summarize solutions we used.

Figures 5.35, 5.36, 5.37, 5.38, 5.39, 5.40 and 5.41 presents key frames that are described by the GDLs from this section. Body joints are taken from NITE. Red marks body joints that are used in the GDLs description, blue—the joints not used in the description.

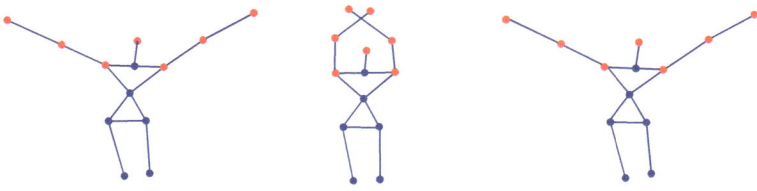

Fig. 5.35 Key frames of the "Jester" gesture

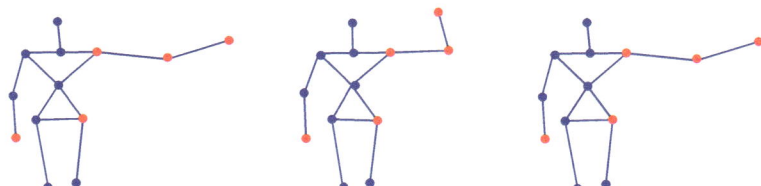

Fig. 5.36 Key frames of the "Waving" gesture

Fig. 5.37 Key frames of the "Clapping" gesture

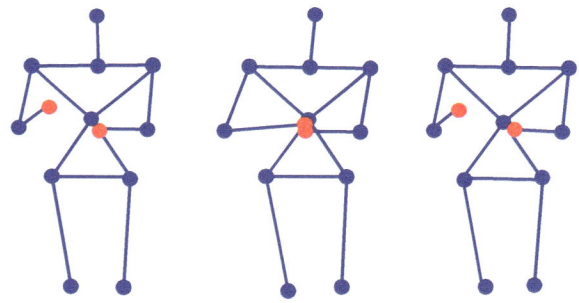

Fig. 5.38 Key frames of "HandOnHead" and "HandsOnHips" gestures

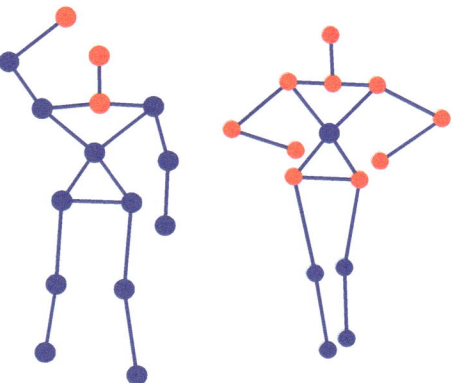

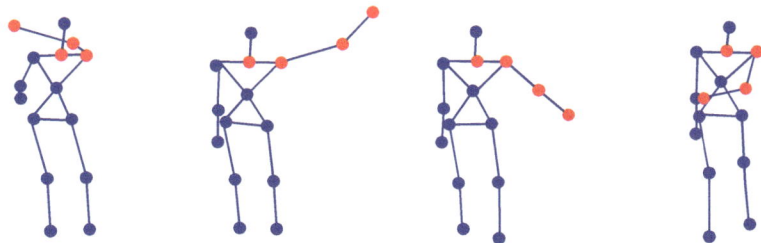

Fig. 5.39 Key frames of the "RotationClockwise" gesture

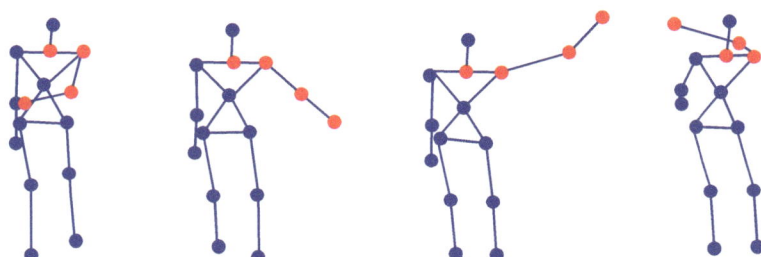

Fig. 5.40 Key frames of the "RotationAntiClockwise" gesture

```
//"Jester" gesture.
RULE distance(RightHand.xyz[0], RightShoulder.xyz[0])
>
    distance(RightHand.xyz[0], LeftShoulder.xyz[0])
    & distance(LeftHand.xyz[0], LeftShoulder.xyz[0])
    > distance(LeftHand.xyz[0], RightShoulder.xyz[0])
    THEN HandsReverse
RULE angle(RightHand.xyz[0] - RightElbow.xyz[0],
    RightShoulder.xyz[0] - RightElbow.xyz[0])  > 140
    & RightHand.y[0] > Head.y[0]
    & abs(RightHand.y[0] - LeftHand.y[0]) < 100
    & not(HandsReverse) THEN jester1
RULE angle(RightHand.xyz[0] - RightElbow.xyz[0],
    RightShoulder.xyz[0] - RightElbow.xyz[0]) > 90
    & RightHand.y[0] > Head.y[0]
    & abs(RightHand.y[0] - LeftHand.y[0]) < 100
    &  HandsReverse THEN jester2
RULE sequenceexists("[jester2,1][jester1,1][jester2,1]")
THEN jester11
RULE sequenceexists("[jester1,1][jester2,1][jester1,1]")
THEN jester22
RULE jester11 | jester22 THEN Jester
```

The "Jester" gesture is represented by three key frames and two sequences. The first key frame is described by the rule that checks if the hands are crossed over the head (see Fig. 5.24. frames 10, 11 and 12)—its conclusion is *HandsReverse*. The second key frame is represented by a rule which is satisfied if both hands are at the same vertical height and spread above the head to the sides (*jester1*). The last key

Fig. 5.41 Key frames of the
"NotMe" gesture

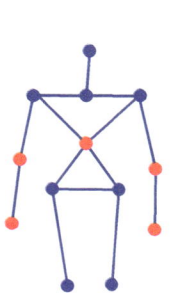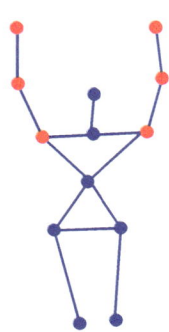

frame checks if the hands are above the head, the arms are bent at elbows and *HandsReverse* is satisfied. The first sequence in the rule with the conclusion *jester11* checks if the conclusions of rules *jester2*, *jester1* and *jester2* are present in the memory stack in the above order within a given time limit. This means that the observed user first spread their hands, then crossed them above their head and then spread them again. The second rule with sequenceexists functions (with the conclusion *jester22*) verifies whether the observed user first crossed their hands, then spread them, and then crossed them again above their head. The last rule recognizes the Jester gesture if any of previous sequences has been detected.

```
//Waving with right hand.
RULE distance(RightHand.xyz[0], LeftHand.xyz[0])
< 200 THEN HandsToClose
RULE RightHand.y[0] < RightHip.y[0]
THEN RightHandUnderHip
RULE abs(angle(RightHand.xyz[0] - RightElbow.xyz[0],
RightShoulder.xyz[0] - RightElbow.xyz[0]) - 90) <= 20
& RightHand.y[0] > RightElbow.y[0]
THEN WavingGestureCenter
RULE angle(RightHand.xyz[0] - RightElbow.xyz[0],
RightShoulder.xyz[0] - RightElbow.xyz[0]) > 110
& RightHand.y[0] > RightElbow.y[0]
THEN WavingGestureRight
RULE
 sequenceexists("[WavingGestureCenter,1][WavingGestureRight,1]")
THEN WavingRight
RULE
sequenceexists("[WavingGestureRight,1][WavingGestureCenter,1]")
THEN WavingLeft
RULE (sequenceexists("[WavingRight,2][WavingLeft,2]")
| sequenceexists("[WavingLeft,2][WavingRight,2]"))
& not(sequenceexists("[HandsReverse,4]"))
& not(sequenceexists("[RightHandUnderHip,3]"))
& not(sequenceexists("[HandsToClose,3]")) THEN Waving
```

While making the "Jester" gesture, the user is simultaneously waving their left and right hands, so as a matter of fact the "Waving" gesture is a subset of the

"Jester" gesture. In order to exclude the possibility of an ambiguous recognition, in our GDL script the memory stack must not contain the *HandsReverse* conclusion for the "Waving" gesture in the previous 4 s. Our observations showed that a person making the "Not me" gesture may 'accidently wave', so we excluded the *RightHandUnderHip* conclusion. Also, a wide clapping may be confused with waving, and therefore the *HandsToClose* conclusion was excluded.

```
//Clapping
RULE distance(RightHand.xyz[0], LeftHand.xyz[0])
< 100 THEN HandsT
RULE distance(RightHand.xyz[0], LeftHand.xyz[0])
>= 100 THEN HandsS
//exclude jester
RULE sequenceexists("[HandsS,0.5][HandsT,0.5][HandsS,0.5]")
& not(sequenceexists("[HandsReverse,1.5]")) THEN Clapping
```

When the hands are close to each other, the tracking software could segment joints incorrectly—hand joints might be crossed as in the "Jester" gesture. For this reason, the *HandsReverse* key frame of the Jester gesture was excluded.

```
//Left hand on head
RULE distance(Head.xyz[0], LeftHand.xyz[0]) <
distance(Head.xyz[0], Neck.xyz[0])
& not(sequenceexists("[HandsReverse,4]"))
THEN HandOnHead
```

This simple rule checks if the hand is touching the head. Because people's heads differ in size, the diameter of the head is estimated as the distance between the joints representing the head and the neck. The hand is very close to the head in the "Jester" gesture, so to exclude the false recognition of the HandOnHead during the "Jester", the HandsReverse position must not appear in the last 4 s.

The distance between head and neck joints proved to be a good estimator of the overall user size and we used it again in the next rule.

```
//Both hands on hips
RULE distance(RightHand.xyz[0], RightHip.xyz[0])
< distance(Head.xyz[0], Neck.xyz[0])
& distance(LeftHand.xyz[0], LeftHip.xyz[0])
< distance(Head.xyz[0], Neck.xyz[0])
& abs(angle(RightHand.xyz[0] - RightElbow.xyz[0],
RightShoulder.xyz[0] - RightElbow.xyz[0])- 90) < 40
& abs(angle(LeftHand.xyz[0] - LeftElbow.xyz[0],
 LeftShoulder.xyz[0] - LeftElbow.xyz[0])- 90) < 40
THEN HandsOnHips
```

This simple rule checks if the hands are on hips. People have different body proportions, so the size of hips is estimated to be proportional to the distance between the joints representing the head and the neck.

```
//Rotation of right hand clockwise
RULE angle(Neck.xyz[1] - RightShoulder.xyz[1],
RightShoulder.xyz[1] - RightElbow.xyz[1])
- angle(Neck.xyz[0] - RightShoulder.xyz[0],
RightShoulder.xyz[0] - RightElbow.xyz[0]) > 0
& angle(Neck.xyz[2] - RightShoulder.xyz[2],
RightShoulder.xyz[2] - RightElbow.xyz[2])
- angle(Neck.xyz[1] - RightShoulder.xyz[1],

RightShoulder.xyz[1] - RightElbow.xyz[1]) > 0
THEN AnglGoesRight
RULE angle(Neck.xyz[1] - RightShoulder.xyz[1],
RightShoulder.xyz[1] - RightElbow.xyz[1])
- angle(Neck.xyz[0] - RightShoulder.xyz[0],
RightShoulder.xyz[0] - RightElbow.xyz[0]) < 0
& angle(Neck.xyz[2] - RightShoulder.xyz[2],
RightShoulder.xyz[2] - RightElbow.xyz[2])
- angle(Neck.xyz[1] - RightShoulder.xyz[1],
RightShoulder.xyz[1] - RightElbow.xyz[1]) < 0
THEN AnglGoesLeft

RULE RightHand.y[0] - RightHand.y[1] > 10
& RightHand.y[1] - RightHand.y[2] > 10
THEN HandGoesUp
RULE RightHand.y[0] - RightHand.y[1] < 10
& RightHand.y[1] - RightHand.y[2] < 10
THEN HandGoesDown

RULE HandGoesUp & AnglGoesRight & RightHand.y[0]
> RightShoulder.y[0]
THEN RotC1
RULE HandGoesDown & AnglGoesRight
& sequenceexists("[RotC1,0.5]")
& RightHand.y[0] > RightShoulder.y[0]
THEN RotC2
RULE HandGoesDown & AnglGoesLeft
& sequenceexists("[RotC2,0.5]")
& RightHand.y[0] < RightShoulder.y[0]
THEN RotC3
RULE HandGoesUp & AnglGoesLeft
& sequenceexists("[RotC3,0.5]")
& RightHand.y[0] < RightShoulder.y[0]
THEN RotationClockwise
RULE sequenceexists("[RotationClockwise,1]")
& not(sequenceexists("[HandsReverse,4]"))
& not(sequenceexists("[handsUp,4]"))
THEN RotationClockwise
```

The above script introduces four rules that are used both to recognize the "RotationClockwise" and the "RotationAntiClockwise" gestures. The rule with the conclusion *AnglGoesRight* checks whether the shoulder muscle is expanding. The rule with the conclusion *AnglGoesLeft*—if the shoulder muscle is contracting. The third rule checks whether the hand is moving up (conlusion *HandGoesUp*) and the fourth checks if the hand is going down (*HandGoesDown*). The clockwise rotation is the sequence of the following conditions:

- Shoulder muscle is expanding while the hand is going up over the shoulder.
- Then the shoulder muscle is expanding while the hand is moving down.
- Then the shoulder muscle is contracting while the hand is going down.
- And finally the shoulder muscle is contracting while the hand is moving up.

After the last rule and if the previous ones were satisfied, the hand can end up in a position similar to that at the beginning, having made a full clockwise circle.

```
// Rotation of right hand anti-clockwise
RULE HandGoesDown & AnglGoesRight & RightHand.y[0]
< RightShoulder.y[0] THEN RotA1
RULE HandGoesUp & AnglGoesRight
& sequenceexists("[RotA1,0.5]")
& RightHand.y[0] < RightShoulder.y[0] THEN RotA2
RULE HandGoesUp & AnglGoesLeft
& sequenceexists("[RotA2,0.5]")
& RightHand.y[0] > RightShoulder.y[0] THEN RotA3
RULE HandGoesDown & AnglGoesLeft
& sequenceexists("[RotA3,0.5]")
& RightHand.y[0] > RightShoulder.y[0]
THEN RotationAntiClockwise
RULE sequenceexists("[RotationAntiClockwise,1]")
& not(sequenceexists("[HandsReverse,4]"))
& not(sequenceexists("[handsUp,4]"))
THEN RotationAntiClockwise
```

This GDL script is very similar to the clockwise rotation but the key frames occur in a different order in the sequences.

```
//"Not me" gesture.
RULE RightHand.y[0] < RightElbow.y[0]
& RightElbow.y[0] < Torso.y[0]
& LeftHand.y[0] < LeftElbow.y[0]
& LeftElbow.y[0] < Torso.y[0] THEN handsDown
RULE RightHand.y[0] > RightElbow.y[0]
& RightHand.y[0] > RightShoulder.y[0]
& LeftHand.y[0] > LeftElbow.y[0]
& LeftHand.y[0] > LeftShoulder.y[0]
THEN handsUp
RULE
sequenceexists("[handsUp,0.5][handsDown,0.5]")
THEN NotMe
```

Fig. 5.42 Key frames of the
"StandStill" (left) and the
"MotoDachi"(right) gestures

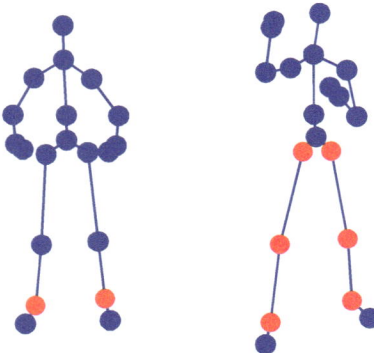

The GDL script description of this gesture is very straightforward. First, the hands should be down along the body, than the hands are raised above the body.

5.10.2 GDL for the Okinawa Shorin-ryu Karate Dataset

This section presents a GDL script for the Kinect SDK set of joints we used to classify Okinawa Shorin-ryu Karate gestures (techniques). It also includes short descriptions that summarize solutions we used.

Figures 5.42, 5.43 and 5.44 present key frames described by the GDLs from this section. Body joints are taken from the Kinect SDK. Red marks body joints that are used in the GDLs description, blue—the joints not used in the description.

```
RULE (distance(AnkleRight.xyz[0], AnkleRight.xyz[1])
< 10
& distance(AnkleRight.xyz[1], AnkleRight.xyz[2]) < 10
& distance(AnkleRight.xyz[2], AnkleRight.xyz[3]) <
10)
& (distance(AnkleLeft.xyz[0], AnkleLeft.xyz[1]) < 10
& distance(AnkleLeft.xyz[1], AnkleLeft.xyz[2]) < 10
& distance(AnkleLeft.xyz[2], AnkleLeft.xyz[3]) < 10)
THEN StandStill
```

During Karate training it is common practice that some movements end in a body position which the athlete holds their body in for a short period of time. The conclusion StandStill is used to find out if the observed user is holding his position for a short interval (about 0.1 s when the tracking frequency is 30 Hz).

Fig. 5.43 Key frames of the
"AgeUke" gesture. It is
apparent that in the second
key frame the instructor is
taking the Moto-dachi stance

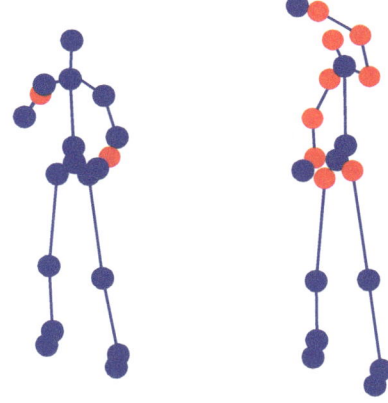

Fig. 5.44 Key frames of the
"MaeGeri" gesture

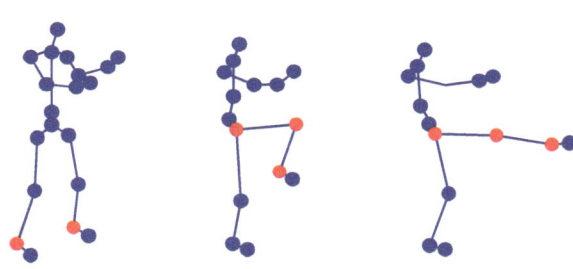

```
RULE angle(HipLeft.xyz[0] - KneeLeft.xyz[0],
HipRight.xyz[0] - KneeRight.xyz[0]) > 5
& angle(HipLeft.xyz[0] - KneeLeft.xyz[0],
HipRight.xyz[0] - KneeRight.xyz[0]) < 45
THEN MotoLegsA
RULE HipRight.z[0] < HipLeft.z[0]
& KneeRight.z[0] < KneeLeft.z[0]
& AnkleRight.z[0] < AnkleLeft.z[0]
THEN MotoLegsZRight
RULE HipRight.z[0] > HipLeft.z[0]
& KneeRight.z[0] > KneeLeft.z[0]
& AnkleRight.z[0] > AnkleLeft.z[0]
THEN MotoLegsZLeft
RULE ABS(AnkleRight.z[0] - AnkleLeft.z[0]) >
ABS(DISTANCE(HipRight.xyz[0], HipLeft.xyz[0]))
THEN MotoStepFront
RULE angle(HipRight.xyz[0] - KneeRight.xyz[0],
AnkleRight.xyz[0] - KneeRight.xyz[0]) > 150
& angle(HipLeft.xyz[0] - KneeLeft.xyz[0],
AnkleLeft.xyz[0] - KneeLeft.xyz[0]) > 150
THEN MotoKnee
RULE  (MotoStepFront & MotoLegsA & MotoKnee)
& (MotoLegsZRight | MotoLegsZLeft) & StandStill
THEN MotoDachi
```

MotoDachi is one of the basic stances. In this stance, the athlete stands in the short stride (we measure the angle between vectors defined by the left and right hips and knees). Both legs are slightly bent. There are also conditions concerning feet positions but due to the limited tracking hardware and software accuracy they cannot be checked.

```
RULE WristRight.y[0] < WristLeft.y[0]
THEN AgeUkeRStart
RULE WristRight.y[0] > WristLeft.y[0]
THEN AgeUkeLStart
RULE angle(WristRight.xyz[0] - ElbowRight.xyz[0],
ShoulderRight.xyz[0] - ElbowRight.xyz[0]) > 80
& Distance(WristRight.xyz[0], HipRight.xyz[0]) < 200
THEN AgeUkeRightHand
RULE angle(WristLeft.xyz[0] - ElbowLeft.xyz[0],
ShoulderLeft.xyz[0] - ElbowLeft.xyz[0]) > 80
& Distance(WristLeft.xyz[0], HipLeft.xyz[0]) < 200
THEN AgeUkeLeftHand
RULE ABS(WristLeft.y[0] - Head.y[0]) < 100
& ABS(WristLeft.x[0] - Head.x[0]) < 100
& angle(WristLeft.xyz[0] - ElbowLeft.xyz[0],
ShoulderLeft.xyz[0] - ElbowLeft.xyz[0]) > 90 &
angle(WristLeft.xyz[0] - ElbowLeft.xyz[0],
ShoulderLeft.xyz[0] - ElbowLeft.xyz[0]) < 150
THEN AgeUkeRightHandLeftHandBlock
RULE ABS(WristRight.y[0] - Head.y[0]) < 100
& ABS(WristRight.x[0] - Head.x[0]) < 100
& angle(WristRight.xyz[0] - ElbowRight.xyz[0],
ShoulderRight.xyz[0] - ElbowRight.xyz[0]) > 90
& angle(WristRight.xyz[0] - ElbowRight.xyz[0],
ShoulderRight.xyz[0] - ElbowRight.xyz[0]) < 150
THEN AgeUkeLeftHandRightHandBlock
RULE (AgeUkeLeftHand & AgeUkeLeftHandRightHandBlock)
THEN AgeUkeRStop
RULE (AgeUkeRightHand & AgeUkeRightHandLeftHandBlock)
THEN AgeUkeLStop
RULE (AgeUkeRStop
& sequenceexists("[AgeUkeRStart,1]"))
| (AgeUkeLStop & sequenceexists("[AgeUkeLStart,1]"))
& StandStill THEN AgeUke
```

The description of the Age-uke ("rising block") contains two key frames. In the first, the hand (wrist) which will be used to block the attack is under the other one. In the second key frame the hand not used for blocking is situated close to the hip with the appropriate angle of the arm. The hand that blocks the punch should be sufficiently close to the head and the angle within that arm should fall within a given interval.

```
RULE ABS(AnkleRight.y[0] - AnkleLeft.y[0]) < 50
THEN MaeStart
RULE (HipRight.y[0] - KneeRight.y[0]) < 100 &
ABS(angle(HipRight.xyz[0] - KneeRight.xyz[0],
AnkleRight.xyz[0] - KneeRight.xyz[0]) - 90) < 30
THEN MaeMiddleRight
RULE (HipRight.y[0] - KneeRight.y[0]) < 200
& angle(HipRight.xyz[0] - KneeRight.xyz[0],
AnkleRight.xyz[0] - KneeRight.xyz[0]) > 150
THEN MaeEndRight
RULE abs(angle(HipLeft.xyz[0] - KneeLeft.xyz[0],
AnkleLeft.xyz[0] - KneeLeft.xyz[0]) - 90) < 30
THEN MaeMiddleLeft
RULE (HipLeft.y[0] - KneeLeft.y[0]) < 200
& angle(HipLeft.xyz[0] - KneeLeft.xyz[0],
AnkleLeft.xyz[0] - KneeLeft.xyz[0]) > 150
THEN MaeEndLeft
RULE
(sequenceexists("[MaeMiddleRight,1][MaeStart,1]")
& MaeEndRight)
| (sequenceexists("[MaeMiddleLeft,1][MaeStart,1]")
& MaeEndLeft)
THEN MaeGeri
```

Mae-geri is a front kick. Its GDLs description is partitioned into three key frames. At first, both feet (ankles) are at the same level—both feet are resting on the ground. In the second key frame, the angle between the thigh and the shin ranges from 60 to 120° and the distance between the hip and the knee is measured. The description of the last key frame is similar to the previous one, but differs by the angle and distance values.

References

1. Flavio LC, Carlos H (2013) Morimoto, improving head movement tolerance of cross-Ratio based eye trackers. Int J Comput Vis 101:459–481. doi:10.1007/s11263-012-0541-8
2. Fanelli G, Dantone M, Gall J, Fossati A, Van Gool L (2013) Random forests for real time 3D face analysis. Int J Comput Vis 101:437–458. doi:10.1007/s11263-012-0549-0
3. Ellis C, Masood SZ, Tappen MF, LaViola Jr JJ, Sukthankar R (2013) Exploring the trade-off between accuracy and observational. Int J Comput Vis 101:420–446. doi:10.1007/s1126-012-0550-7
4. Lehment N, Kaiser M, Rigoll G (2013) Using segmented 3D point clouds for accurate likelihood approximation in human pose tracking. Int J Comput Vis 101:482–497. doi:10.1007/s11263-012-0557-0
5. Pisharady PK, Vadakkepat P, Loh AP (2013) Int J Comput Vis. Attention based detection and recognition of hand postures against complex backgrounds 101:403–419. doi:10.1007/s11263-012-0560-5
6. Derboven J, Roeck DD, Verstraete M (2012) Semiotic analysis of multi-touch interface design: the MuTable case study. Int. J Human-Computer Studies 70:714–728

7. Francisco V, Hervás R, Peinado F, Gervás P (2012) EmoTales: creating a corpus of folk tales with emotional annotations. Lang Resour Eval 46:341–381. doi:10.1007/s10579-011-9140-5

8. Seo DW, Lee JY (2013) Direct hand touchable interactions in augmented reality environments for natural and intuitive user experiences. Expert Syst Appl 40:3784–3793

9. Zhang Y, Kambhamettu C (2002) 3D headtracking under partial occlusion. Pattern Recogn 35:1545–1557

10. Portet F, Vacher M, Golanski C, Roux C, Meillon B (2013) Design and evaluation of a smart home voice interface for the elderly: acceptability and objection aspects. Pers Ubiquit Comput 17:127–144. doi:10.1007/s00779-011-0470-5

11. Metze F, Black A, Polzehl T (2011) A review of personality in voice-based man machine interaction. Human-computer interaction. interaction techniques and environments. Lecture notes in computer science, vol 6762, pp 358–367

12. Cohen MH, Giangola JP, Balogh J (2004) Voice user interface design. Addison-Wesley Professional (February, 2004), ISBN-13: 978-0321185761

13. Glowacz A, Glowacz W (2008) Sound recognition of DC machine with application of LPC and metrics, In: 2008 Conference on human system interaction, vol 1 and 2 Book Series: Eurographics Technical Report Series, pp 328–333

14. Glowacz A (2010) Diagnostics of dc machine based on sound recognition with application of LPC and GSDM, Przeglad Elektrotechniczny. In: 10th international school on nonsinusoidal currents and compensation, vol 86, no 6, pp 243–246

15. Glowacz A, Glowacz W (2008) Dc machine diagnostics based on sound recognition with application of FFT and fuzzy logic, Przeglad Elektrotechniczny, vol 84, no 12, pp 43–46

16. Hachaj T, Ogiela MR (2013) Nowadays and future computer application in medicine. IT CoNvergence PRActice (INPRA), vol 1, no 1, pp 13–27

17. Johnson PT, Zimmerman SL, Heath D, Eng J, Horton KM, Scott WW, Fishman EK (2012) The iPad as a mobile device for CT display and interpretation: diagnostic accuracy for identification of pulmonary embolism. Emergency Radiology, vol 19, no 4, pp 323–327, August 2012

18. Hachaj T, Ogiela MR (2012) Framework for cognitive analysis of dynamic perfusion computed tomography with visualization of large volumetric data. J Electron Imaging 21(4). doi:10.1117/1.JEI.21.4.043017 (Article Number: 043017)

19. Kotter E, Baumann T, Jäger D, Langer M (2006) Technologies for image distribution in hospitals. European Radiology, vol 16, no 6, pp 1270–1279, June 06

20. Elvins TT (1996) Volume visualization in a collaborative computing environment. Computers and Graphics, vol 20, no 2, March–April 1996, pp 9–222

21. Hancock DJ, Hubbold RJ (1997) Distributed parallel volume rendering on shared memory systems. High-performance computing and networking. Lect Notes Comput Sci 1225:157–164

22. Renambot L, van der Schaafa T, Bala HE, Germansb D, Spoelderb HJW (2003) Griz: experience with remote visualization over an optical grid. Future Gener Comput Syst 19(6):871–882

23. Schulze JP, Lang U (2003) The parallelized perspective shear-warp algorithm for volume rendering. Parallel Comput 29(3):339–354

24. Liang XH, Zhao QP, He ZY, Xie K, Liu YB (2009) A point-based rendering approach for real-time interaction on mobile devices. Sci China F: Inform Sci 52(8):1335–1345

25. Paravati G, Sanna A, Lamberti F, Ciminiera L (2010) An adaptive control system for interactive virtual environment content delivery to handheld devices. User centric media. Lect Notes of the Inst Comput Sci, Soc Inform Telecommun Eng 40:169–178

26. Okamoto Y, Oishi T, Ikeuchi K (2011) Image-based network rendering of large meshes for cloud computing. Int J Comput Vision 94(1):12–22

27. Chen Y-Y, Lu J-C, Jan J-K (2012) A secure EHR system based on hybrid clouds. J Med Syst 36(5):3375–3384

28. Jeong S-J, Kaufman AE (2007) Interactive wireless virtual colonoscopy. Vis Comput 23(8):545–557

29. Parka S, Kimb W, Ihm I (2008) Mobile collaborative medical display system. Comput Methods Programs Biomed 89(3):248–260
30. Wua Q, Gaob J, Chenc Z (2009) Pipelining parallel image compositing and delivery for efficient remote visualization. J Parallel Distrib Comput 69(3):230–238
31. Hachaj T (2014) Real time exploration and management of large medical volumetric datasets on small mobile devices—evaluation of remote volume rendering approach. Int J Inf Manage 34:336–343. doi:10.1016/j.ijinfomgt.2013.11.005
32. Kato H, Billinghurst M (1999) Marker tracking and HMD calibration for a video-based augmented reality conferencing system. In: IWAR '99 proceedings of the 2nd IEEE and ACM international workshop on augmented reality
33. Yang G, Jiang T (2004) Medical imaging and augmented reality, In: 2nd international workshop on MIAR
34. Soler L, Forest C, Nicolau S, Vayssiere C, Wattiez A, Marescaux J (2006) Computer-assisted operative procedure: from preoperative planning to simulation. Eur Clin Obstet Gynaecol 2(4):201–208. doi:10.1007/s11296-006-0055-4
35. Marmulla R, Hoppe H, Mühling J, Eggers G (2005) An augmented reality system for image-guided surgery. Int J Oral Maxillofac Surg 34(6):594–596
36. Denis K et al (2006) Integrated medical workflow for augmented reality applications. In: International workshop on augmented environments for medical imaging and computer-aided surgery (AMI-ARCS)
37. ARToolkit website http://www.hitl.washington.edu/artoolkit/
38. Hachaj T, Ogiela MR (2012) Visualization of perfusion abnormalities with GPU-based volume rendering. Comput Graphics 36(3):163–169
39. Microsoft Developer Network website msdn.microsoft.com
40. Khoshelham K (2011) Accuracy analysis of kinect depth data. In: ISPRS workshop laser scanning 2011, Calgary, Lichti DD, Habib AF (ed) international society for photogrammetry and remote sensing (ISPRS),(International archives of photogrammetry and remote sensing: IAPRS; ISPRS; XXXVIII-5/W12) Canada, pp 29–31, August 2011
41. Khoshelham K, Oude Elberink SJ (2012) Accuracy and resolution of Kinect depth data for indoor mapping applications. In: Sensors : journal on the science and technology of sensors and biosensors : open access, vol 12, no 2, pp 1437–1454
42. Schwarz LA, Mkhitaryan A, Mateus D, Navab N (2011) Human skeleton tracking from depth data using geodesic distances and optical flow, Image and vision computing. Best Autom Face Gesture Recognit 30(3):217–226
43. Shotton F et al (2011) Real-time human pose recognition in parts from single depth images. CVPR 3
44. Prime Sensor™ NITE 1.3 Algorithms notes, Version 1.0, PrimeSense Inc. (2010) http://pr.cs. cornell.edu/humanactivities/data/NITE.pdf
45. Zhang Q, Song X, Shao X, Shibasaki R, Zhao H (2013) Unsupervised skeleton extraction and motion capture from 3D deformable matching. Neurocomputing 100:170–182
46. Catuhe D (2012) Programming with the Kinect for windows software development kit. Microsoft Press, ISBN: 978-0-7356-6681-8
47. Liu Y, Huang Q, Ma S, Zhao D, Gao W (2009) Joint video/depth rate allocation for 3D video coding based on view synthesis distortion model. Sig Process Image Commun 24(8):666–681
48. Ruppert GC, Reis LO, Amorim PH, de Moraes TF, da Silva JV (2012) Touchless gesture user interface for interactive image visualization in urological surgery, World J Urol 30(5):687–691. doi: 10.1007/s00345-012-0879-0 (Epub 2012 May 12)
49. Chang Y-J, Chen S-F, Huang J-D (2011) A Kinect-based system for physical rehabilitation: a pilot study for young adults with motor disabilities. Res Dev Disabil 32:2566–2570
50. Clark RA, Pua Y-H, Fortin K, Ritchie C, Webster KE, Denehy L, Bryant AL (2012) Validity of the microsoft Kinect for assessment of postural control. Gait Posture 36:372–377
51. Du Y, Chen F, Xu W, Zhang W (2008) Activity recognition through multi-scale motion detail analysis. Neurocomputing 71:3561–3574

52. Gamage N, Kuang YC, Akmeliawati R, Demidenko S (2011) Gaussian process dynamical models for hand gesture interpretation in sign language. Pattern Recogn Lett 32:2009–2014
53. Kang J, Zhong K, Qin S, Wang H, Wright D (2013) Instant 3D design concept generation and visualization by real-time hand gesture recognition. Comput Ind 64(7):785–797
54. López-Méndez A, Casas JR (2012) Model-based recognition of human actions by trajectory matching in phase spaces. Image Vis Comput 30:808–816
55. Gupta S, Jaafar J, Ahmad WFW (2012) Static hand gesture recognition using local gabor. Procedia Eng 41:827–832
56. Zhu F, Shao L, Lin M (2013) Multi-view action recognition using local similarity random forests and sensor fusion. Pattern Recogn Lett 34:20–24
57. Ray SJ, Teizer J (2012) Real-time construction worker posture analysis for ergonomics training. Adv Eng Inform 26:439–455
58. Kapuscinski T, Oszust M, Wysocki M (2013) Recognition of signed dynamic expressions observed by ToF camera. In: SPA 2013 signal processing algorithms, architectures, arrangements, and applications—conference proceedings, Poznan, pp 291–296
59. Venkatesh Babu R, Ramakrishnan KR (2004) Recognition of human actions using motion history information extracted from the compressed video. Image Vis Comput 22:597–607
60. Augsburg University (2011) Full body interaction framework. http://hcm-lab.de/fubi.html
61. Kistler F, Endrass B, Damian I, Dang CT, André E (2012) Natural interaction with culturally adaptive virtual characters. J Multimodal User Interfaces 6(1–2):39–47
62. Wobbrock JO, Wilson AD, Li Y (2007) Gestures without libraries, toolkits or training: a $1 recognizer for user interface prototypes. In: Proceeding UIST '07 proceedings of the 20th annual ACM symposium on user interface software and technology. ACM, New York, pp 159–168
63. Allevard T, Benoit E, Foulloy L (2003) Fuzzy glove for gesture recognition, 17th IMEKO world congress. Croatia, Dubrovnik, pp 2026–2031
64. Elakkiya R, Selvamai K, Velumadhava Rao R, Kannan A () Fuzzy hand gesture recognition based human computer interface intelligent system. In: UACEE international journal of advances in computer networks and its security, vol 2, no 1, pp 29–33
65. Chen Q, Georganas ND, Petriu EM (2007) Real-time Vision-based hand gesture recognition using haar-like features. In: Instrumentation and measurement technology conference proceedings, pp 1–6
66. Arulkarthick VJ, Sangeetha D, Umamaheswari S (2012) Sign language recognition using K-Means clustered Haar-like features and a stochastic context free grammar. Eur J Sci Res 78(1):74–84 (ISSN 1450-216X)
67. Bickerstaffe A, Lane A, Meyer B, Marriott K (2008) Developing domain-specific gesture recognizers for smart diagram environments graphics recognition. Recent advances and new opportunities. Springer, Berlin, pp 145–156
68. Kettebekov S, Sharma R (2001) Toward natural gesture/speech control of a large display. In: EHCI '01 proceedings of the 8th IFIP international conference on engineering for human-computer interaction. Springer, London, pp 221–234
69. Yeasin M, Chaudhuri S (2000) Visual understanding of dynamic hand gestures. Pattern Recogn 33:1805–1817
70. Suma AE, Krum DM, Lange B, Koenig S, Rizzo A, Bolas M (2013) Adapting user interfaces for gestural interaction with the flexible action and articulated skeleton toolkit. Comput and Graphics 37:193–201
71. Hachaj T, Ogiela MR (2012) Recognition of human body poses and gesture sequences with gesture description language. J Med Inf Technol 20:129–135
72. Hachaj T, Ogiela MR (2012) Semantic description and recognition of human body poses and movement sequences with gesture description language. Computer Applications for Biotechnology, Multimedia, and Ubiquitous City, Communications in Computer and Information Science 353:1–8
73. Hachaj T, Ogiela MR (2014) Rule-based approach to recognizing human body poses and gestures in real time. Multimedia Systems 20(1), pp 81–99. doi:10.1007/s00530-013-0332-2

74. Official website of GDL technology with available implementations for download: http://www.cci.up.krakow.pl/gdl/
75. Official website of the Laboratory of Cryptography and Cognitive Informatics: http://www.cci.up.krakow.pl/
76. Hachaj T, Ogiela MR, Piekarczyk M (2013) Dependence of Kinect sensors number and position on gestures recognition with gesture description language semantic classifier, In: Proceedings of the 2013 federated conference on computer science and information systems (FedCSIS 2013) Ganzha M, Maciaszek L, Paprzycki M (eds), ISBN 9-1-4673-4471-5, IEEE Catalog Number CFP1385 N-ART, IEEE Computer Society Press, 8–11 September 2013. Kraków, Poland, pp 571–575
77. Obdrzalek S, Kurillo G, Ofli F, Bajcsy R, Seto E, Jimison H, Pavel M (2012) Accuracy and robustness of Kinect pose estimation in the context of coaching of elderly population. In: Annual international conference of the IEEE engineering in medicine and biology society, pp 1188–1193, August 2012
78. Hachaj T, Ogiela MR (2013) Computer karate trainer in tasks of personal and homeland security defense. Lect Notes Comput Sci 8128:430–441
79. Hachaj T, Ogiela MR, Piekarczyk M (2014) Real-time recognition of selected karate techniques using GDL approach. Adv Intell Syst Comput 233:99–106. doi:10.1007/978-3-319-01622-1_12

Chapter 6
Summary

In recent years, pattern recognition techniques have undergone rapid development, in terms of both inventing and improving new algorithmic and technical solutions, which allow computers to be used to increasingly keenly and precisely observe the world around us. Image analysis and recognition systems allow micro-world structures to be visualized, e.g., those with the size of cells, but they can also reach into the macro-world and allow satellite images to be explored. Image recognition algorithms as well as vision systems of computers and robots have begun to play such a major role in both scientific research and everyday life that it seems they will not only gain in significance in the future, but also there will be no going back or giving up the ability to use scientific achievements in this regard.

The pattern recognition methods currently under development constitute an incredibly interesting field of research due to their one very characteristic feature. These techniques are increasingly frequently developed at the interface of informatics and cognitive science. This makes them more and more interdisciplinary, not only because of the wide-ranging opportunities to use them in various scientific disciplines, but also due to the influence of other disciplines on the newly developed algorithmic and technical solutions in the field of computer image recognition systems. The greatest such influence comes mainly from cognitive science and neurobiology [1]. Previous years have seen the overlapping of these fields with informatics thanks to the definition and use of artificial neural networks in image recognition. Today, we are witnessing attempts at adapting many other, biologically inspired solutions and models of visual information processing [2]. This was made possible by the development of cognitive science and cognitive informatics which allow new solutions aimed at the semantic analysis and interpretation of the examined images, patterns, scenes, and even situations and referring to the context of the recognition system to be introduced into image recognition algorithms.

This is the spirit in which this monograph has been written, combining aspects of practical uses of pattern recognition methods with original scientific achievements in a further development of cognitive systems for recognizing and interpreting image patterns. In this book, we tried to cover the entire spectrum of

M. R. Ogiela and T. Hachaj, *Natural User Interfaces in Medical Image Analysis*,
Advances in Computer Vision and Pattern Recognition,
DOI: 10.1007/978-3-319-07800-7_6,
© Springer International Publishing Switzerland 2015

subjects connected with advanced computer pattern recognition systems, and in particular the areas of computer vision, biologically inspired perception, image processing and analysis, biomedical engineering, multimedia and augmented reality, neural networks, medical imaging, computer-aided diagnosis and man–machine interfaces.

The above areas are closely connected to the topic of this book, which presents practical solutions supporting the semantic interpretation of brain tissue lesions [3–5] and morphological changes of carotid arteries [6, 7]. The semantic analysis of such medical conditions has become possible thanks to the use of a series of pattern recognition techniques and methods of their semantic computer interpretation. Both well-known methods of initial image analysis and a series of heuristics solutions enabling the diagnostic interpretation of the type of lesion detected and the consequences of their presence for further therapeutic procedures have been used for this purpose. Apart from practical implementations of procedures for the semantic analysis of brain perfusion and carotid vessel images, this monograph also reviews initial image analysis and recognition techniques. Methods of computer image analysis based on cognitive resonance processes have been discussed [1]. Medical imaging standards have been presented as having basic image algebra and 3D image rendering operations. Also presented are the most recent achievements in algorithms for creating augmented reality and their use not only to produce and interpret medical images, but also their mobile applications. Another important element was to demonstrate innovative solutions for man–machine interfaces and define an original solution called the Gesture Description Language (GDL) [8, 9], based on methods originating from mathematical linguistics.

The originality and universality of the presented solutions also allow us to indicate the directions of future development of the methods proposed in this publication; these directions should focus on the following subjects:

- Enhancing cognitive resonance processes by adding the ability to learn and extend knowledge bases that are used to interpret the meaning of image patterns.
- Extend the presented paradigm of computer understanding of images to the analysis of complex scenes and situations taking into account the context in which the examined image, scene, or the recognizing system are located.
- Developing and improving the GDL gesture recognition technology by adding the ability to analyze various gestures and motions that can help interpret the behavior of people, their education, recreation, and rehabilitation, and also enable contactless interaction with IT systems.
- Giving a recognition system founded on the GDL technology the ability to automatically learn by analyzing new, unknown motion sequences.
- Applying the developed methods to new types of images and scenes.

It seems that these subjects will play a major role in the scientific research conducted by the authors of this monograph. The results of such research can once again contribute to the development of contemporary pattern recognition methods and may turn out to be very useful when building mobile humanoid robots, which will analyze the world around them using cognitive resonance processes and will act in an adaptive way depending on the environment in which they find themselves.

References

1. Ogiela L, Ogiela, MR (2009) Cognitive techniques in visual data interpretation. Studies in computational intelligence 228. Springer, Berlin
2. Ogiela L, Ogiela MR (2012) Advances in cognitive information systems. Cognitive systems monographs 17. Springer, Berlin
3. Hachaj T, Ogiela MR (2011) A system for detecting and describing pathological changes using dynamic perfusion computer tomography brain maps. Comput Biol Med 41(6):402–410. doi:10.1016/j.compbiomed.2011.04.002
4. Hachaj T, Ogiela MR (2012) Visualization of perfusion abnormalities with GPU-based volume rendering. Comput Graph UK 36(3):163–169. doi:10.1016/j.cag.2012.01.002
5. Hachaj T, Ogiela MR (2013) Application of neural networks in detection of abnormal brain perfusion regions. Neurocomputing 122:33–42. doi:10.1016/j.neucom.2013.04.030
6. Hachaj T, Ogiela MR (2012) Evaluation of carotid artery segmentation with centerline detection and active contours without edges algorithm. Lect Notes Comput Sci 7465:469–479
7. Ogiela MR, Hachaj T (2013) Automatic segmentation of the carotid artery bifurcation region with a region-growing approach. J Electron Imaging 22(3):033029, doi: 10.111/1.JEI.22.3. 033029
8. Hachaj T, Ogiela MR (2012) Semantic description and recognition of human body poses and movement sequences with Gesture Description Language. Commun Comput Inf Sci 353:1–8
9. Hachaj T, Ogiela MR (2014) Rule-based approach to recognizing human body poses and gestures in real time. Multimedia Syst 20:81–99. doi:10.1007/s00530-013-0332-2

Index